Fundamentals of Dental Radiography

Fundamentals of Dental Radiography

LINCOLN R. MANSON-HING, D.M.D., M.S.

Professor Emeritus of Dentistry
School of Dentistry
University of Alabama at Birmingham

with Contributor
Dennis E. Clark, D.D.S., M.S.
Assistant Professor of Dentistry
School of Dentistry
Loma Linda University
California

THIRD EDITION

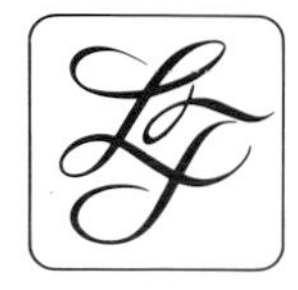

Lea & Febiger 1990 *Philadelphia • London*

Lea & Febiger
600 Washington Square
Philadelphia, Pennsylvania 19106-4198
U.S.A.
(215) 922-1330

Lea & Febiger (UK) Ltd.
145a Croydon Road
Beckenham, Kent BR3 3RB
U.K.

First Edition, 1979
Reprinted, 1980

Second Edition, 1985
Third Edition, 1990

Library of Congress Cataloging-in-Publication Data

Manson-Hing, Lincoln R.
Fundamentals of dental radiography / Lincoln R. Manson-Hing; with contributor, Dennis E. Clark.—3rd ed.
p. cm.
Includes bibliographies and index.
ISBN 0-8121-1253-9
1. Teeth—Radiography. I. Clark, Dennis E., 1956–
II. Title.
[DNLM: 1. Radiography, Dental. WN 230 M289f]
RK309.M35 1989
617.6'07572—dc20
DNLM/DLC
for Library of Congress
89-7971
CIP

PRINTED IN THE UNITED STATES OF AMERICA

Print Number 5 4 3 2 1

To Caitlin

Preface

Improperly used, ionizing radiation can be harmful to both patient and operator. Properly applied, it can be very helpful in alleviating much suffering. The basic danger of large doses of x rays and other forms of ionizing radiations to humans has been known for many years. With the rapidly increasing health needs of the population, the greatly increased use of ionizing radiations by industry, and the use of many radiation-producing devices in the home, the environment of modern man is now polluted with ionizing radiations. Governmental agencies are concerned with the radiologic health of the population, and all persons working with radiation-producing materials or devices are required to be properly trained. The contents of this book attend to guidelines for the training of persons making dental radiographs.

The major source of harmful radiation in the dental office is the x-ray machine. All operators of this machine, be they dentist, dental hygienist, dental assistant, or other auxiliary, must be knowledgeable of the properties of x rays and the technics of radiography. This knowledge is essential if good diagnostic quality radiographs are to be made safely and efficiently. In recent years, the control of infection in the dental office has become of great concern and thus a chapter on this subject is included in this edition. The material is contributed by Dr. Dennis Clark who teaches, practices and has graduate credentials in dental radiology.

In-depth knowledge of the subject would require many books to present the information. This book is written to provide the fundamental information needed for clinical dental radiography in a concise manner to assist the reader in maintaining maximum contact with the discipline at all times. Many illustrations are used to clarify the subject. A relatively large page size is used to keep text and related illustrations on the same or adjacent pages. This form also permits the reader to observe many subject areas on two opposing or adjacent pages. The material is organized to present information as closely as possible in a parallel teaching sequence of text and illustrations that has a high degree of flexibility useful to many types of dental radiographers. It can be used effectively not only in beginning radiography courses but also in short or continuing education programs involving trained participants. Some parts are made concise in order to present an overview of some subjects to the beginner; for example, changes taking place in the film during processing, the basic parts of the darkroom and principles of radiographic image formation. Radiography requirements vary between different parts of the country and between countries. In addition, radiographic technic and equipment used vary greatly between users. This book does not seek to promote any particular radiographic system but attempts to present information useful to the many diverse groups of radiographers. Previously trained persons can easily and quickly obtain refresher information through use of the many illustrations. The primary objective of this book is to provide student and experienced dental radiographers with basic information for the safe and effective use of x rays in the dentist's office.

Birmingham, Alabama LINCOLN R. MANSON-HING

Contents

Chapter 1

Physical Foundation of Radiography

Dental radiology includes the use of x-ray machines and radioactive materials in diagnosis and research. Usually the practicing dentist is concerned only with diagnostic radiography. The dentist makes an x-ray picture (radiograph) that shows shadows of the internal structures of the patient to gain essential diagnostic information. Modern dentistry is seldom practiced without radiography. It should be noted that the radiograph is an important part of the patient's record.

X RADIATION

X rays are a form of energy. Like visible light, radar and radio waves they belong to a group called electromagnetic radiations (Figure 1–1). They were discovered by Wilhelm Conrad Roentgen in 1895 and are sometimes called roentgen rays. Roentgen found that these invisible rays could cast shadows of internal body tissues. Because of the unknown nature of the rays he called them x rays.

Electromagnetic radiations are made of units of pure energy called photons or quanta. They have no mass or weight and thus are different from corpuscular radiations that consist of bits of matter or subatomic particles that have mass and weight. Examples of corpuscles are protons, neutrons, electrons, and alpha particles. All photons of electromagnetic radiation travel at the speed of 186,000 miles per second, move through space in a straight line, and have a wave form (Figure 1–2). The greater the energy a photon has, the shorter is the photon's wavelength. Some long wavelength photons of the electromagnetic family can be as long as thousands of miles; some with very short wavelengths can be much shorter than the width of an atom. In the x-ray region of the electromagnetic spectrum, the shorter the wavelength of the photon the easier it is for the photon to pass through matter. When much material must be penetrated by x rays, the x rays used must have great energy and

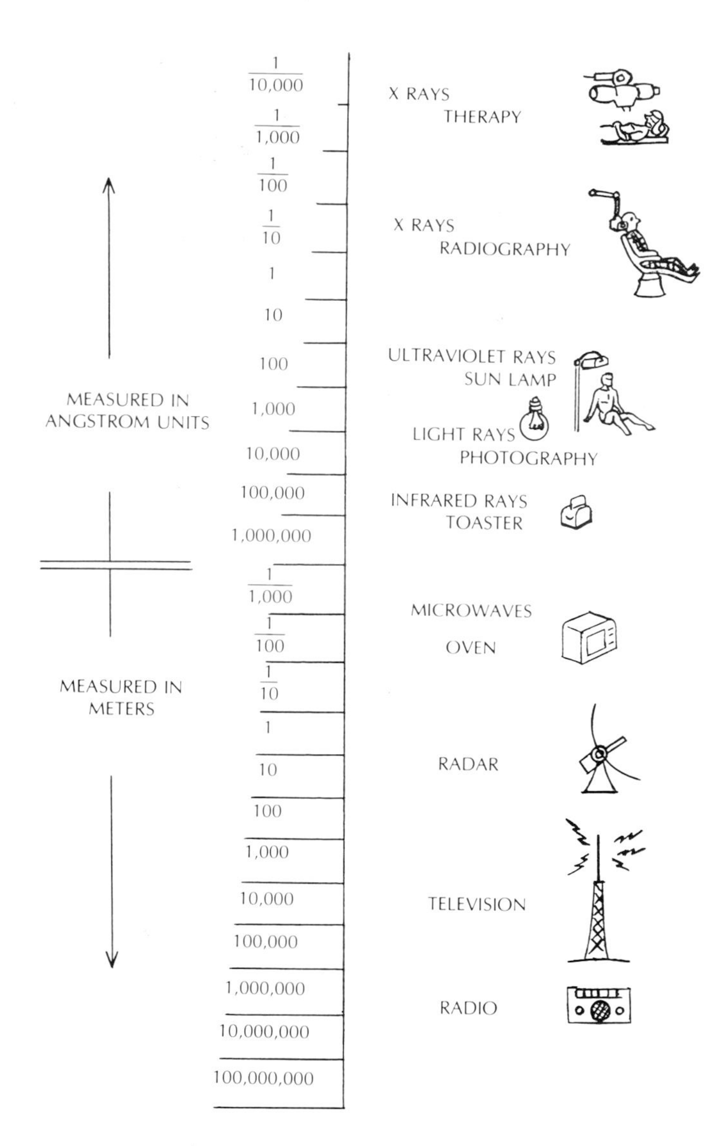

Figure 1–1. Electromagnetic spectrum. An angstrom unit is $\frac{1}{10,000,000,000}$ meter.

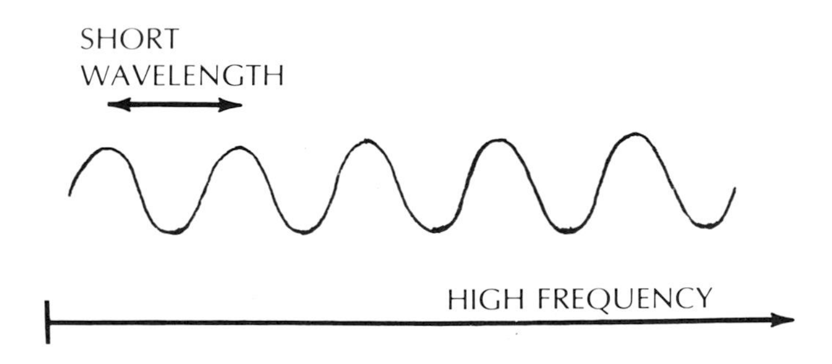

Figure 1–2. Diagrams of long wavelength photon (above) and short wavelength photon (below). Over a given time or distance there are more wave cycles or oscillations with short wavelength photons and thus such photons have higher frequency.

short wavelengths to have great penetrating power. Such photons are sometimes called "hard x rays." Long wavelength, low energy, poorly penetrating rays are called "soft x rays."

Since x rays travel in straight lines and move away in all directions from the point where they are produced in an x-ray tube, their intensity (or number of photons arriving at a given area) becomes less with greater distance from the x-ray source. In addition, the number of photons arriving at a given area will spread to an area four times as large when the distance from the source is doubled (Figure 1–3). This relationship is evidenced in the "Inverse Square Law" which states that "the intensity of radiation is inversely proportional to the square of the distance measured from the source of radiation." Note that radiation intensity decreases rapidly as distance from the radiation source is increased.

The exact nature of x radiation, like that of other forms of energy, is unknown. However, much is known of the behavior and effect of these rays. X rays behave like light in many ways. They cast similar shadows (Figure 1–4). Photographic film and radiographic film are exposed by both types of radiation; however, light sensitive film is more sensitive to light photons than to x-ray photons. X-ray films are more sensitive to x-ray photons than to light photons. X rays are invisible. They can penetrate materials that are opaque to light, ionize atoms, and produce fluorescence and phosphorescence. These properties are used in crystallography, radiation biology, radiation therapy, photo chemistry, and other scientific fields.

MATTER

Matter is composed of atoms (Figure 1–5A). Different atoms make up the different elements such as hydrogen, fluorine, iron, oxygen, aluminum, and lead. Atoms differ in the number of subatomic particles. The centrally located nucleus of an atom has protons, each having one unit of positive electrical charge, neutrons with no electrical charge, and many other particles. The nucleus is surrounded by electrons traveling in different orbits or shells. Each electron has one unit of negative electrical charge. A neutral atom

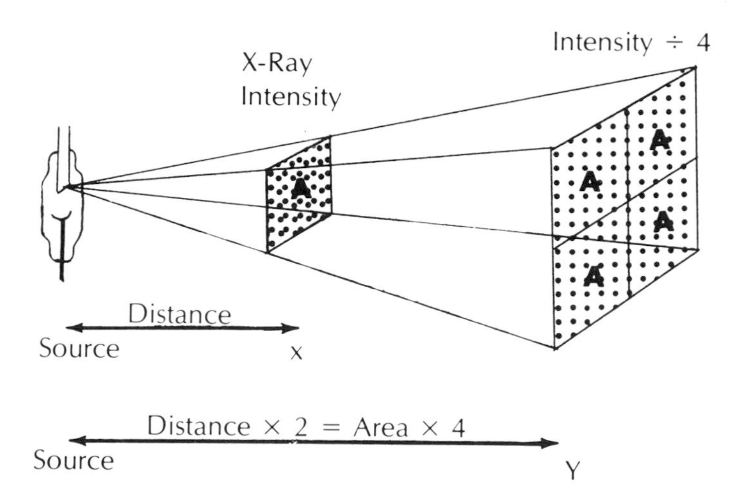

Figure 1–3. Diagram showing effect of distance upon x-ray photon intensity as described in the inverse square law. The formula showing this relationship is $\frac{\text{Intensity at X}}{\text{Intensity at Y}} = \frac{(\text{Distance Y})^2}{(\text{Distance X})^2}$.

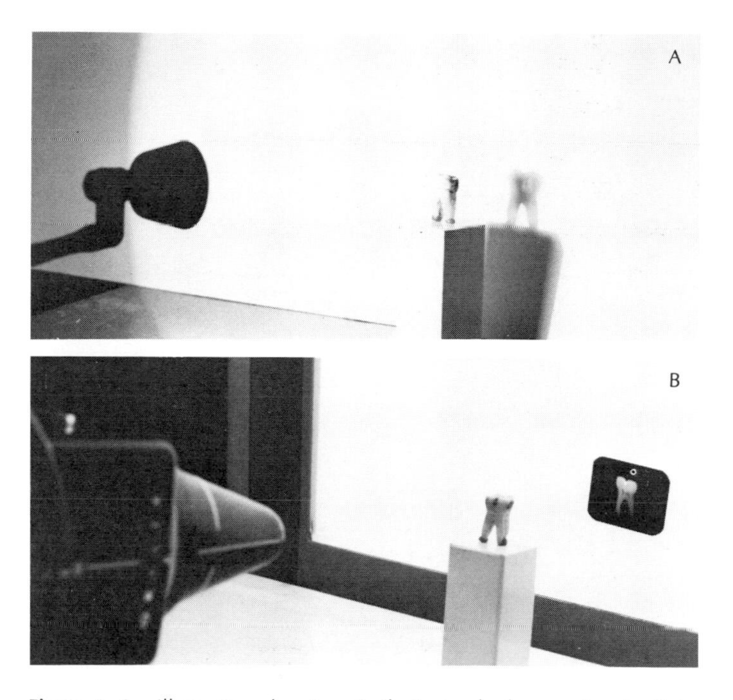

Figure 1–4. Illustration showing similarity in shadow casting by light and x rays. A, Light shadows show the outlines of opaque objects. B, A radiograph shows the internal structures of the object.

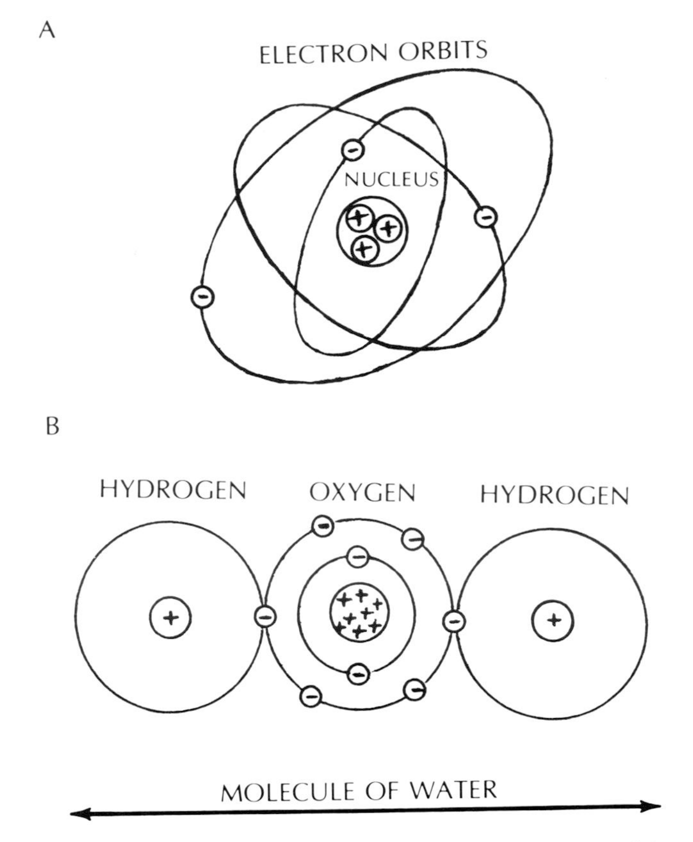

Figure 1–5. A, Diagram of atom that has three protons (+) and three orbiting electrons (−). B, Diagram of molecule of water (H_2O) consisting of two atoms of hydrogen connected to one atom of oxygen.

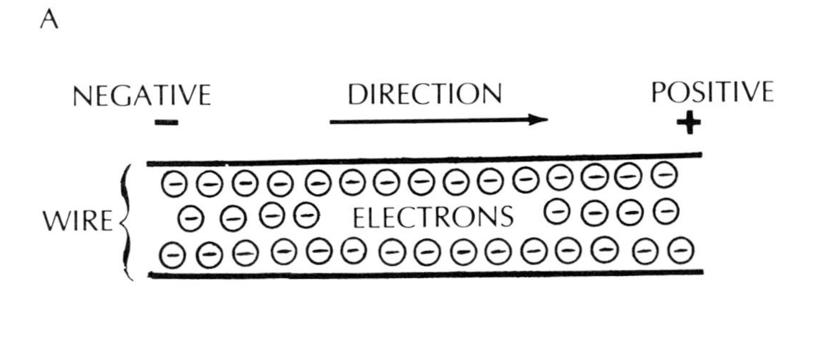

Figure 1–6. A, Flow of electrical energy in wire in one direction from negatively charged pole to positive pole. B, Alternating electric current that flows in one direction for short time then reverses itself and flows in opposite direction.

has equal numbers of protons and electrons. The space occupied by the mass of the nucleus and electrons is a small part of the space traveled by the outermost electron; it is like a football in the stadium. Because an atom consists mostly of empty space, short wavelength photons and subatomic particles can pass through an atom without interacting with the nucleus or electrons of the atom. Unstable atoms emit or eject subatomic particles or x rays to achieve stability. The subatomic particles from unstable or radioactive atoms are called particulate radiations and may be comprised of electrons, proton, neutrons, or alpha particles. Atoms of different elements join together by their electrons to form chemicals. The smallest chemical unit or molecule of water (H_2O) is shown in Figure 1–5B. Complex chemicals can be made up of hundreds of atoms.

ELECTRICITY

Electricity is the energy used to make x rays. Electrical energy can be thought of as a flow or current of electrons in a wire similar to the flow of water in a pipe (Figure 1–6). Voltage is the term used for electrical pressure and the unit of measurement is the volt (V). One *kilovolt* (kV) is equal to 1,000 volts. As large or small amounts of water can flow through large or small pipes under the same pressure, so can large and small amounts of electricity flow through wires at the same voltage. *Amperage* is the term used for amounts of electrical energy and the unit of measurement is the *ampere* (A). One milliampere (mA) is equal to $\frac{1}{1,000}$ ampere. The electric current flows from the negative side of the electric circuit to the positive side. If the flow is only in one direction, it is called a *direct current* (DC). If the flow travels in one direction, stops and then reverses its direction, it is called an *alternating current* (AC).

If an alternating current's voltage is plotted on a graph that also shows time, a sine wave shape is shown (Figure 1–7). Voltage in one direction of current is plotted above the horizontal line and in the other direction below the horizontal line. From a time when there is no current in the wire, the *voltage* builds up to a maximum or *peak* (Vp). It must then return to zero before changing direction.

When the current goes from zero to zero and has traveled in both directions, it is said to have completed one cycle. Most AC currents in the United States of America complete 60 cycles every second. X-ray machines and household electrical appliances usually have this requirement (60 cycles AC). In many foreign countries a 50-cycle AC is used.

A *transformer* is a device that changes the voltage of an electric current (Figure 1–8). It consists of two coils of wire insulated from each other and connected by a magnetic conductor. Voltage of the current put into (input) the device is proportioned to the voltage of the current emerging on the other side of the transformer (output) in relation to the number of coils of each wire. Transformers can be made to increase (step up) or decrease (step down) the voltage of an electric current.

A *rheostat* is a device that places varying degrees of resistance to flow of an electric current in a wire (Figure 1–9). It therefore controls the amount or amperage of electricity in an electric circuit. A common use of a rheostat is to control the speed of a sewing machine's motor or the motor of a belt-driven laboratory hand piece. With greater depression of the pedal on the rheostat less electrical resistance is obtained, more energy reaches the machine's motor, and the machine goes faster.

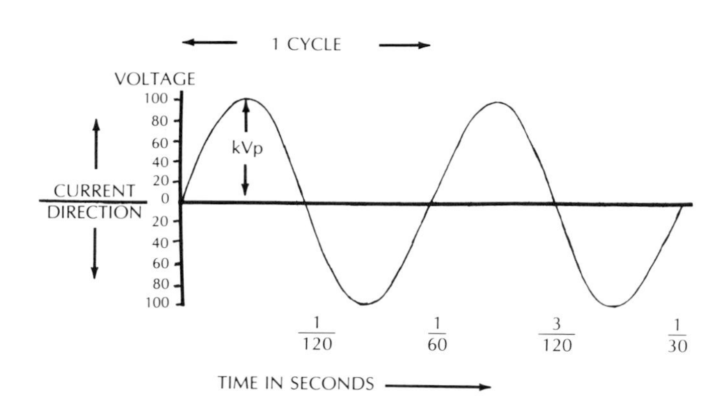

Figure 1–7. Diagram of sine wave of 60-cycle AC current operating at maximum voltage of 100 volts.

THE X-RAY TUBE

The x-ray tube is situated in the head of the x-ray machine. It consists of a glass enclosure from which all the air has been removed to produce a vacuum (Figure 1–10). The *anode* and *cathode* are separated in the tube by a gap. The cathode and anode are supplied with a high voltage electric current (60 to 100 kVp) from a step-up transformer situated in the tubehead of the x-ray machine. The cathode contains a filament, similar to the filament in a light bulb, that is connected to a separate electric circuit of low voltage and very little amperage (10 to 15 milliamperes).

The filament current heats the filament to produce a cloud of electrons around the filament (Figure 1–11). When a high voltage is applied to the anode and the cathode, the electrons are driven from the cathode to the anode. The beam of electrons is sometimes

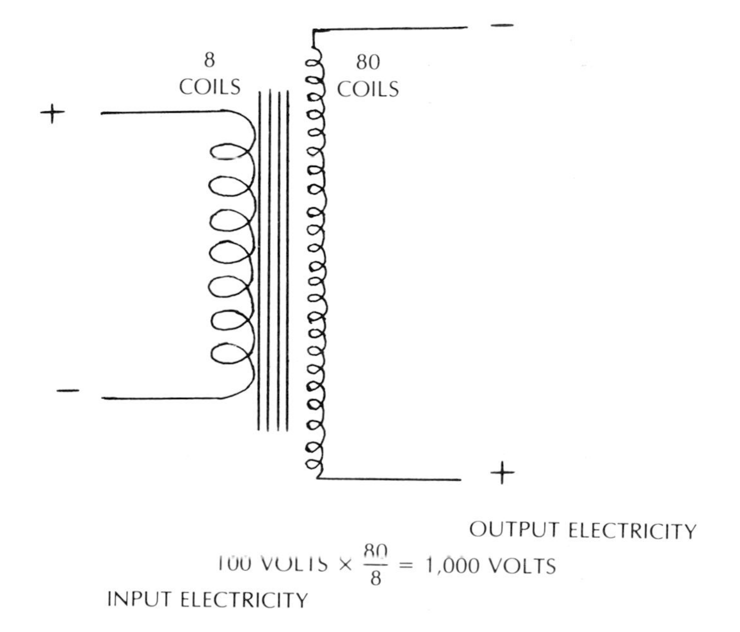

Figure 1–8. Step-up transformer, with 10 times the number of coils on output side, changing 100-volt electric current to a 1,000-volt current.

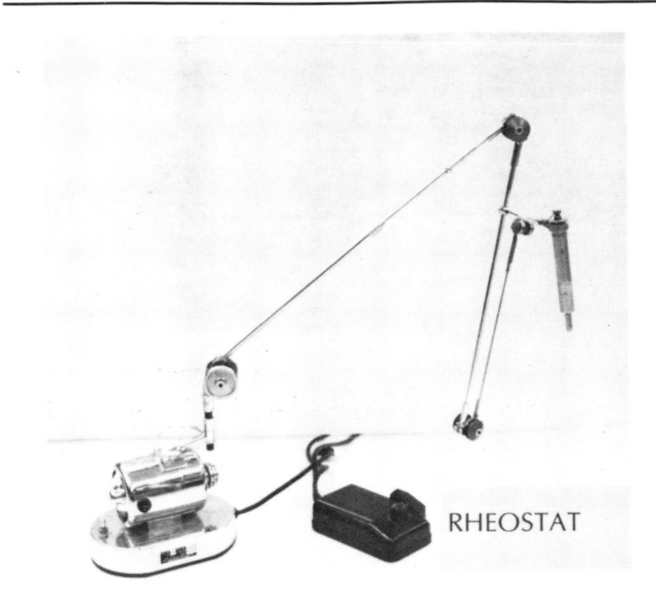

Figure 1–9. Photograph of belt-driven laboratory motor showing rheostat that controls speed of motor.

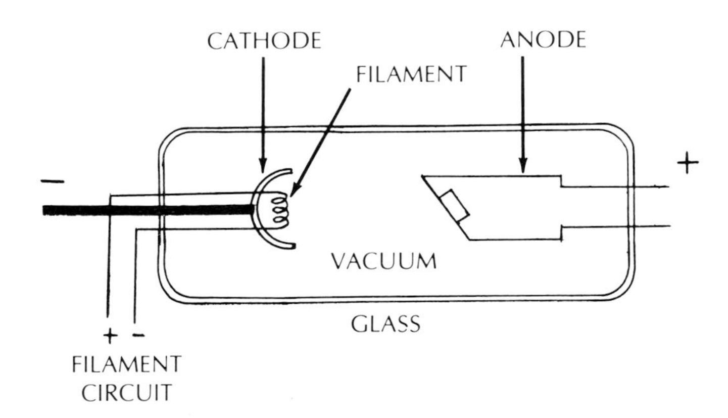

Figure 1–10. X-ray tube.

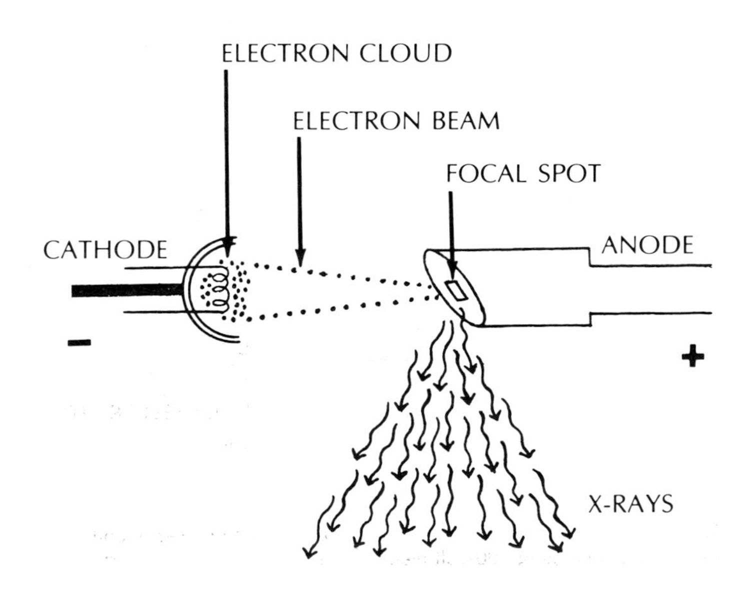

Figure 1–11. Diagram depicting electrical energy conversion into high speed electron beam into x radiation.

called a cathode ray. The speed of the electrons depends on the difference in energy potential (voltage) between the cathode and anode. When the electrons encounter the hard solid anode, they are suddenly stopped and the kinetic energy of speed or motion is converted into heat and electromagnetic radiation. The electrons are focused or directed to a small area on the anode called the *focal spot.* A small focal spot is desirable in dental x-ray machines.

Different voltage potentials between the anode and the cathode exist at different times during each cycle of the alternating current, resulting in different electron speeds between the cathode and the anode, and thus different energy x-ray photons are produced. X-ray photons of different wavelengths also result from individual electrons converting all their kinetic energy into one or more x-ray photons, in one step into one photon or in many steps into many photons, when they encounter the atoms of the anode. Thus the x-ray beam consists of photons of many wavelengths (Figure 1–12). The maximum energy or shortest wavelength photon produced is determined by the kVp of the electric current of the anode-cathode circuit.

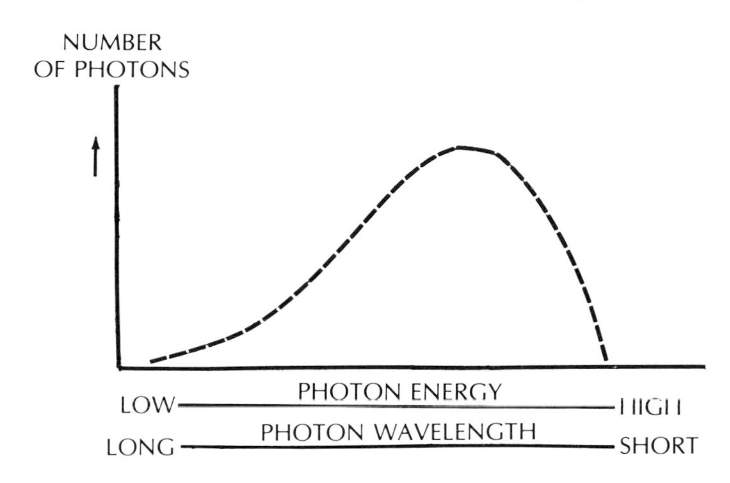

Figure 1–12. Spectrum of x-ray beam.

BASIC X-RAY MACHINE OPERATION

The dental x-ray machine consists of two basic parts: a control panel and a tubehead (Figure 1–13). The two parts can be in one unit or separated from each other. In addition, one control panel can be designed to control more than one tubehead. The tubehead is supported by an extension arm and is provided with horizontal and vertical rotation movements to allow the x-ray beam to be aimed in any direction. Control panels vary greatly among the various machines manufactured. The on/off switch may activate a light. The exposure timer selects the amount of time that x rays are to be produced. The timer switch starts the exposure. The amperage regulator (mA) controls the amount of electricity supplied to the filament and thus the number of electrons produced in the electron cloud which in turn controls the amount or number of x rays produced; the amperage is read on the mA meter. The mA meter is only activated when x rays are being created. The kVp regulator controls the

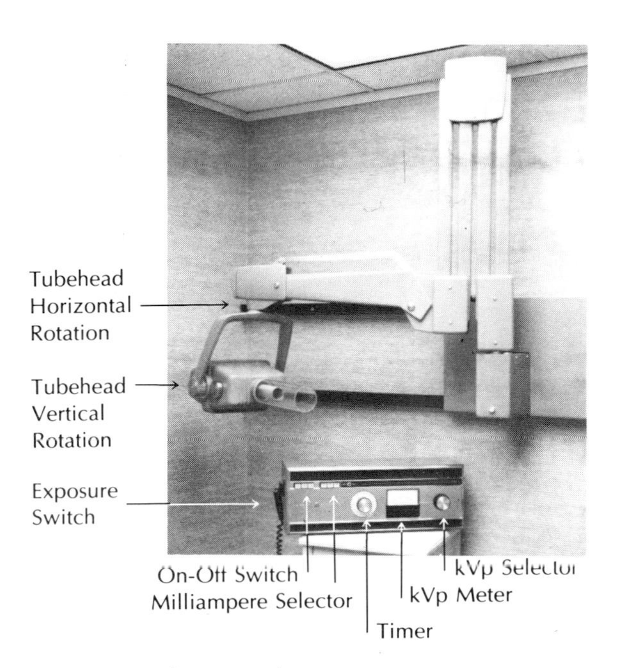

Figure 1–13. Dental x-ray machine.

voltage sent to the step-up transformer attached to the anode-cathode circuit of the x-ray tube. It regulates the speed of the electrons between the cathode and anode; this speed affects the amount of energy of the individual x-ray photons produced. High kVp produces more energetic, more penetrating x rays.

A clearer understanding of how an x-ray machine works is obtained if a study is made of the two basic electric circuits of the machine (Figure 1–14). The kVp selector adjusts the desired voltage to the step-up transformer; note that the voltmeter is activated immediately without x rays being created. The high voltage between the anode and cathode is not produced until the timer switch is activated. No electric current will flow from cathode to anode if no electron cloud is available to carry the energy across the gap; thus no amperage control is needed in the anode-cathode circuit. The milliampere meter in the anode-cathode circuit measures the amount of electricity flowing through the circuit; this current flow is controlled by the number of electrons supplied by the filament. Since the number of electrons used controls the number of x-ray pho-

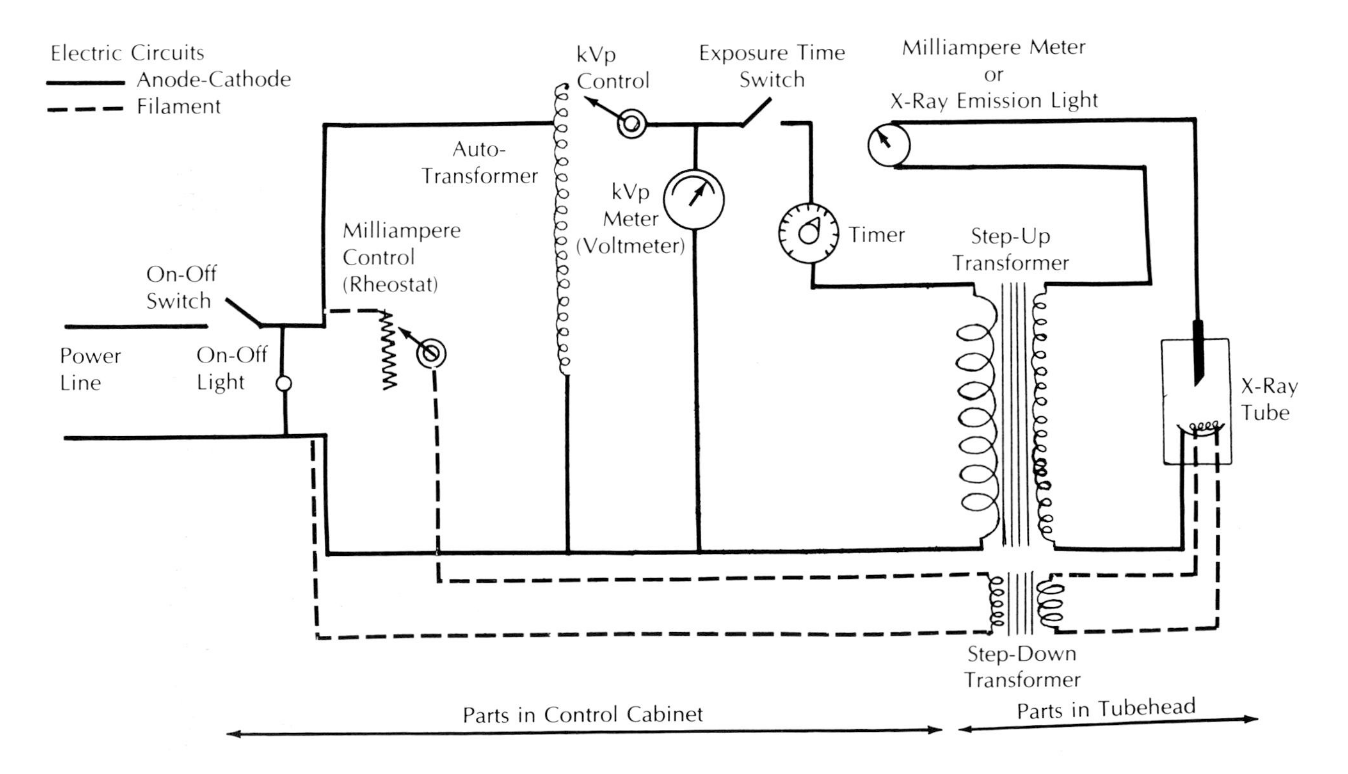

Figure 1–14. Basic electric circuits of x-ray machine.

tons produced, the milliampere meter indicates the amount of x rays that are being produced. The filament is supplied with a low voltage current by a step-down transformer; the circuit has an amperage regulator (mA) that controls the amount of electricity sent to the filament. The mA regulator controls the number of electrons created by the filament that are subsequently used to transport energy between the cathode and anode. This feature explains why the milliampere meter is activated only when x rays are being produced and why the mA can only be adjusted for non-push-button systems when the machine is operating.

THE EXPOSURE TIMER

The exposure switch activates the high voltage between the cathode and anode and starts the production of x rays (Figure 1–15). The switch is of the "dead man" type which means that it must be continually depressed to maintain x-ray production. Release of the switch stops the production of x rays. An audible sound usually accompanies the activation of the anode-cathode circuit to indicate when the machine is producing x rays.

The timer starts when the x-ray exposure begins with the closing of the exposure switch and terminates the x-ray production at the selected time. Most timers automatically reset themselves to the last used exposure time. Timers are calibrated in seconds at or above one second (Figure 1–16). Below one second most timers are calibrated in impulses. There are 60 impulses in each second when the machine is attached to an electric supply that is a 60-cycle AC current. Exposure time is measured in impulses because x rays are not created in a continuous stream of photons but in bursts or pulses of x rays. X rays are created only when the cathode is charged electrically negative and the anode electrically positive; this means that x rays are created only half of the time during each cycle of an AC electric current (x rays are not created when the anode is negative and the cathode positive because there are no electrons at the anode to carry the electric energy across the gap). When an alternating electric current is made to flow only in one direction, it is said to be "rectified." A dental x-ray tube rectifies the high voltage electric circuit and

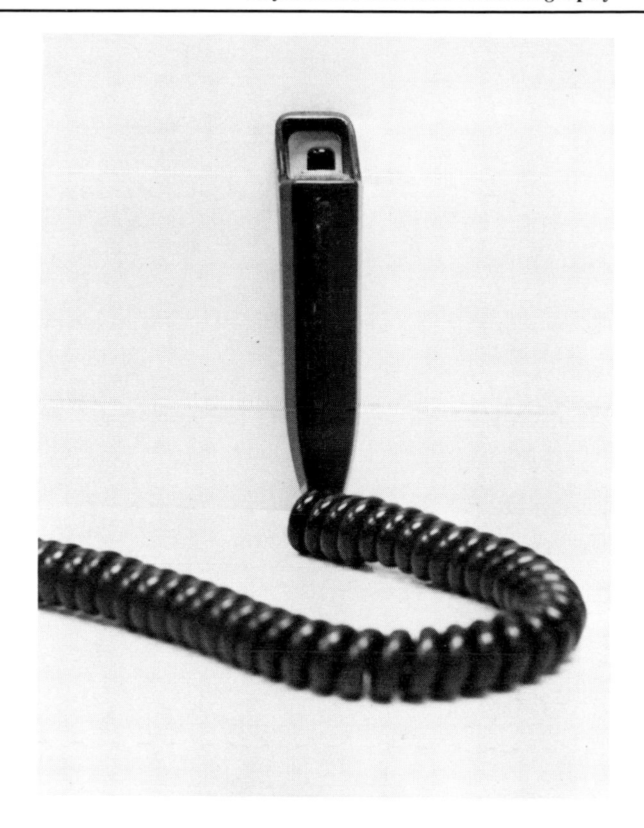

Figure 1–15. Exposure switch.

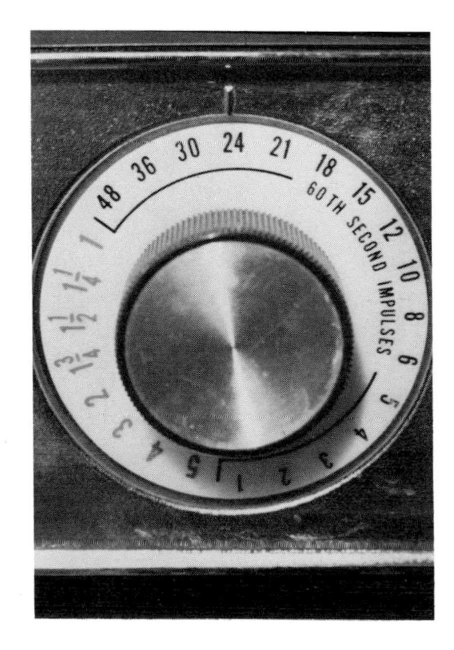

Figure 1–16. X-ray timer.

A

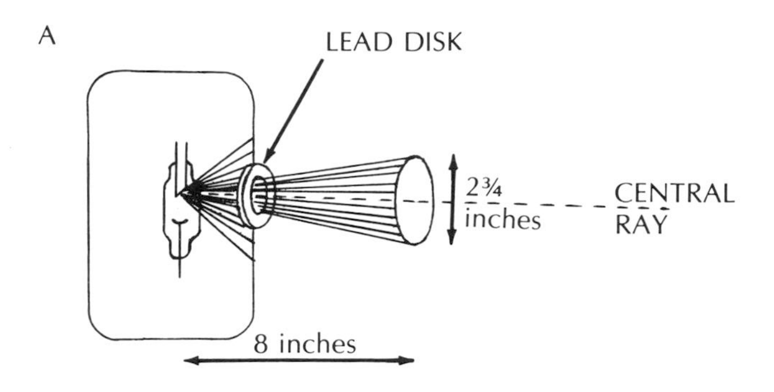

B

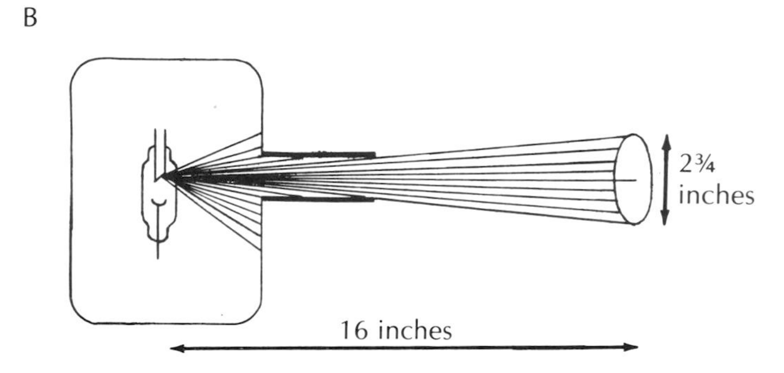

Figure 1–17. A, Lead diaphragm type of collimator producing x-ray beam with diameter of 2¼ inches at 8 inches from x-ray tube. B, Cylinder type of collimator producing x-ray beam with diameter of 2¼ inches at 16 inches from x-ray tube.

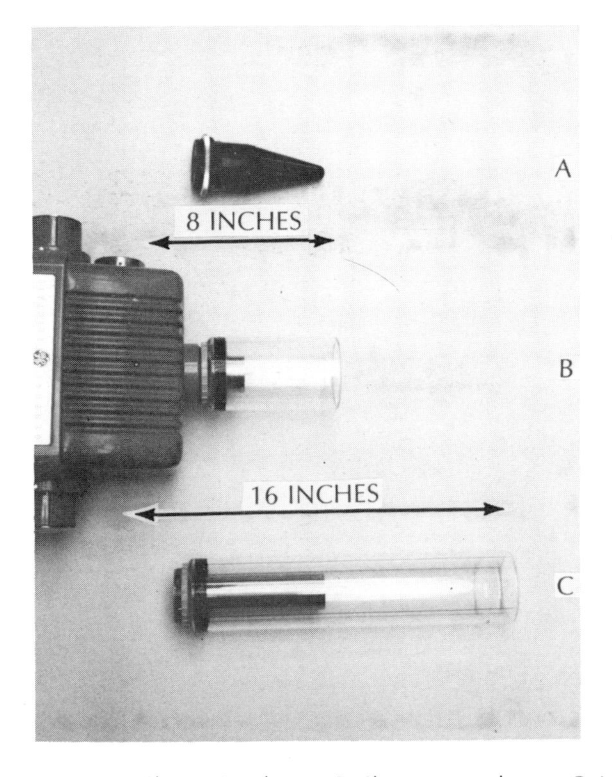

Figure 1–18. A, Short pointed cone. B, Short open-end cone. C, Long open-end cone with cylinder collimator.

is therefore called a "self-rectified x-ray tube."

Some machines use a continuous direct current flowing from the cathode to the anode. These machines produce a continuous stream of x rays instead of pulses. The timers of these machines may employ a decimal timing system.

COLLIMATION

Collimation is the term used to indicate shaping of the x rays coming from the tubehead into a column or beam of x rays. The collimator may be a metal cylinder or lead washer with a hole in the center (Figure 1–17). Some x rays are blocked while others are permitted to pass through the hole in the cylinder or diaphragm. The x-ray beam can be shaped to any desired shape or size at any distance from the patient by an appropriate collimator. Most dental machines have collimators that produce a cone-shaped beam of x rays that start at the x-ray tube's focal spot and spread to a circular area 2¾ inches in diameter on the patient's skin. The x rays traveling along the center of the cone are called the central ray. The term *central ray* is commonly used to indicate the location or direction of the x-ray beam, e.g., the central ray was aimed at ____.

The shape of the x-ray beam is also affected by the position of the x-ray tube in the machine tubehead. When the tube is placed in the back of the tubehead the x-ray beam at 4 to 6 inches in front of the tubehead can be similar to the beam at 12 to 14 inches from the tubehead when the x-ray tube is in the front of the tubehead.

CONES

Cones are x-ray beam locating devices (Figure 1–18). They are sometimes called position indicating devices (PID). Most cones are made of plastic, a material easily penetrated by x rays. A cone is often constructed with a collimator in the base. There are two types of cones, open-end and pointed cones. The open-end cone indicates the position and size of the x-ray beam at the end of the cone. The x-ray beam does not strike the plastic cylinder of the open-end cone. The pointed cone indicates the position of the central ray at the point of the cone and the position where the x-ray beam diameter is 2¾ inches wide. With a pointed cone the x-ray beam must pass through the plastic material and in so doing it produces a small amount of scattered x rays; for this reason, most machines are sold equipped with open-end cones.

FILTRATION

The x-ray beam produced by the x-ray tube consists of photons of many different wavelengths. The long wavelength, poorly penetrating x rays cannot easily pass through teeth and bone. These x rays are not useful in making dental radiographs and can be absorbed by the patient's living tissues. They are therefore removed or filtered out of the x-ray beam by passing the beam through one or more sheets of aluminum (Figure 1–19). The thickness of aluminum used is increased until all parts of the tubehead that the x rays pass through to reach the patient filter the x-ray beam similar to the filtration of 1.5 mm of aluminum (2.5 mm above 70 kVp). The x-ray beam is thus filtered with 1.5 mm Al "equivalent" when the machine is operated at 70 or lower kVp. Filtration produces an x-ray beam with a greater percentage of short wavelength x rays. The x-ray beam is said to be "hardened." The beam is also attenuated (reduced in energy) through the absorption of some x rays by the filter. Filters are located in the x-ray tubehead behind the collimator. This design permits the collimator to assist in blocking the small amount of scattered radiation (produced when the x-ray beam passes through the filter) from reaching the patient.

HALF VALUE LAYER

When an x-ray beam is filtered, the amount of energy in the beam is reduced. The thickness of the aluminum filter that reduces the beam energy by 50% is called the half value layer (HVL). When the x-ray beam has more short wavelength photons (for example, at high kVp) it is more penetrating and the thickness of aluminum needed to reduce the beam energy by 50% is greater. Dental x-ray machines are required to have a minimum HVL of 1.5 mm of aluminum when operated

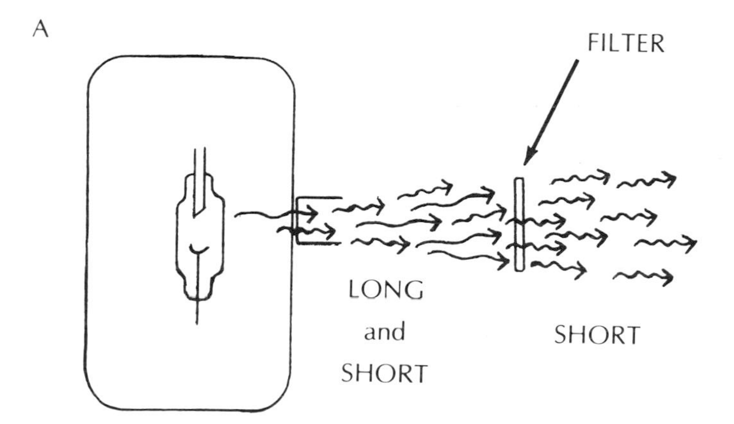

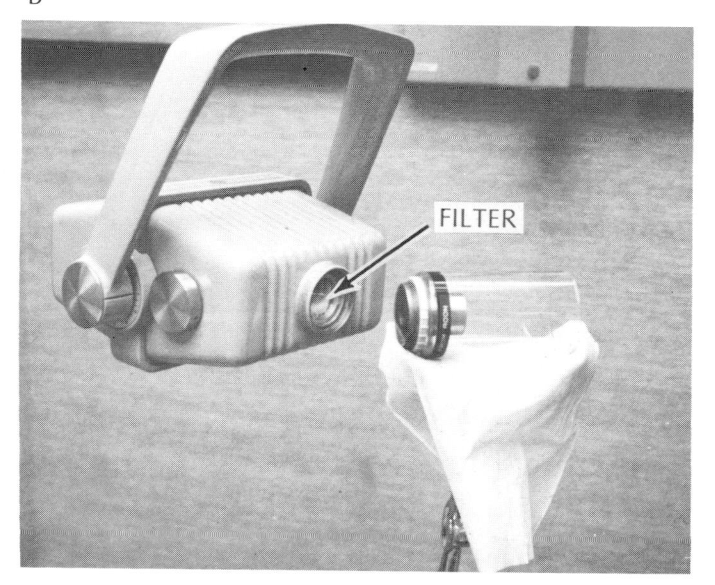

Figure 1–19. A, Diagrammatic representation of removal of long wavelength, low energy, poorly penetrating x rays by aluminum filter. B, Location of filter behind collimator in x-ray machine.

at or below 70 kVp. Above 70 kVp the required HVL gradually increases. These requirements are usually satisfied when the machine is filtered with 1.5 mm aluminum at 70 (or below) kVp and with 2.5 mm aluminum at kilovoltages above 70 kVp. The requirements are established to prevent the use of x-ray beams that do not readily penetrate dental tissues to reach the film and thus prevent unnecessary patient exposure to x rays. The HVL measures the penetrating quality of an x-ray beam.

X-RAY ABSORPTION AND SCATTERED X RAYS

X rays produce changes in an object when they are absorbed by the atoms of the object and give up energy when they encounter the electrons of atoms (Figure 1–20A). A photon may give up all its energy to a single electron and disappear. This process is called photoelectric absorption and results in a single high speed electron. The photon may interact with many electrons a little at a time. This process is called Compton scattering and results in many electrons traveling at lesser speeds. X rays have enough energy to push electrons out of their orbits and produce ions (atoms or molecules with a positive or negative electric charge). Thus, x rays belong to the group of ionizing radiations. Dental x rays cannot affect the tightly bound nucleus of an atom and are only changed in their direction or scattered (Figure 1–20B). They cannot make atoms radioactive; thus patients do not give off x rays after the x-ray machine stops producing x rays. The electrons removed from atoms by x rays may be moving with considerable speed; they give up energy by removing the electrons of other atoms, thus creating more ions until all their energy of motion is dissipated. X rays in the x-ray beam coming from the machine are commonly called primary x rays; photons changed in direction after interacting with atoms are often called scattered or secondary x rays.

The more electrons available in an absorbing material, the more x rays are absorbed. Heavy materials such as lead, gold, and amalgam easily absorb x rays and are thus difficult for x rays to penetrate. Likewise, lightweight materials such as acrylic and human

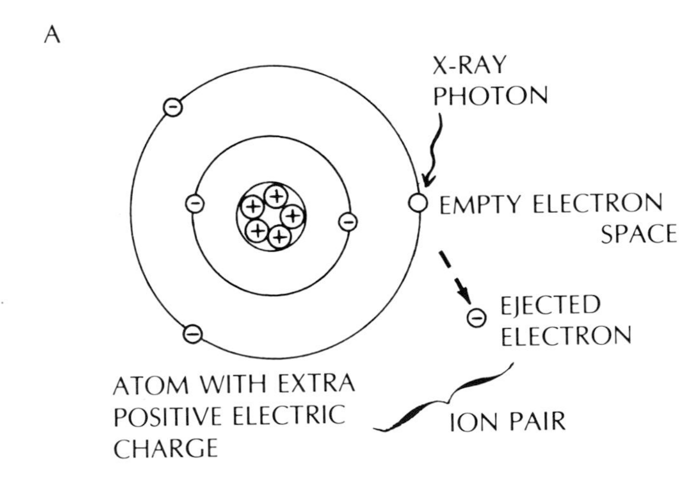

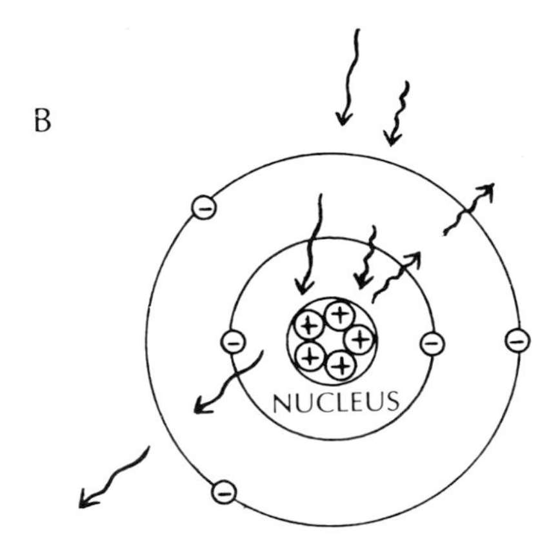

Figure 1–20. A, X-ray photon giving its energy to electron, resulting in pair of ions consisting of freely moving negatively charged electron and positively charged atom. B, X-ray photons scattered by nucleus of atom.

soft tissue are easily penetrated (Figure 1–21A). Lead and similar materials are said to be radiopaque; acrylic and soft tissues are radiolucent.

The thicker the material that an x-ray beam has to penetrate, the more x rays are absorbed. Thus a small amount of a radiopaque material may absorb the same number of x rays as a large amount of radiolucent material (Figure 1–21B).

DETECTION AND MEASUREMENT OF X RAYS

X rays are not detected by any human sensory system such as eyes, ears, nose, and taste, pressure and temperature organs. The radiation is thus detected by devices responding to the radiation in a manner that the human senses can evaluate. Responses of detection instruments can be the blackening of a film, the movement of a dial, the illumination of a light bulb or emitting of a sound.

Instruments are also made to measure the amount of radiation. X rays are measured in roentgen units or exposure units. A roentgen (R) is the amount of x rays that produces 1 electrostatic unit of electricity (2.08×10^9 ion pairs) in 1 cubic centimeter of air at standard conditions of temperature and pressure (Figure 1–22A). It utilizes the ability of x rays to separate electrons from their atoms, i.e., ionize and produce ion pairs. The roentgen is useful in describing the energy of an x-ray beam at a given spot and is used in dentistry to quantitate x-ray exposure at the skin of the patient. In dentistry the amounts of radiation are small and are often measured in milliroentgens (mR) or thousandths of a roentgen.

The roentgen is measured in air and a different unit is needed for tissues, since tissues are more dense than air and also vary in density among themselves. A measurement of the energy deposited in a tissue is important because the effect of x rays upon tissue is dependent upon the amount of energy it absorbs from the x-ray beam. The radiation unit used for tissues is the Rad or roentgen absorbed dose (Figure 1–22B). It is the production of 100 ergs of energy in 1 gram of tissue by any form of ionizing radiation. An Erg is a small fraction (10^{-7}) of a Joule which is a unit measuring the work done by a force

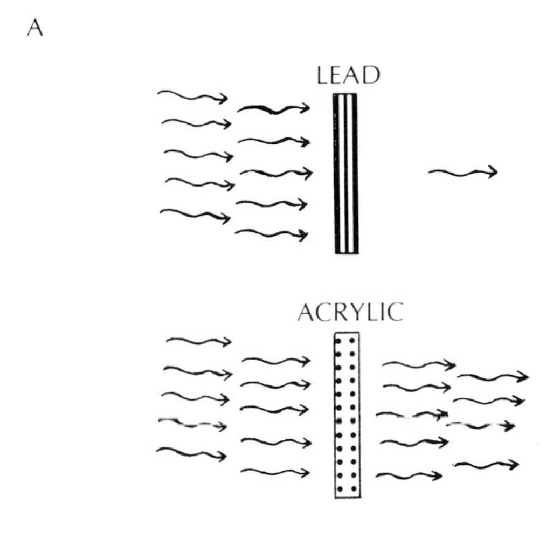

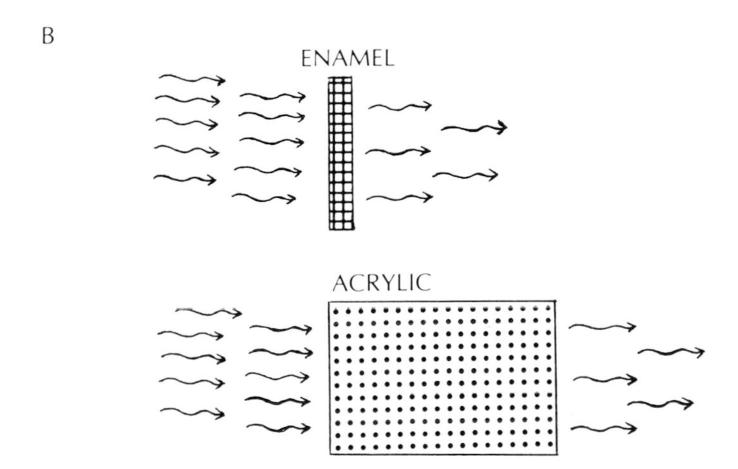

Figure 1–21. A, Different amounts of x-ray absorption by similar thickness of radiopaque (lead) and radiolucent (acrylic) material. B, Similar amounts of x rays absorbed from x-ray beam by small amount of enamel and large amount of acrylic.

A

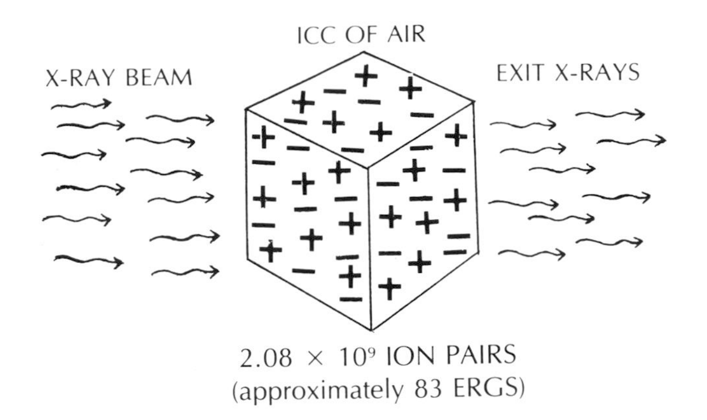

B

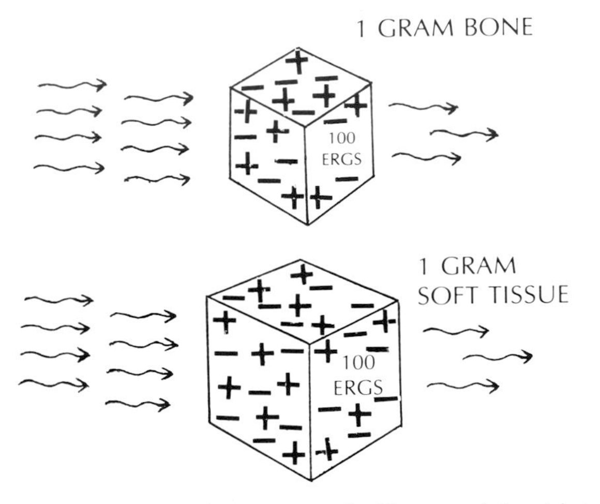

Figure 1–22. A, Diagram of 1 roentgen. B, Diagram of 1 rad being produced in bone and soft tissues.

Measurement	*Unit*
Exposure	Roentgen (R) 1 ESU/1 cc Air
Dose	RAD 100 Ergs/1 gram of any material
Dose equivalent	REM Rads × QF of radiation used
Integral dose	Gram-Rad

Figure 1–23. International radiation measurement units prior to 1985.

Old Unit		*New Unit*
1 Roentgen	=	2.58×10^{-4} Exposure Units
3.88×10^{3} Roentgens	=	1 Exposure Unit
1 RAD	=	0.01 Gray (Gy) = 1 c Gy
100 RADS	=	1 Gray
1 REM	=	0.01 Sievert (Sv)
100 REM	=	1 Sievert

Figure 1–24. Relationship of new (1985) and old radiation measurement units.

(0.225 pound or 1 newton) exerted for a distance of 1 meter. The rad is basically similar in energy to a roentgen (approximately 83 ergs). The roentgen is the measuring unit of x-ray exposure and the rad the measuring unit of dose.

Different types of radiation (e.g., x rays, electrons, protons and alpha particles) produce different degrees of biologic effect in tissue with the same dose or amount of energy deposited in the tissue. In order to measure all types of radiation for biologic effects with the same measurement a separate unit, called a REM, is used. The rem is the product of multiplying the dose (in rads) by the relative effectiveness (Quality Factor or QF) of the type of radiation used compared to x rays in producing biologic effects. The rem is an equivalent dose (Figure 1–23) that compensates for different types of radiation. When x rays are used the dose in rads and rems is the same.

A radiation dose expressed in rads or rems only measures what has occurred in a particular gram of tissue. It does not measure the total amount of energy absorbed by a person. The total energy is obtained by adding the energy deposited in each gram of irradiated tissue. The individual gram doses are thus integrated and the total is called the integral absorbed dose. The measuring unit of this dose is the *gram-rad.*

International radiation measuring units use the metric system (Systeme International or S.I. Units). These units were adopted in the year 1985. The international unit for radiation exposure that replaced the roentgen is the *exposure unit* which is defined as the amount of x rays producing one coulomb per kilogram of air. The exposure unit is equal to approximately 3.88×10^3 roentgens. For absorbed radiation the measurement unit is the Gray which is 1 joule of energy in 1 kilogram of any material. One Gray is thus equivalent to 100 rads. Similarly the equivalent dose in rems is replaced by Sievert units. The relationships of the two systems of radiation measurement units are shown in Figure 1–24.

Devices that measure radiation include the film badge, ionization chambers, and ratemeters (Figure 1–25). A film badge utilizes a dental-type film in a package containing various metal filters. When the film is developed, the blackness or density of the film indicates the amount of radiation reaching the film. The amounts of radiation reaching film areas underneath the filters indicate the penetrating ability of the radiation.

An ionization chamber is an electrically charged chamber that collects the ions created in the chamber when the chamber is exposed to x rays. The amount of electricity produced by the collected ions is read through a microscope in the same instrument that charges the chamber (charger reader), in terms of roentgens or milliroentgens.

A ratemeter has an ion collection chamber that is continually being charged by a battery. The instrument constantly measures the amount of ionization taking place in the air within the chamber. It measures a rate of radiation exposure in terms of roentgens or milliroentgens per minute or hour.

Some crystals, such as lithium fluoride and calcium fluoride, have the ability to absorb x rays and trap the energy. The energy is released in the form of visible light when the crystal is heated and thus this measurement system is called thermo-luminescence dosimetry. The crystals can be used as a single piece or in a powder form (Figure 1–26). This system is useful since the crystals absorb x rays similar to soft tissue, the dosimeter can be small and response of the crystals is proportional to the x-ray dose over a wide range of amounts of radiation.

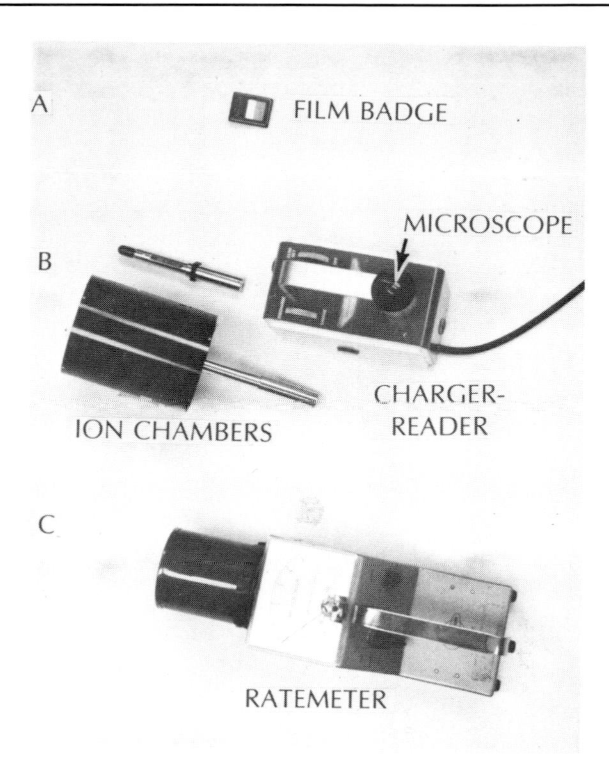

Figure 1–25. A, Film badge. B, Ion-collecting chambers of different sizes used to measure different intensities of x-ray exposures with charger-reader that operates on electricity. C, Battery-operated ratemeter used to measure rate of x rays per minute or hour.

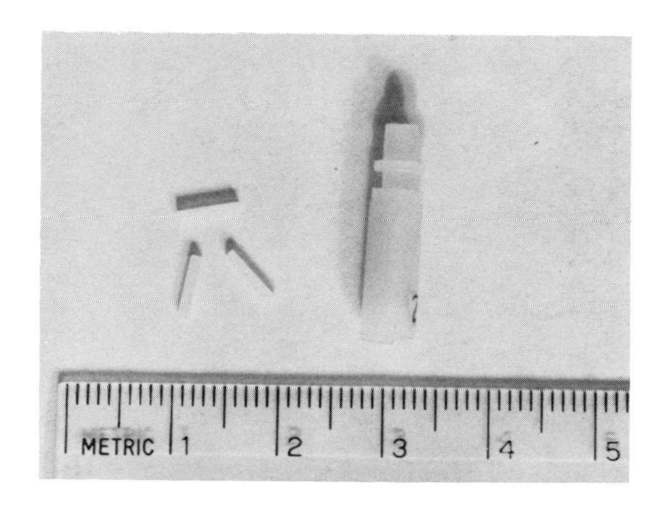

Figure 1–26. Thermoluminescent dosimeters in the form of three rod-shaped crystals and powder in a capsule.

Chapter 2

Films, Processing, Darkroom, and Duplicating

The dental radiograph is made by exposing the patient's jaws to a beam of x rays and capturing the x-ray image on a film placed in the patient's mouth (Figure 2–1A). The captured image is not visible and is thus called a *latent image.* To make the image visible the film is processed in a light tight room (usually called a darkroom) or in a light tight film processing machine (Figure 2–1B). After the processed film or radiograph has been dried, the image is viewed by the operator (radiographer) and the dental region depicted in the radiograph is identified. The radiograph is then mounted in its proper position in a *film mount* and is ready to be viewed and interpreted by the dentist (Figure 2–1C). Lay persons and some dental personnel incorrectly refer to the radiograph as "an x-ray." One should not confuse x rays, which are electromagnetic photons, with a radiograph or x-ray picture.

FILMS

Radiographic films are of two basic types, screen and non-screen film. Non-screen films are exposed directly to the x rays. Screen films are exposed mainly to the light given off by fluorescent screens that capture the x rays and convert the energy into visible light which subsequently exposes the film. Radiographic films can be classified not only as screen or non-screen but also as intraoral or extraoral film.

Intraoral Film

The intraoral dental film is a non-screen film that consists of an emulsion spread on both sides of a relatively rigid but flexible film base (Figure 2–2). The emulsion consists of x-ray sensitive crystals of silver bromide embedded in gelatin. It has a protective coating on the outer surface. Because the emulsion is also sensitive to light, the film is placed in an opaque light tight packet that is also waterproof enough to prevent a pa-

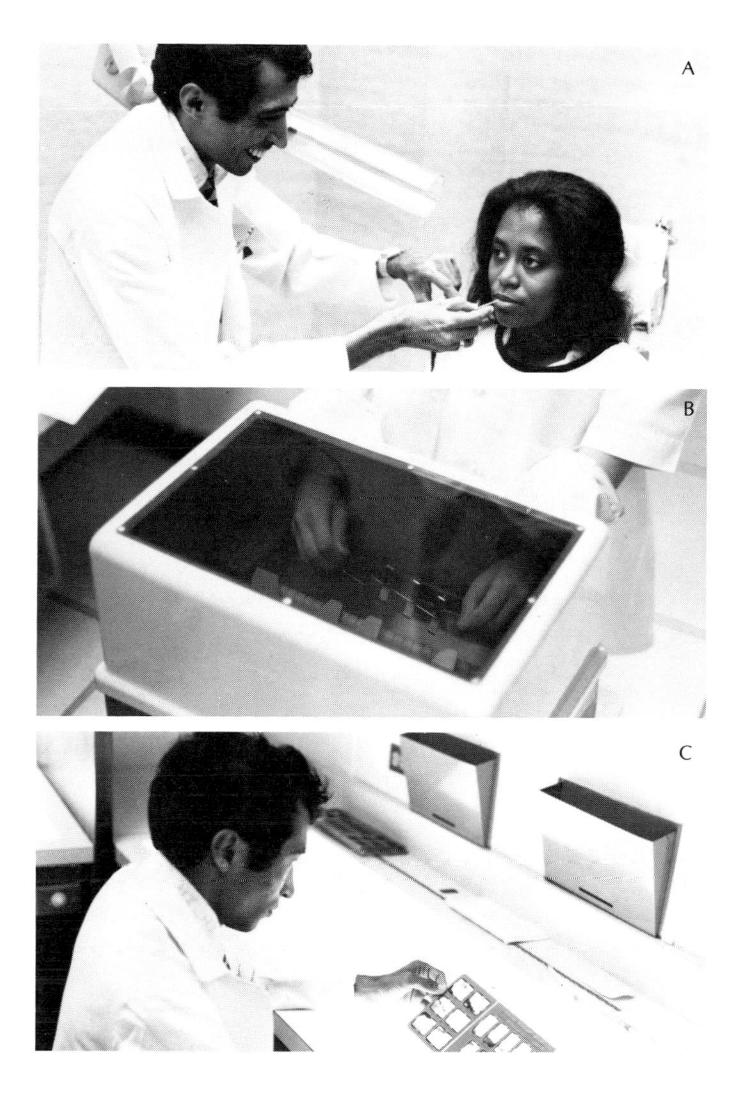

Figure 2–1. Basic processes involved in making set of dental radiographs: A, exposing films: B, processing films; C, identifying and mounting films for viewing.

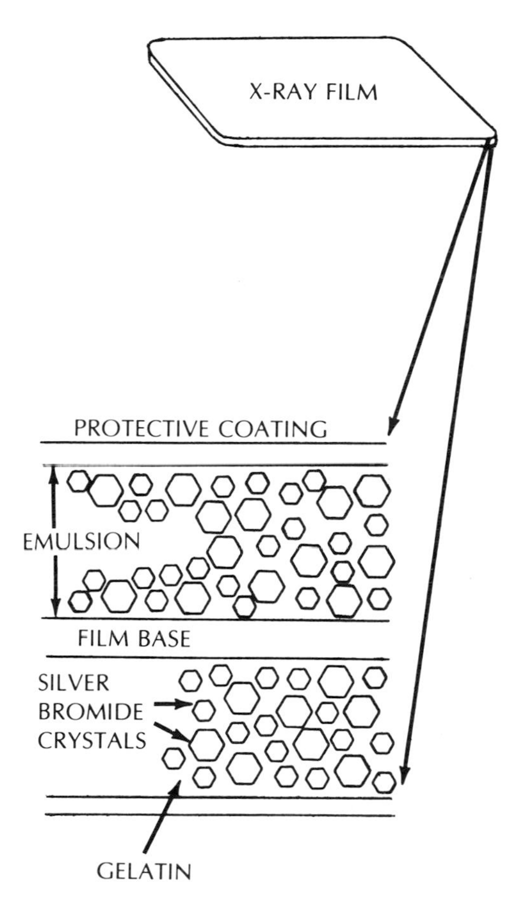

Figure 2–2. Section of dental film showing base and double emulsions.

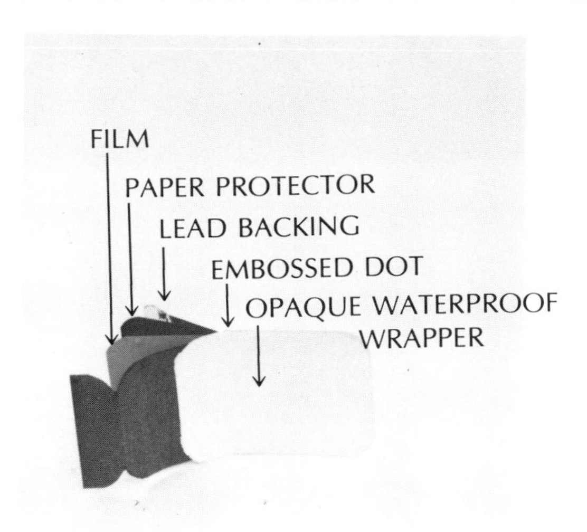

Figure 2–3. Contents of intraoral dental film package.

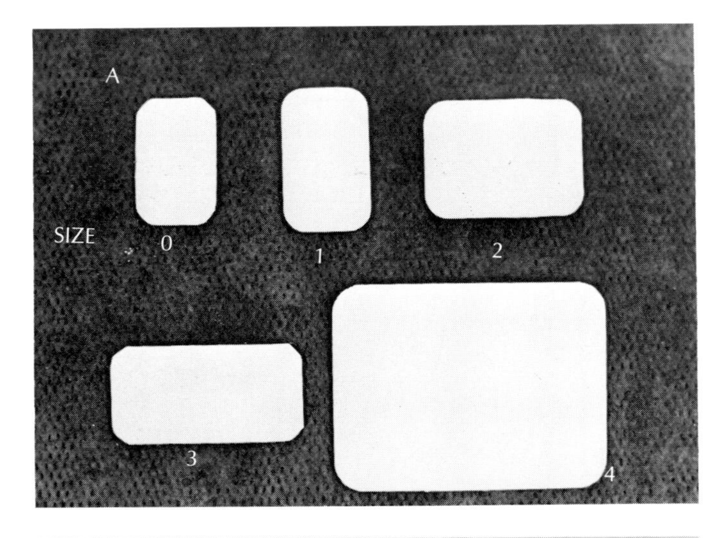

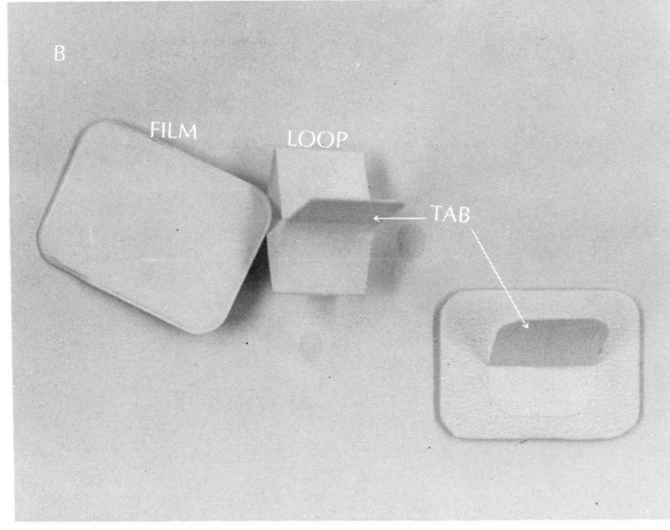

Figure 2–4. A, Intraoral films of different sizes. B, Examples of bitewing films with attached bite tabs and with bitewing loop.

tient's saliva from quickly penetrating the package (Figure 2–3). The film is protected by paper sheets and is backed by a thin sheet of lead. The lead sheet absorbs most of the x rays that pass through the film (thus protecting the patient) and also prevents scattered x rays originating in the patient's tissue behind the film from reaching the film and causing an increase in film fog. Film fog is a small exposure of the entire film and results in a radiograph that is slightly increased in density or darker. The overall increased density tends to hide or obscure the image the dentist wishes to see.

The lead backing has a pattern stamped into it; this pattern appears on the finished radiograph if the film is exposed from the wrong side. The film has an embossed dot stamped into it that appears as a bump on the exposure surface and as a depression on the opposite side.

Intraoral films are manufactured with one or two films in a package (single or double film packets). Double film packets are used when duplicate radiographs are desired or when the dentist wishes a fully processed and an underprocessed radiograph of the same area.

Intraoral films are made to be exposed while positioned in the oral cavity. Intraoral films are numbered according to their use in the mouth and the size of the film. A decimal point is used to separate the two numbers. The whole number in front of the decimal point indicates periapical radiography use (1), bite-wing radiography use (2) or occlusal radiography use (3). Numbers following the decimal point indicate film size. Intraoral films are manufactured in different sizes (Figure 2–4A). Smaller films are needed for children. Size number 1.00 is 0.812 × 1.250 inches, size 1.0 is 0.875 × 1.375 inches, size 1.1 is 0.938 × 1.562 inches, and size 1.2 is 1.219 × 1.609 inches.* These intraoral films are ordinarily used for showing detailed images of teeth and are commonly referred to as periapical films. The No. 1.2 film is often called the standard film, since it is the most commonly used intraoral film. These intraoral films are commonly referred to as double zero, zero, one, and two.

*The American National Standards Institute (ANSI) classification with proprietary sponsorship of the American Dental Association.

Bitewing films are manufactured with bite tabs attached to the film packets, or are constructed from periapical films and bitewing loops (Figure 2–4B). Film size ANSI No. 2.3 measures 2.109 × 1.047 inches and is only made as a bitewing film. Film size ANSI No. 3.4 (2.250 × 3.000 inches) is called an occlusal film because it is usually positioned in the occlusal plane of the patient.

When a film is exposed to radiation and processed the sensitive film becomes opaque (dark to transmitted light). The opacity or density of the film is related to the amount of radiation the film receives. However, the response of the film varies with the same increase in radiation exposure, and the density to exposure relationship is seen as a curve. Figure 2–5 shows the sensitometric or characteristic curve of an intraoral film. The graph is sometimes referred to as a Hurter-Driffield curve and is named after two early investigators of film sensitometry.

Intraoral films vary in speed. Fast films need less x radiation to become exposed and are a major factor in reducing patient exposure to x rays. Film speed is affected by the size and shape of the silver bromide crystals. Speed groups are A, B, C, D, E, and F, with A being the slowest film and each subsequent group being approximately twice as fast as the preceding group. Group D films are considered fast films, group C intermediate speed films, and groups A and B are called slow films. At the present time group D film appears to be the most common type film manufactured and there is some speed E film available.

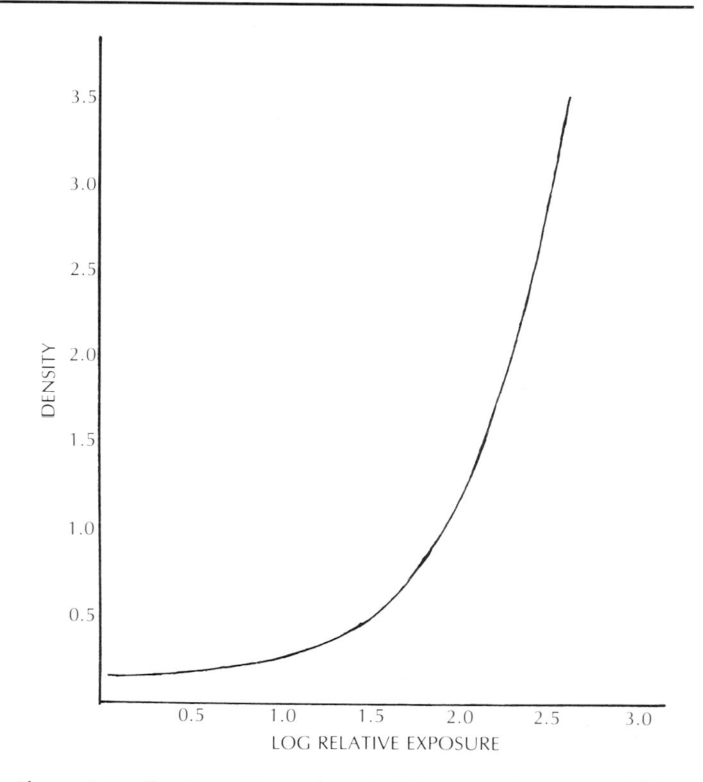

Figure 2–5. Sensitometric or characteristic curve of an intraoral film. The curve is also called a Hurter-Driffield or H and D curve.

Extraoral Film

Extraoral films are made to be exposed while positioned outside of the oral cavity. They are 5 × 7 inches or larger and the film's emulsion is made to be sensitive mainly to the light given off by screens when x rays are absorbed by the screens (Figure 2–6). This system requires fewer x rays to expose the film, since screens are much more efficient than films in absorbing x-ray photons. The screens immediately give up the absorbed energy in the form of light photons (i.e., they fluoresce) which are now easily absorbed by the film. The active ingredients of a screen

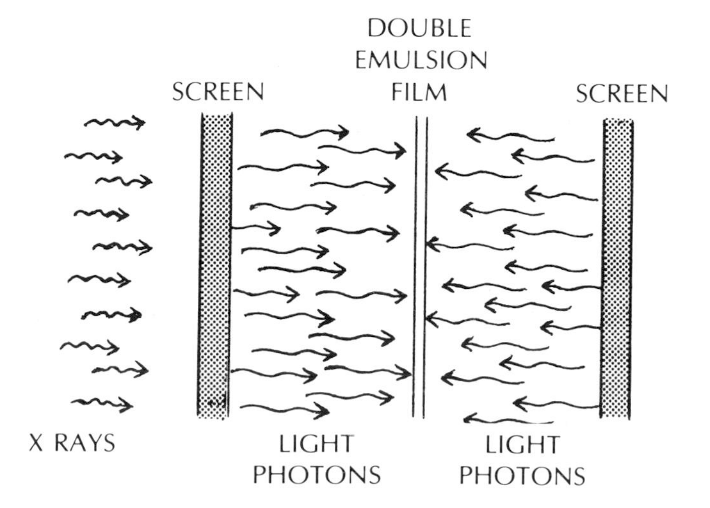

Figure 2–6. Conversion of x rays into light photons by screens.

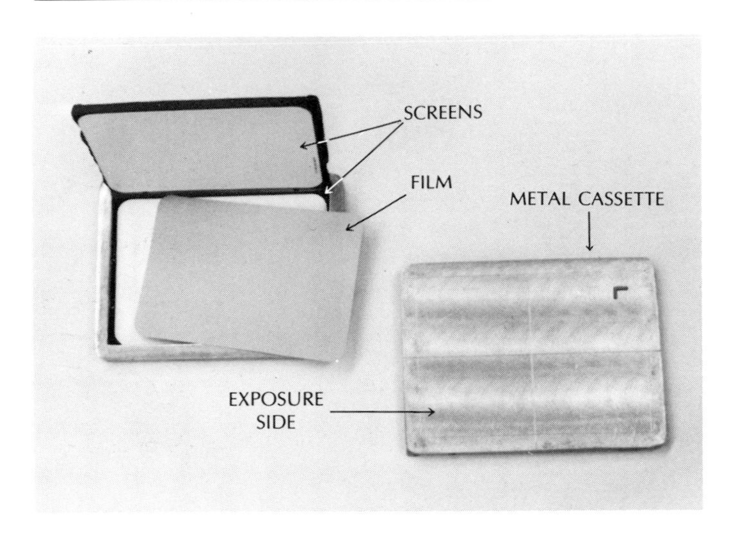

Figure 2–7. Cassette. Opened to show screen film sandwiched between pair of screens (left) and closed cassette (right).

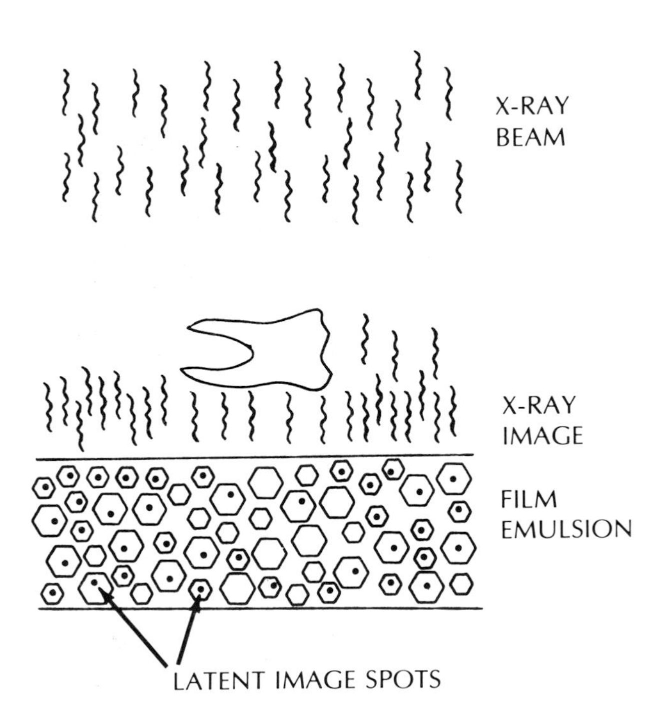

Figure 2–8. Diagram of formation of latent image of tooth in form of specks or spots of silver on exposed crystals in film emulsion.

are x-ray absorbing crystals. Larger crystals or thicker crystal layers absorb more x rays and thus screens, like films, vary in speed.

Screens were made for many years with calcium tungstate crystals that emitted a blue light when struck by x rays. In recent years screens made with different atoms or elements have been manufactured. These elements, crystals or phosphors capture x rays more efficiently than calcium tungstate crystals and screens made with these new crystals are thus faster or more efficient. Many of these elements are not commonly found in the earth and the screens are called rare earth screens. These screens may emit light that is green or another color. Films used with screens are made to be specifically sensitive to the color light emitted by the screen. Screen-film compatibility must always be correct or the speed of the combination will be greatly reduced.

Screen film usually is placed between two screens in a light tight box called a cassette (Figure 2–7). The exposure side of the cassette is radiolucent and the opposite side radiopaque. Clamps or some other means are used to provide contact between film and screen, since the light photons from one spot of the screen must be transmitted to the corresponding spot on the film without spreading to produce an accurate radiographic image.

Extraoral films usually have double emulsions, but unlike intraoral films do not have the embossed dot or bump to indicate the surface facing the x-ray beam. They are used in film holders or cassettes that have the letter R or L (to indicate the right or left side of the patient) made of lead on the exposure side of the cassette. The letter is radiopaque and appears in the finished radiograph.

THE LATENT IMAGE

When a beam of x rays passes through an object, some x rays are absorbed by the object. The x-ray beam now has an image of the object. When this image in x-ray form passes through the film's emulsion, some photosensitive crystals are exposed by x-ray photons and others are not; there are more exposed crystals where there are more photons. Some silver and bromine atoms are separated in the ionized exposed crystals; the silver atoms collect as a speck or spot in each exposed crystal (Figure 2–8). Collectively the crystals with silver specks form an image of the object that cannot be seen visually. It is thus called a latent image. Latent images can also be produced by applying other forms of energy to the film, such as bending the film, producing static electricity on the film, or having chemicals touch the film.

FILM PROCESSING

To make the exposed film into a radiograph the film is removed from its packet or cassette in a darkroom or under similar safe darkroom conditions. It is then passed through a series of solutions that process the latent image into a visible image useful for diagnosis.

Film Development

To see the x-ray image in a film the latent image must be developed. This process must be done in a darkroom under light-safe conditions. The film is removed from its packet or cassette and placed in a developing solution (Figure 2–9). There are five basic chemicals in the radiographic developer. An activator chemical provides the necessary alkaline medium and softens the gelatin of the emulsion. The two developing chemicals act on the exposed crystals that have silver specks and precipitate all the silver in these crystals; they do not easily affect the unexposed crystals (Figure 2–10A).

One developing agent quickly makes the image visible; this chemical is not affected by the temperature of the developing solution. The other developing agent slowly builds contrast between the heavily and lightly x-ray exposed areas of the films; this chemical is temperature sensitive. If the developing solution has a high temperature (80°F or more), the film will be developed quickly, but the radiographic image will have high contrast or a more black and white appearance. At low developer temperatures (60°F or below) the film is developed slowly and has less contrast or a gray shadow image. Films are best developed at 68° to 70°F for 5 minutes.

Other chemicals in the developer solution are a restrainer to prevent chemical fog

DEVELOPER SOLUTION

Chemical	*Action*
Developing Agents	
1. Elon or Metol	Builds image quickly
2. Hydroquinone	Builds contrast slowly
Preservative	
Sodium sulfite	Prevents oxidation
Activator	
Sodium carbonate	Provides alkaline medium Softens gelatin
Restrainer	
Potassium bromide	Prevents chemical fog

Figure 2–9. List of active agents in radiographic developer and their action on film emulsion.

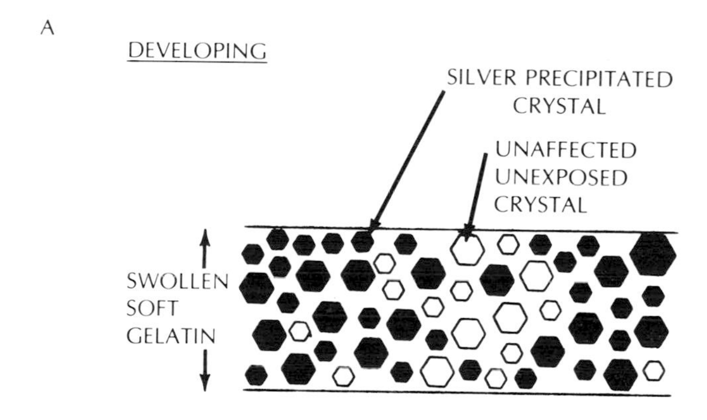

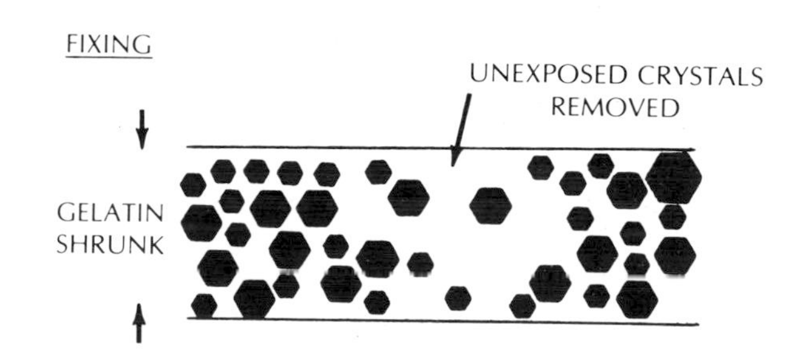

Figure 2–10. A, Diagram of result of film development. B, Diagram of result of film fixing.

FIXER SOLUTION

Chemical	*Action*
Fixing Agent	
Sodium thiosulfate (hypo)	Removes unexposed crystals
Preservative	
Sodium sulfite	Prevents deterioration of hypo
Hardening Agent	
Potassium alum	Shrinks and hardens the gelatin
Acidifier	
Acetic acid	Provides acid medium

Figure 2–11. List of active agents in radiographic fixer and their action on film emulsion.

which occurs when the developer chemicals act on the unexposed crystals and a preservative to prevent oxidation of the developer solution. Oxidation through interaction with oxygen in the air weakens the developer solution. Film processing must be conducted in a manner that minimizes solution oxidation.

Film Rinsing

After developing, the film is rinsed for 20 seconds and then placed in the fixer solution. Rinsing removes the alkaline developer solution from the film and prevents this solution from mixing with the acid fixer and weakening the fixer solution.

Film Fixing

There are four active chemicals in a radiographic fixer solution (Figure 2–11). Sodium thiosulfate (commonly called "hypo") removes the unexposed crystals in the emulsion, allowing light to pass through the film and permitting viewing of the radiographic image on a view-box. A hardening agent shrinks and hardens the gelatin of the emulsion. The fixing solution also has a preservative to prevent oxidation, and an acidifier to provide the necessary acid medium.

The effect of fixer on the film emulsion is shown in Figure 2–10B. The fixing process takes approximately 10 minutes. Most of the crystals are removed in the first 2 minutes of fixing and the film can be viewed in a lighted area at this time; however, it must be returned to the fixer to complete the "fixing" process or some crystals will remain in the emulsion and darken or stain the radiograph months later.

Film Washing

To complete processing, the film is washed for 20 minutes in running water to remove the fixer solution; then it is dried in a dust-free area. The processed film is now called a *radiograph.*

THE DARKROOM

The darkroom must not only be light tight but must also be ventilated, well equipped,

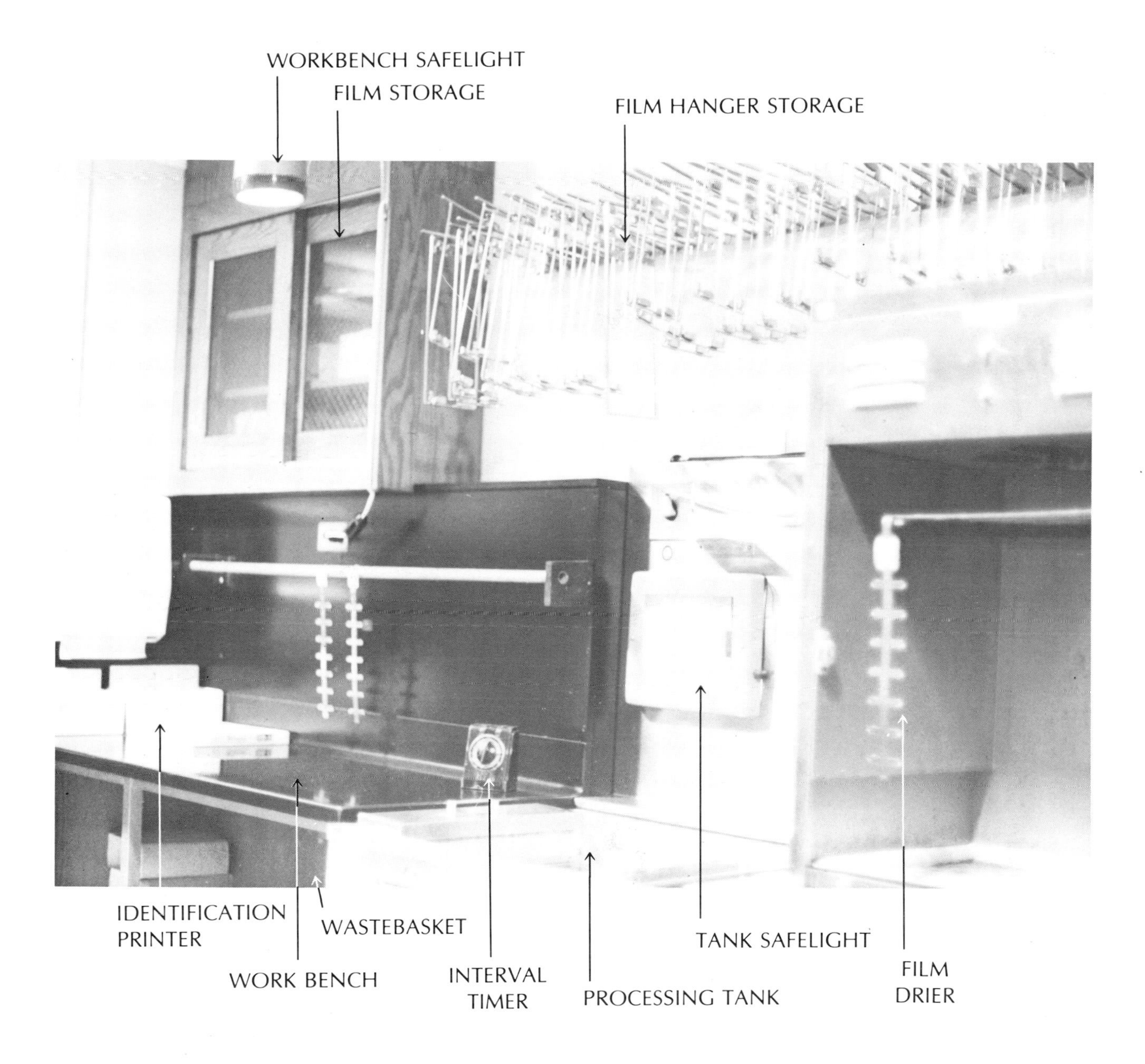
WORKBENCH SAFELIGHT
FILM STORAGE
FILM HANGER STORAGE
IDENTIFICATION PRINTER
WASTEBASKET
WORK BENCH
INTERVAL TIMER
PROCESSING TANK
TANK SAFELIGHT
FILM DRIER

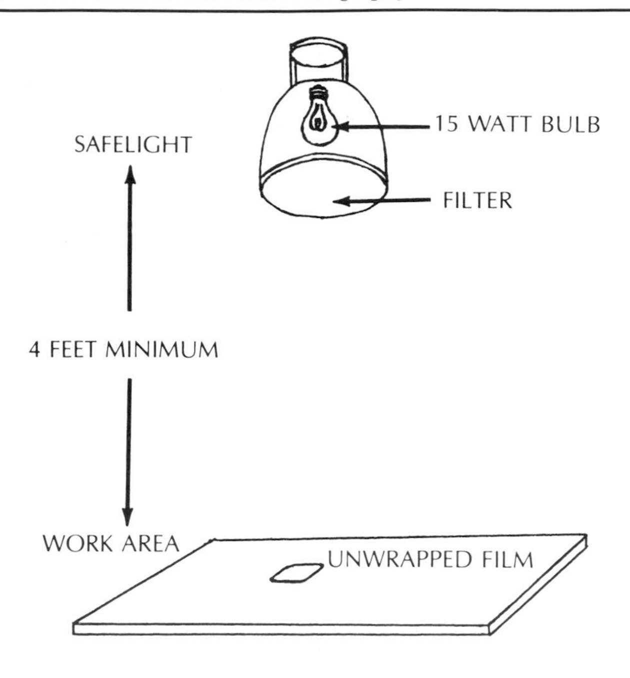

Figure 2–13. Darkroom safelight and its location.

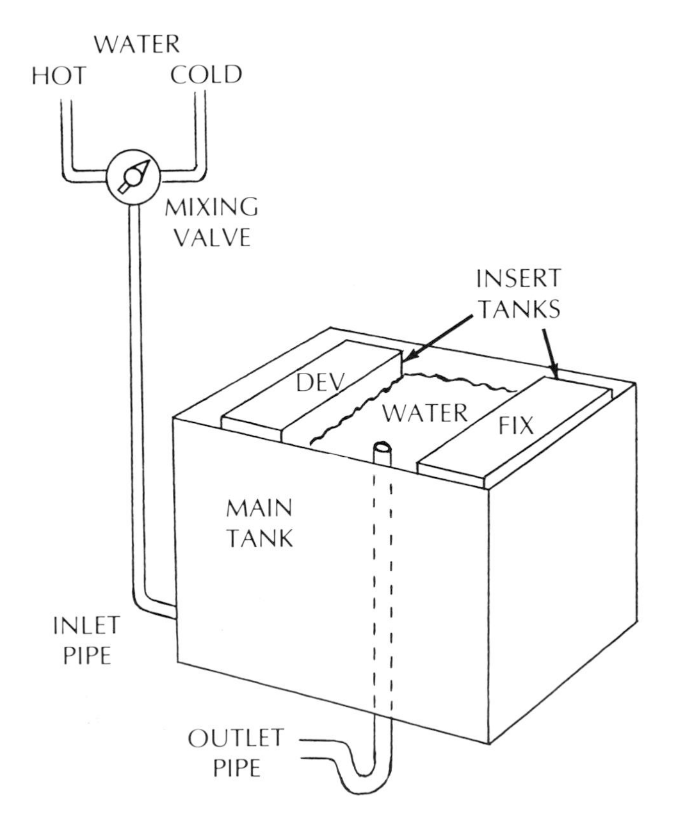

Figure 2–14. Dental processing tank.

clean, and efficient (Figure 2–12). It should be at least 4 × 5 feet and be located as close as possible to the x-ray exposure or radiograph reading area. A light tight darkroom does not mean that the room walls must be painted black; walls should be a light, pleasant color to reflect the room illumination. The darkroom should have a worktable area, both safelight and whitelight, tanks for processing solutions, hot and cold running water, a thermometer, an interval timer, a radiograph viewer, and a film-drying rack.

The Safelight

A safelight recommended by the film manufacturer must be used in the darkroom (Figure 2–13). Different safelight filters are usually used for screen and intraoral films; for example, a Morlite 2 (ML 2) filter is used with Kodak intraoral films. All safelights produce a small amount of unsafe light and thus the light is used with a specified wattage bulb (usually 15 W) at a specific minimum distance (usually 4 feet) from the worktable where films are unwrapped. When the safelight is positioned farther from the unwrapped films, a stronger bulb can be used. Specifications of bulb wattage and distance satisfies darkroom light safety for normal working times. If working time is short a stronger bulb can be used. For example, a 25 watt bulb can be used with a GBX filter for some screen film if the film handling time is not more than 1 minute.

The Processing Tank, Thermometer, and Timer

Tank processing is a simple, accurate, and trouble-free method of processing films. The most practical tank consists of a large tank with intake and outlet connections for running water and two smaller insert tanks for developer and fixer solutions (Figure 2–14). The tanks should be made of stainless steel to resist corrosion and permit easy cleaning. The tank is set into the worktable or with its top at the edge of the worktable. Hot and cold water are mixed and supplied to the bottom of the tank. An overflow pipe is connected to the waste line plumbing of the office. The sizes of the tanks depend upon the number of films to be processed daily. The average single dentist's office uses one-gallon developer and fixer tanks. Insert tanks should be covered whenever possible to minimize oxidation of the solution by air.

Proper film processing requires accurate measurement of developer temperature and developing time. A good thermometer is indispensable (Figure 2–15). The thermometer, either the floating type or one clipped to the side of the developing tank, should be placed in the developing solution, since temperature greatly affects the activity of this solution.

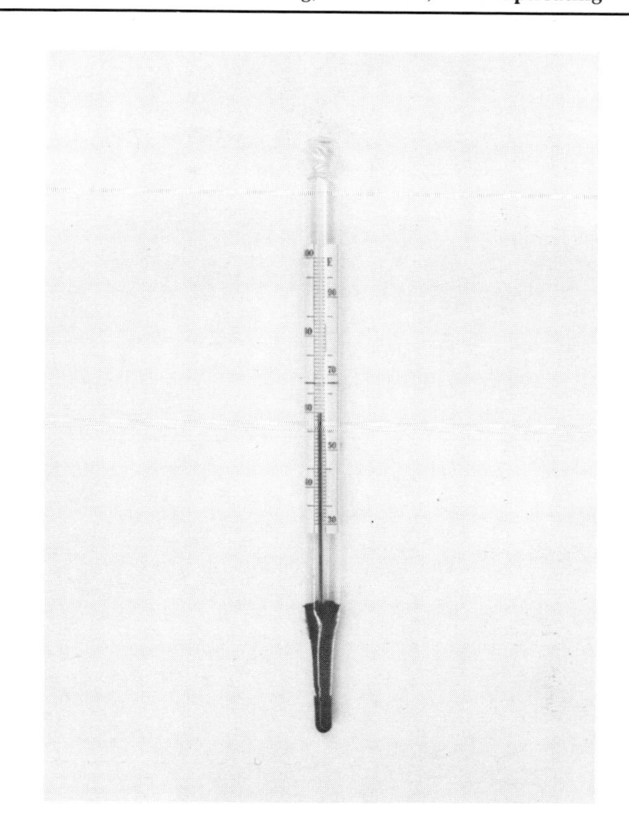

Figure 2–15. Thermometer made to float in water or developer solution.

An interval timer is needed to measure the time a film is in the developer or fixer solution (Figure 2–16). These times are indicated in the instructions of the solution manufacturer. Underdevelopment will produce light density radiographs and underfixing will produce cloudy, partially opaque radiographs. Greatly prolonged overdevelopment will produce chemically fogged radiographs and greatly prolonged overfixing will produce light density radiographs. Some radiographers tend to judge the development of a film by sight. This is not a good procedure, since consistently good quality radiographs cannot be produced in this manner. However, sight-development is useful when a film is known to be accidentally overexposed and a reduced developing time is needed to obtain a usable density radiograph and avoid repeated x-ray exposure of the patient.

Preparing Processing Solutions

Developer and fixer chemicals come in powder form, as ready-mixed solutions, or in liquid concentrates (Figure 2–17). The processing solutions must be of the type required by the processing equipment and the films to be processed. Powdered chemicals must be mixed slowly with distilled water. Mixed solutions stored for later use must be kept in tightly stoppered brown bottles. Liquid concentrates are convenient for most offices; they are usually of good strength, occupy little storage space, and are quickly mixed with water.

Processing solutions are changed when they become exhausted and prolonged processing time is needed to completely develop and fix the exposed film. A weakened developer will not fully develop the latent im-

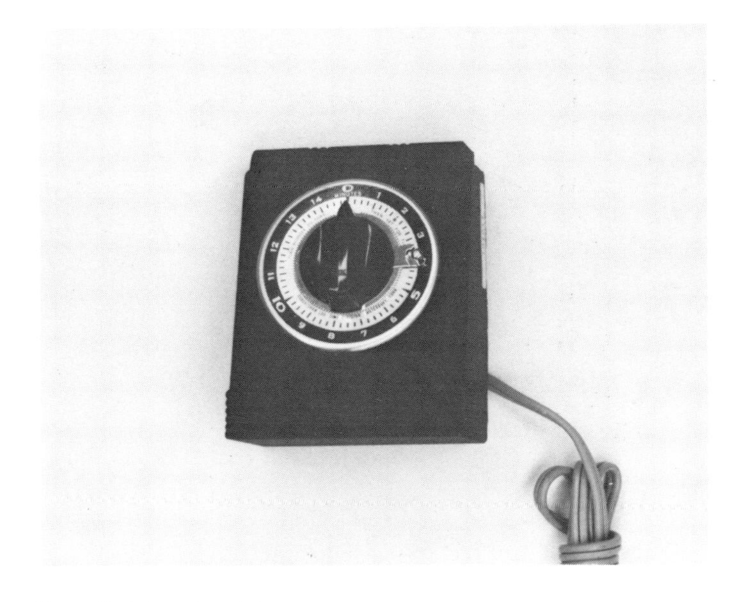

Figure 2–16. Interval timer.

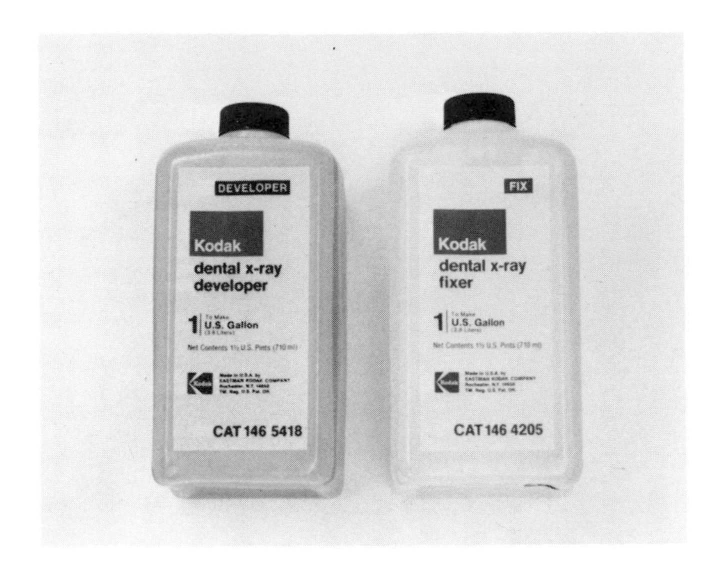

Figure 2–17. Liquid concentrates of developer and fixer.

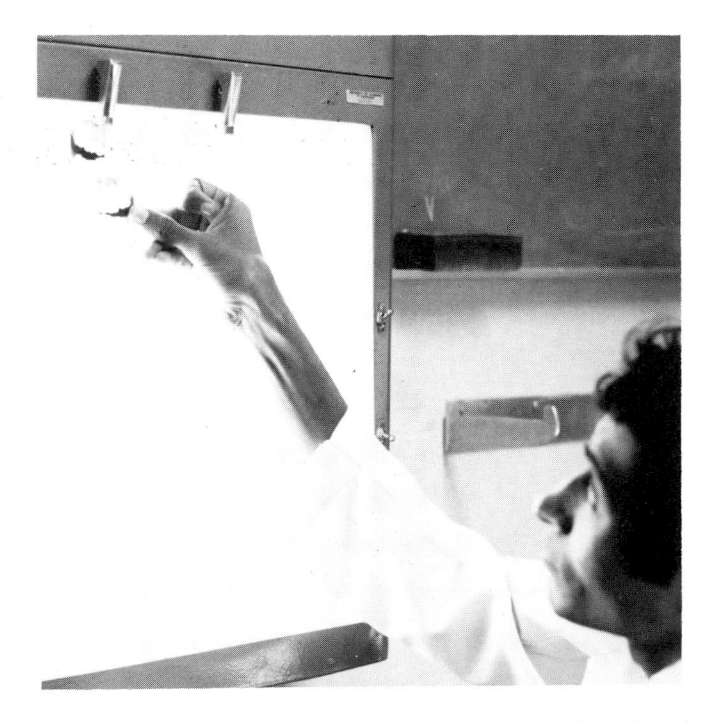

Figure 2–18. Matching of densities of new processed radiograph with density of previously properly exposed and processed radiograph.

age in the usual time, and the density of the radiograph will be too light. It is difficult to establish a specific time period between solution changes for any dental office because many factors affect the strength of the developer solution, for example, the temperature of the developer, the number of films processed, the amount of time the developer tank is left uncovered, forceful agitation of the film holder thus oxidizing the solution, and spillage of fixer chemicals into the developer. However, a rough indication of a weak developer solution can be obtained by placing an unwanted good density radiograph, made on an average-sized patient when the solutions are at full strength, on a corner of the viewbox; later processed radiographs, made of the same dental region of other average-sized patients, are matched for density with the first radiograph. Less density that can be easily seen in a later radiograph indicates a weakened developer solution and signals the need for changing the solution (Figure 2–18). More accurate tests for processing solution strength are described in the chapter on quality control in the dental office. Weakened fixer solution is easily identified when the film takes more than 2 minutes to clear.

Instead of changing weakened processing solutions, the strength of the solution can be restored by adding a replenishing solution (Figure 2–19). Replenishing is usually done according to the number of films processed in the solution. Manufacturer's instructions must be followed.

PROCESSING TECHNIC AND ARTIFACTS

With the darkroom white light "off" and the safelight "on" the film is removed from its packet (Figure 2–20). Too forceful opening of the packet, especially when the room air is dry, can produce static electricity which appears as characteristic dark streaks on the processed radiograph (Figure 2–21A). The film should be held by the edges to prevent crimping or fingernail pressure on the sensitive emulsion; fingernail pressure appears as a crescent-shaped artifact (Figure 2–21B). Bending the film can produce a white undeveloped area or a black line (Figure 2–21C). The operator's fingers must be

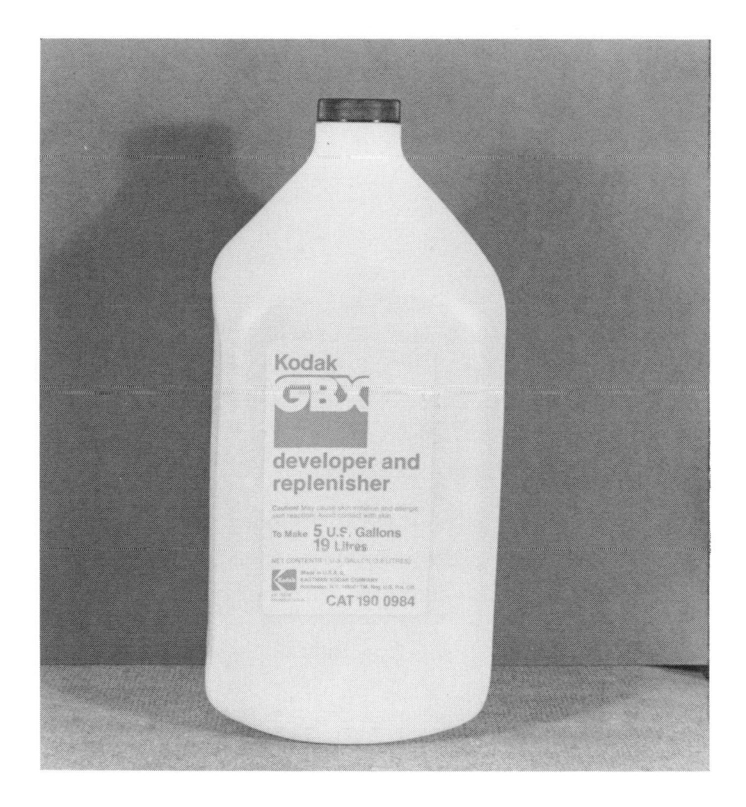

Figure 2–19. Developer replenisher.

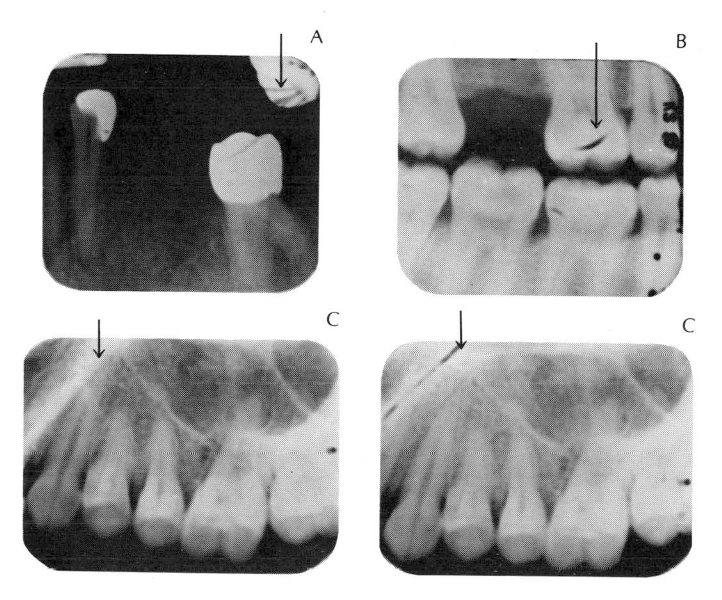

Figure 2–21. A, Dark streaks produced by static electricity. B, Crescent-shaped artifact caused by emulsion crimping. C, White and black lines produced by film bending.

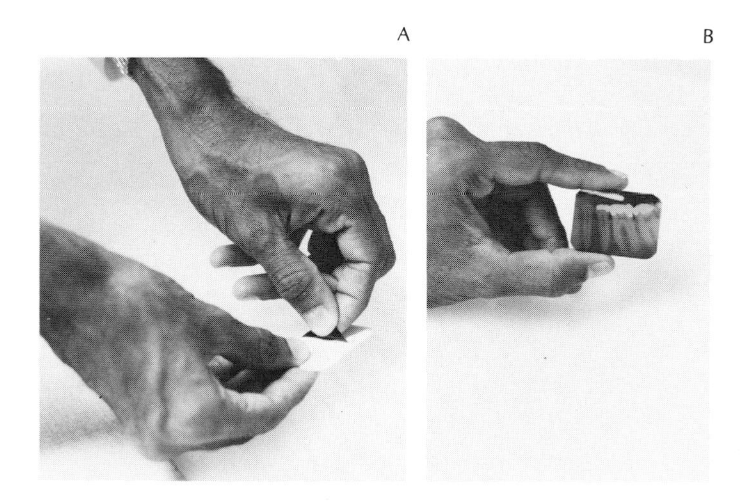

Figure 2–20. Removal of film from film packet: A, opening film packet; B, holding film by edges.

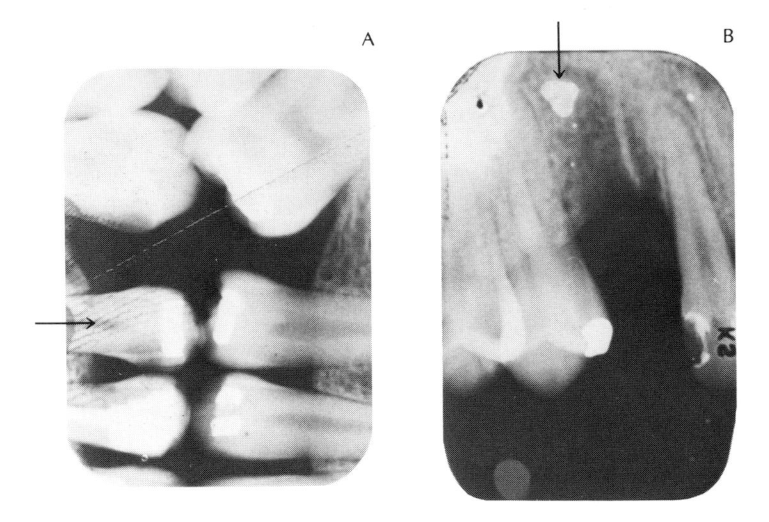

Figure 2–22. A, Fingermarks produced by photosensitizing chemicals. B, Drop of fixer splashed on film prior to development.

DEVELOPING

Temperature	*Time (minutes)*
80°F (26.5°C)	2½
76°F (24°C)	3
72°F (22°C)	4
70°F (21°C)	4½
68°F (20°C)	5
65°F (18.5°C)	6

Figure 2–23. Commonly recommended developer times and temperatures for manual processing of intraoral films. Developing times can be different for extraoral films; follow film manufacturer's instructions.

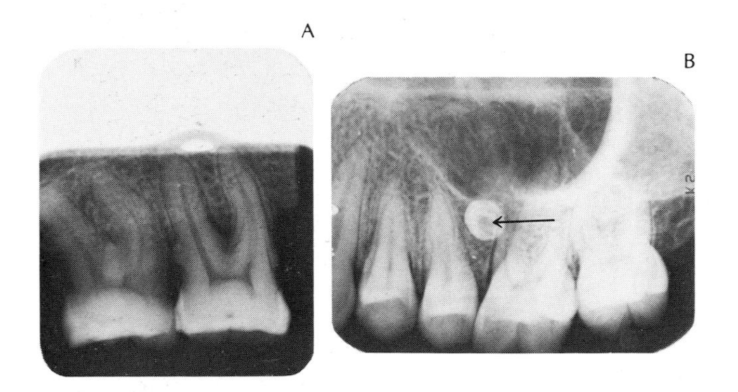

Figure 2–24. A, Film partially immersed in developing solution. B, White spot produced by air bubble in developer.

clean and free of chemicals such as fluoride or fixer. Such chemicals can produce a latent image which appears as fingerprints in the processed radiograph (Figure 2–22A). If the darkroom is not kept clean or the operator is careless, fixer solution can be splashed on the film prior to development and the crystals may be removed from that area of the emulsion (Figure 2–22B).

The film is placed in the clip of a film hanger. The temperature of the developer is read, the developing times are selected (Figure 2–23), and the interval timer is set. Higher developer temperatures need less developing time; however, a high contrast radiograph is produced. The optimum temperature is 68°F and the water temperature of the large tank should be adjusted prior to use of the darkroom to be as close to 68°F as is practical.

The film hanger is placed in the developing solution and the interval timer is started. A check should be made to see that the film is completely immersed in solution. Evaporation can lower the level of the solution, and a partially immersed film will result in partial area development (Figure 2–24A). The film hanger is agitated to remove air bubbles clinging to the film which prevent the developer solution from acting on the emulsion (Figure 2–24B). If the clips of the film hanger contain fixer chemicals from improper washing of the film hanger after a previous film was processed, the chemicals will produce streaks or lines on the radiograph (Figure 2–25A).

When the interval timer indicates that the proper developing time has elapsed, the latent image is now fully developed. The film hanger is removed from the developer and rinsed in the running water of the main tank for 20 seconds. Rinsing removes the alkaline developer solution clinging to the film and hanger and prevents its weakening the acid fixer solution. If the developing is done at a high temperature and the film is rinsed in very cold water in another tank, the sudden change in temperature may cause the swollen emulsion to shrink quickly and produce a wrinkled appearance called *reticulation* (Figure 2–25B).

After rinsing, the film is placed in the fixing solution for 10 minutes for proper fixing and hardening of the emulsion. Most of the

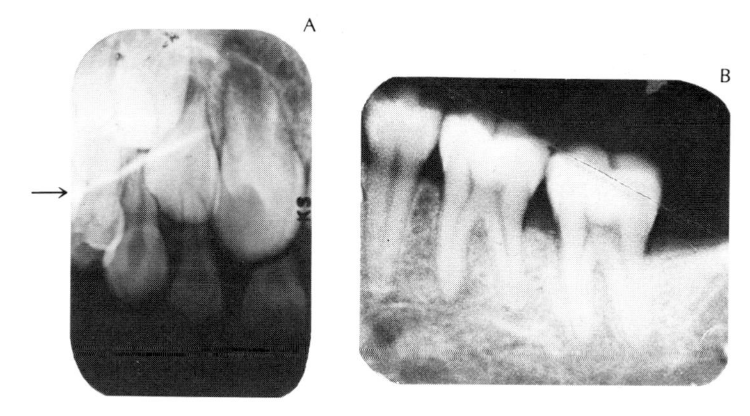

Figure 2–25. A, Line produced by fixer left under film hanger clip after improper washing. B, Reticulation.

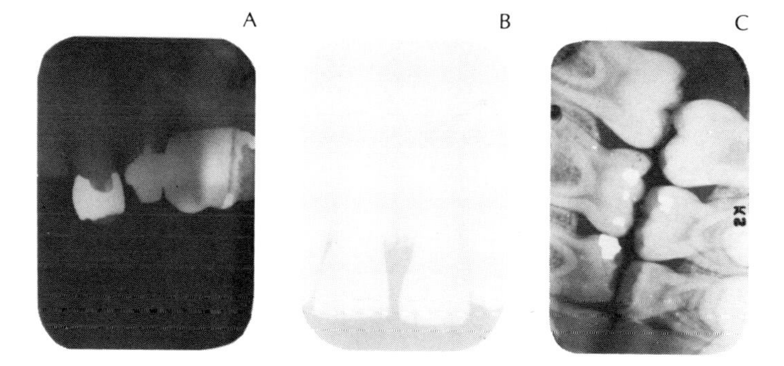

Figure 2–26. A, Stained film from incomplete fixing or incomplete washing. B, Light image film due to overfixing. C, Clear spots caused by undissolved fixer chemicals.

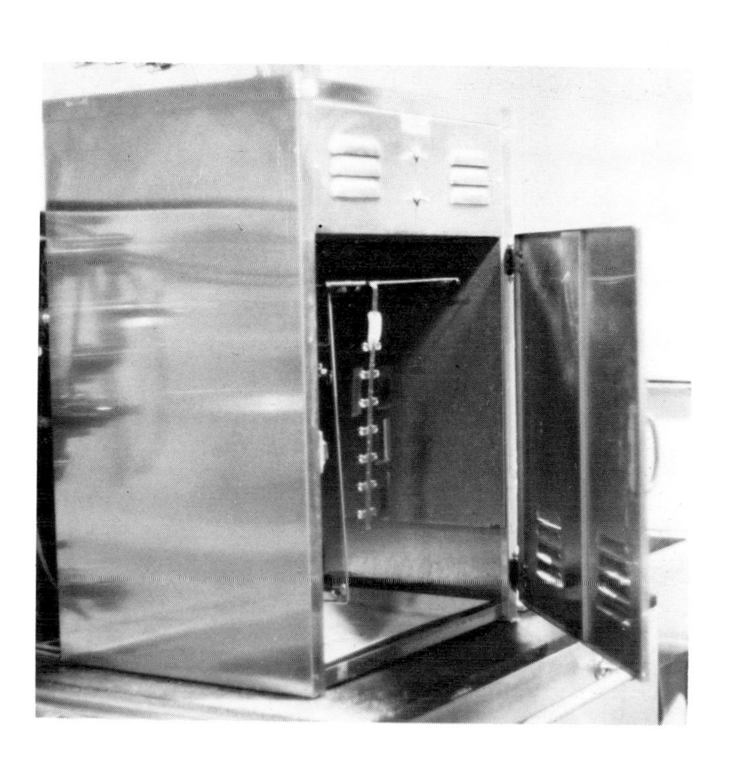

Figure 2–27. Film drier.

unexposed undeveloped crystals will be removed in the first 2 minutes and the film will become transparent. The radiograph can be rinsed and viewed in white light at this time (wet viewing) but must be kept moist and must be returned to the fixer to complete the fixing process. Failure to fully fix a film will result in the radiograph's becoming stained and semiopaque in later weeks or months (Figure 2–26A). If the film is left in the fixer for a prolonged period, such as one or more hours, the fixer will remove some of the developed image and the density of the radiograph will be light (Figure 2–26B). When powdered fixer chemicals are used, the chemicals must be totally dissolved or powder particles may adhere to the emulsion and remove the image where they touch the emulsion (Figure 2–26C).

After fixing, the film is washed in running water to remove fixer chemicals from the emulsion. Failure to completely wash results in chemical stain appearing in the radiograph at a later date. The stain is similar to that due to incomplete fixing (Figure 2–26A).

After washing, the film is hung in a clean, dust-free area to dry. Commercial driers are available to reduce drying time (Figure 2–27). The dried film is now a radiograph and is ready for viewing and interpretation.

A review of the steps in manual film processing is shown in Figure 2–28.

1. Stir processing solutions.
2. Measure developer temperature.
3. Check time-temperature chart.
4. Set timer.
5. Label film holder.
6. Turn on safelight and turn off room light.
7. Open film packet.
8. Attach film to film holder.
9. Immerse film in developer.
10. Tap film holder to tank.
11. Activate timer.
12. Agitate film holder.
13. Remove film from developer.
14. Rinse film in water.
15. Place film in fixer.
16. Optional wet reading.
17. Return film to fixer.
18. Wash film.
19. Dry film.
20. Record, mount and store.

Figure 2–28. Check-list for manual film processing.

FILM IDENTIFICATION

Radiographs must be identified to properly assign them to their respective patient's charts. Small intraoral films are clipped to film hangers that are numbered or have the patient's name written on a reusable plastic tab (Figure 2–29). Large films have the patient's name, date, and other pertinent information photographically printed on a small unused area of the radiograph. The film cassette has a small lead sheet in one corner of the exposure surface to prevent film exposure of this area when radiographing the patient. The patient's name and other information are written on a semitransparent card and printed into the unexposed film area in the darkroom when the film is removed from the cassette (Figure 2–30). The white-light printed latent image is developed along with the radiographic image during film process-

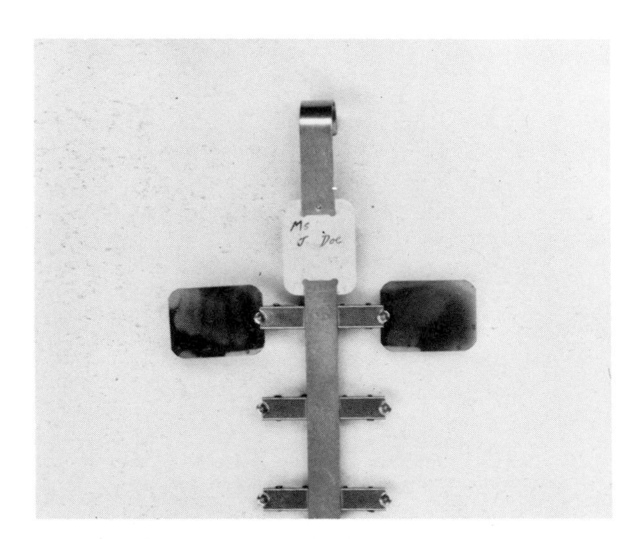

Figure 2–29. Intraoral film hanger with patient's name written on plastic tab.

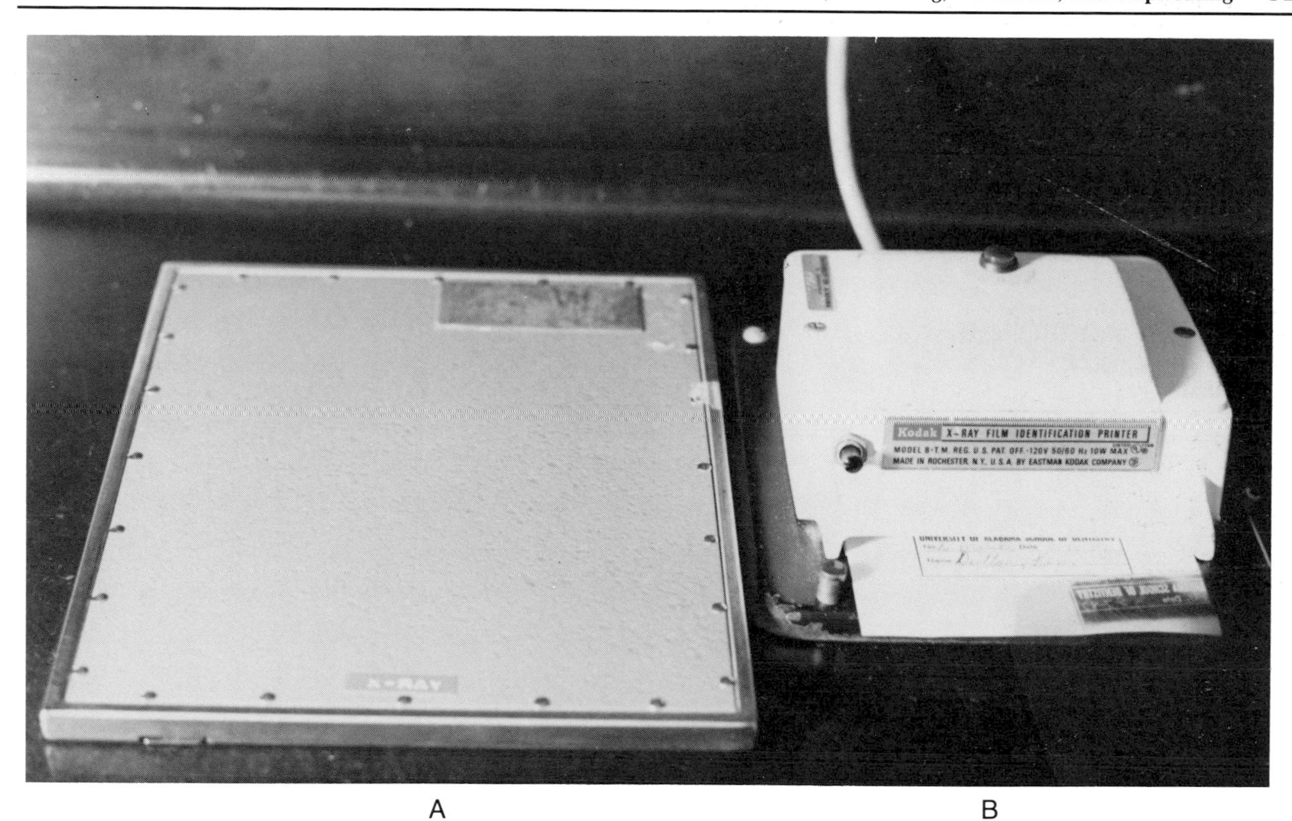

Figure 2–30. A, Exposure surface of cassette with lead sheet and R lead letter. B, Printer with identification card. C, Radiograph with information about patient.

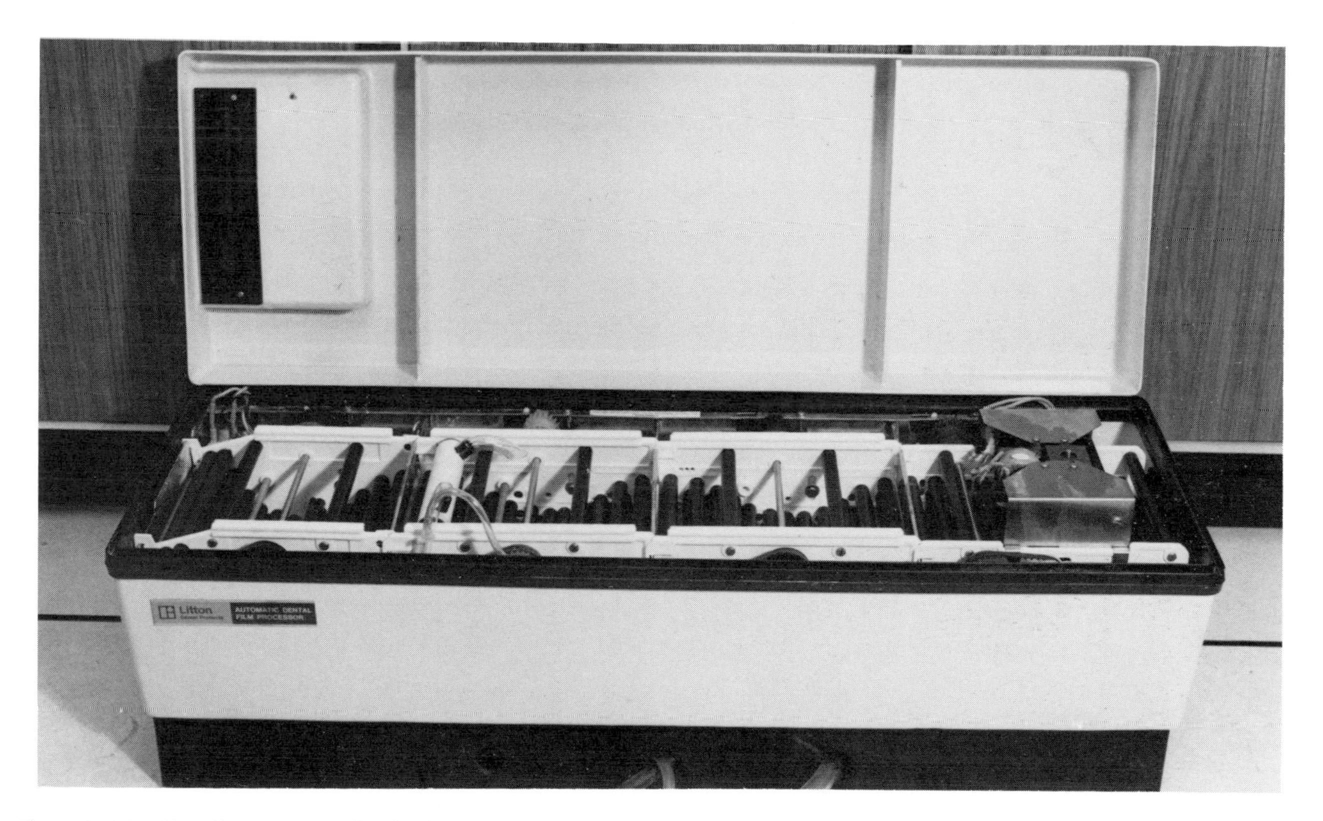

Figure 2–31. Hope® processor. Tubes lead to under-table automatic replenishing solution reservoirs. Films are processed in a dry to dry cycle.

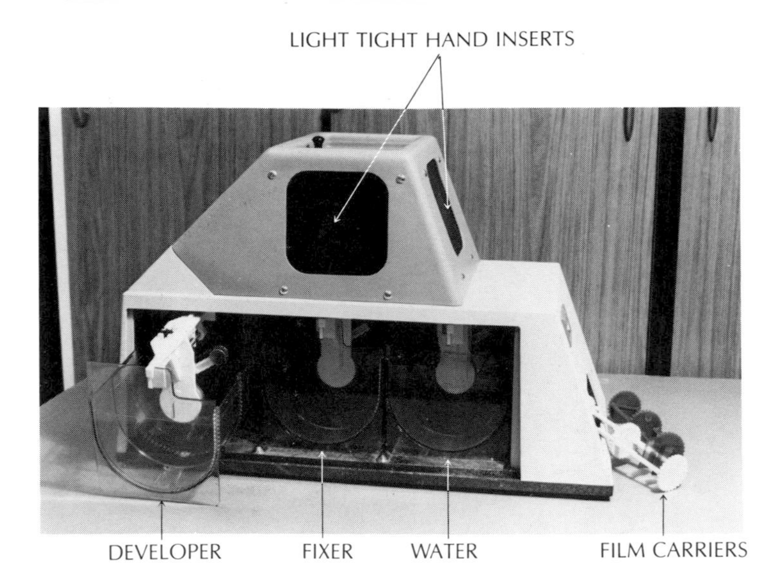

Figure 2–32. Phillips 4–10 automatic processor, unattached to plumbing, with nonreplenishment of solutions. Unit accepts only intraoral films.

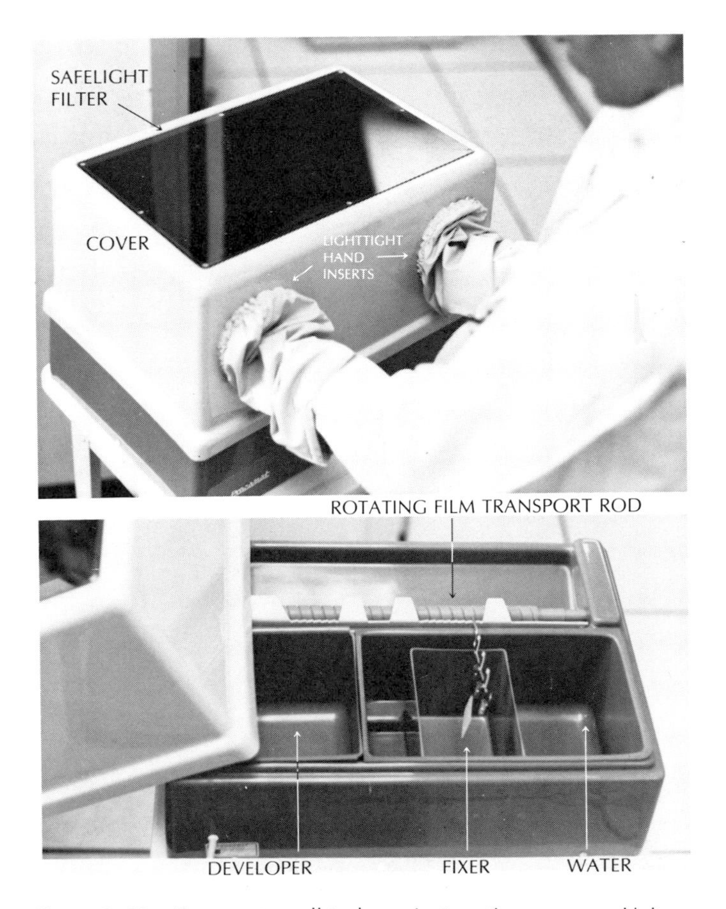

Figure 2–33. Procomat small-tank semiautomatic processor. Unit accepts intraoral films and delivers wet radiograph.

ing. Large radiographs need identification of the left and right sides of the patient. This is accomplished by placing a letter R or L made of lead on the exposure surface of the cassette. The unexposed film area appears as a printed R or L in the processed radiograph (Figure 2–30A and C).

AUTOMATIC PROCESSING

Automatic processors are manufactured with a variety of capabilities. Some processors accept only small intraoral films, whereas others accept films up to 10 inches wide. Some process films to a dry radiograph; others produce a wet radiograph. When a film is processed, the developer and fixer are weakened; some processors automatically replenish solutions from attached reservoirs, some require the operator to replenish solutions manually, and some do not replenish the solutions (Figures 2–31 and 2–32). Most automatic processors use high concentration solutions to develop films quickly. Some processors also heat the developer to 80°F or above. Automatic processors reduce the time between film exposure and viewing the dry radiograph. They can be useful in dental offices with high workloads; they eliminate the need for film hangers and reduce processing solution drip in the office. Most automatic processors use a roller system to transport film from one solution to the next. The transport mechanism requires regular careful cleaning and maintenance if the unit is to function properly.

A fully automated film processor with solution replenishment ability is a complex machine. It requires an efficient water supply system that controls both the flow and temperature of the water in the automatic processor. The processing cycle control programs the processing speed of the film from the time it enters to the time it leaves the processor. The processing time is affected by the solution's temperature, solution's concentration and the type of film being processed; failure to adjust for any of these variables can result in very poor quality radiographs. Both daily and periodic maintenance procedures are established by machine manufacturers. The procedures vary between types of processors but must be routinely performed or uniform quality radiographs will not be obtained and life expectancy of the processor will be shortened. Bent or crimped film can slip between the small rollers of a dental automatic processor. Such films must be made flat before being inserted into the processor and it is advisable to enter the film by the unbent edge of the film.

Many small tank, non-solution-replenishing units are also available with a variety of different film transport systems (Figure 2–33). These units, without attached plumbing, can process a small number of intraoral films between solution changes. Most units usually utilize a daylight loader with a built-in safelight type of filter and can be used in the x-ray exposure room. The light filter in a daylight loader is only safe for intraoral film. When screen film is used in a daylight loader a light tight cover must be placed over the filter. Many small semiautomatic processors deliver a wet film; such film often needs additional fixing and washing to produce archival quality radiographs necessary for record keeping. Operators using small tank processors must exercise care in counting the number of films processed, since solution strengths are easily weakened and underdevelopment or underfixing of films can result if the solutions are not changed often.

QUICK PROCESSING

Film processing times can be reduced by processing at high temperatures, using concentrated solutions, or rapidly agitating the film during processing. The first two methods are more effective and can reduce developing and fixing time to approximately one minute. High temperatures tend to produce chemical fog in the radiograph and rapidly deteriorate the strength of solutions. Concentrated solutions do not increase fog levels much at temperatures below 80°F; however, they also deteriorate in a few days when exposed to air. Quick processing is not recommended for routine film processing because less radiographic density is produced from the latent image by this technic. There are a number of commercially available concentrated rapid processing solutions (Figure 2–34).

If a concentrated developer replenisher solution is used in the dental office, it can be prepared as a quick developing solution by

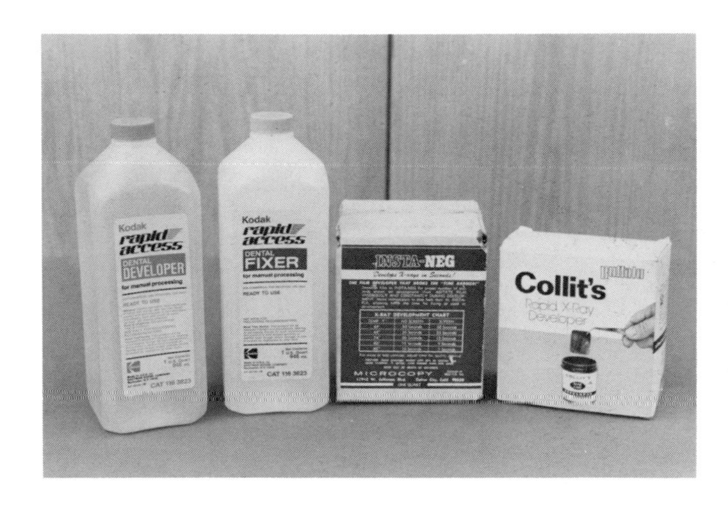

Figure 2–34. Some available rapid processing solutions.

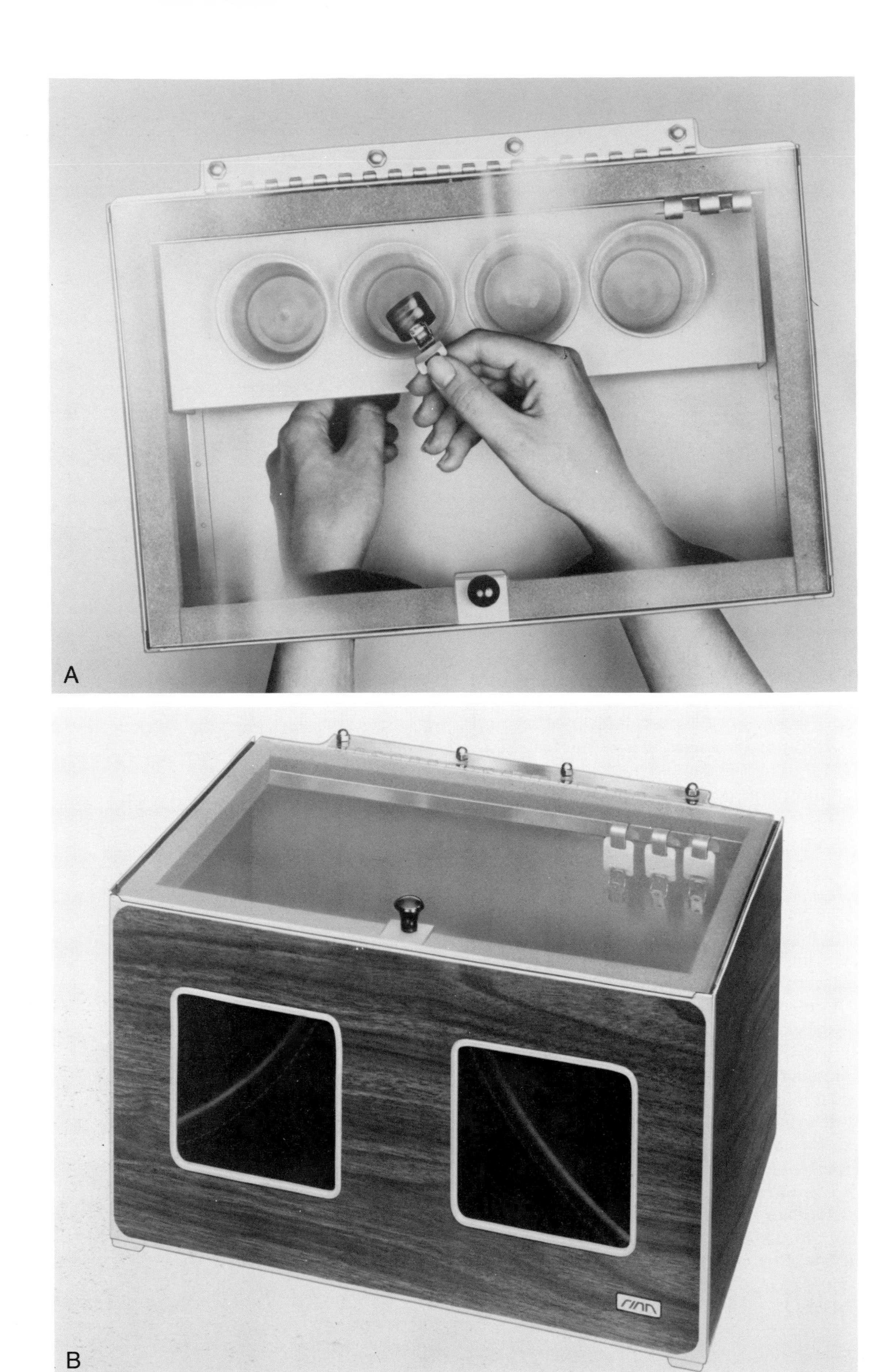

Figure 2–35. A and B, Small film processor used for processing single intraoral dental films.

diluting with 50 to 75% less water than is normally recommended for preparation of the replenisher solution. A developer replenisher solution does not contain some chemicals found in the normal developer solution that restrain the activity of the developer chemicals. Fixer concentrate can also be prepared as a rapid fixing solution by diluting it with less water than is recommended for preparing normal fixer solution.

Quick processing of single radiographs can be accomplished in the operatory through the use of a small box-type processor. These processors use a light-safe see-through filter and light-safe hand inserts (Figure 2–35).

SILVER RECOVERY

Silver can be recovered from dental film processing solutions. Recovery systems vary from simply exchanging the silver for a base metal (by placing the metal in the solution) to electrolytic equipment requiring an electrical supply. Silver recovery is usually practical only in group practices using a large number of radiographs since it takes about 3,500 intraoral or 120 panoramic films to produce 1 ounce of silver. Economic feasibility depends on the amount of silver in the films used, the number of films processed, the percentage of silver recovered from the solutions by the recovery system used, the cost of the recovery system and the price of silver.

XERORADIOGRAPHY

Xeroradiography uses the same x-ray machine and exposure technic as conventional radiography. The system differs in the image receptor. Conventional radiography uses x-ray film as the image receptor while xeroradiography uses a rigid selenium plate. Instead of sensitive silver halide crystals in an emulsion, the plate is made sensitive with a uniform electric charge on the surface of the plate. When exposed to x rays in the patient's mouth, a latent image is formed as electric charges are removed by the x rays. The remaining electric image is processed in a special small processing machine using a system similar to the xerox office copying machine that duplicates the pages of a book. In the machine, the electric image attracts a powder to make a visible image which is then trans-

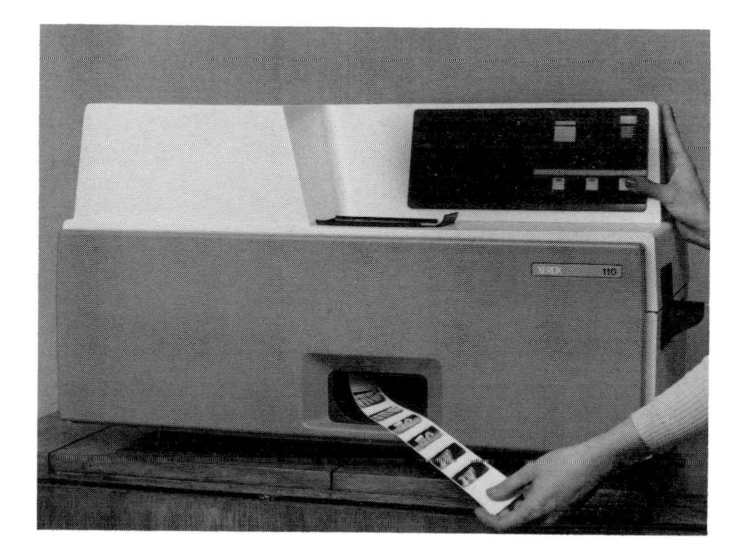

Figure 2–36. The Xerox dental radiographic imaging system.

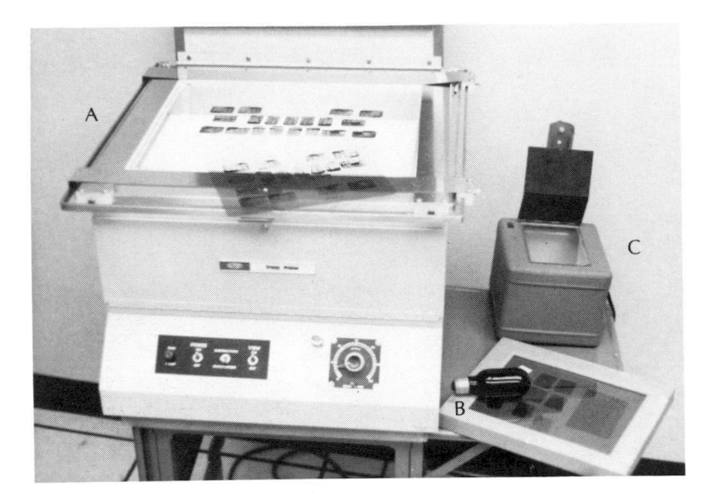

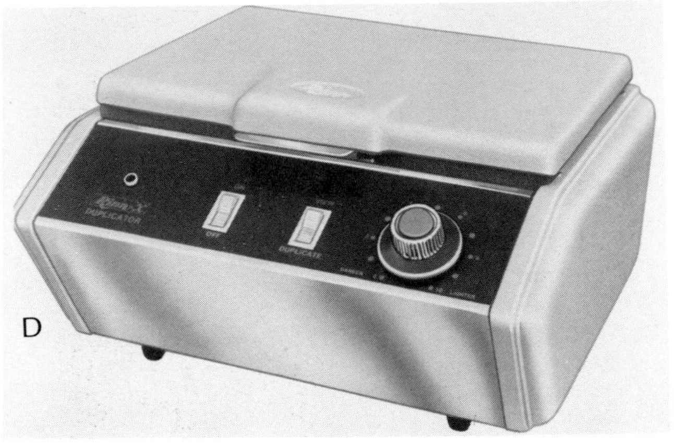

Figure 2–37. A, Large radiographic duplicator; B, printing frame and ultraviolet bulb; C, small photographic contact printer. D, Rinn duplicator for dental size films.

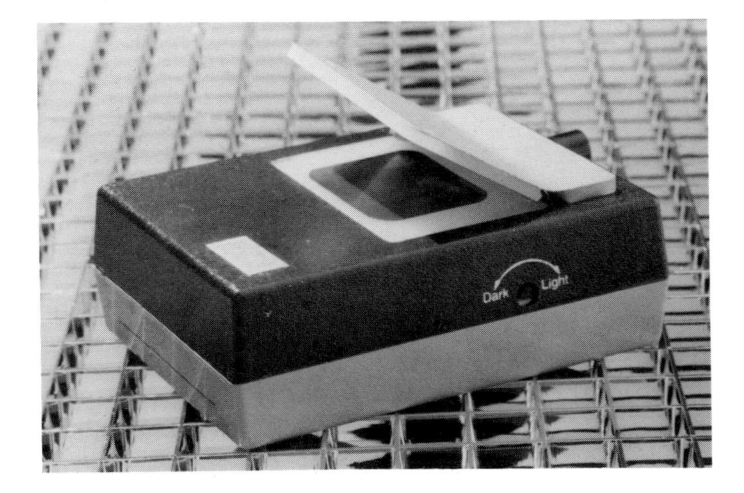

Figure 2–38. Small battery powered duplicator designed to use periapical No. 2 size duplicating film.

ferred to a paper or transparent strip (Figure 2–36). The image can be viewed like a photograph or a radiograph. The selenium plates can be sterilized, recharged and used repeatedly.

DUPLICATING RADIOGRAPHS

The need for duplicate radiographs has increased in the last decade. Duplicate radiographs are used for separate patient records, insurance company or third party requirements, supplying patients with a private record when they move from the dental practice, patient education and teaching. Duplicates of radiographs can be made in the darkroom with special duplicating film that is sensitive to ultraviolet light (black light). A screen film type of safelight can be used in the darkroom. Large and small radiographic duplicators are available (Figure 2–37). A small photographic printer, available in photographic stores, can be used if the bulb is replaced with an ultraviolet bulb. (The system will also work with a regular low wattage white-light bulb, but the duplicated radiograph will not be of the best quality.)

An inexpensive photographic printing frame with an ultraviolet bulb located a few feet away can also be used. The radiograph is placed between the light source and the duplicating film. Intimate contact between the radiograph and the duplicating film is mandatory for sharp reproductions; contact is obtained by clamps. Radiographs must not be reproduced in film mounts because the mounts prevent good contact between the films.

A small duplicator for single intraoral radiographs can be used in the daylight loader of an automatic processing machine or small box type processor (Figure 2–38). The duplicator can be hand held and is powered by a battery.

Exposure time varies with bulb light intensity and bulb film distance (most commercial duplicators use 3 to 5 seconds). Overexposure produces a light-density duplicate and underexposure a darker duplicate radiograph. The exposed duplicate radiograph is processed in a regular x-ray developer and fixer according to the film manufacturer's recommended time and temperature. Developing time is usually less than that required for dental films and the film must be agitated during the rinsing in water between the developer and fixer solutions. Since the developing time is less than for dental films the duplicating film is usually overdeveloped in automatic processors. In such intances, a useful but more contrasting image results in the duplicate radiograph.

Duplicating film is supplied in various sizes. There is only one emulsion on the film and the emulsion must contact the radiograph. When intraoral radiographs are duplicated on large films, there will be no orientation bubble in the duplicate and thus the duplicate must be marked with an R or L to indicate the right or left side of the patient that the radiograph depicts.

When duplicate extraoral radiographs are known to be needed prior to making the radiograph, two screen films can be placed in the cassette. The films should have a single emulsion and care must be taken to place each emulsion side in contact with the opposing screens. The same exposure factors can be used if the single emulsion has twice the speed of the double emulsion film normally used.

When duplicate intraoral radiographs are known to be needed prior to making the radiograph, the use of double film packets is recommended. The exposure of two films in a single film packet in the patient's mouth does not increase the patient's exposure to x rays.

Single intraoral radiographs can be duplicated on similar size No. 2 duplicating film that have a similar raised dot as the original radiograph. Special care must be taken to place the correct emulsion side of both films in contact with each other during the duplicating process. If this is not done, the duplicate can be interpreted as being a radiograph of the other side of the patient. The duplicate image may show less sharpness but can still be considered of acceptable quality if the image in the original radiograph was sharp (Figure 2–39).

The person who makes a duplicate should always check to see that the duplicate is accurate and correctly labeled. Improperly exposed or incorrectly labeled duplicates are easily recognized if one is looking at both the original radiograph and the duplicate. How-

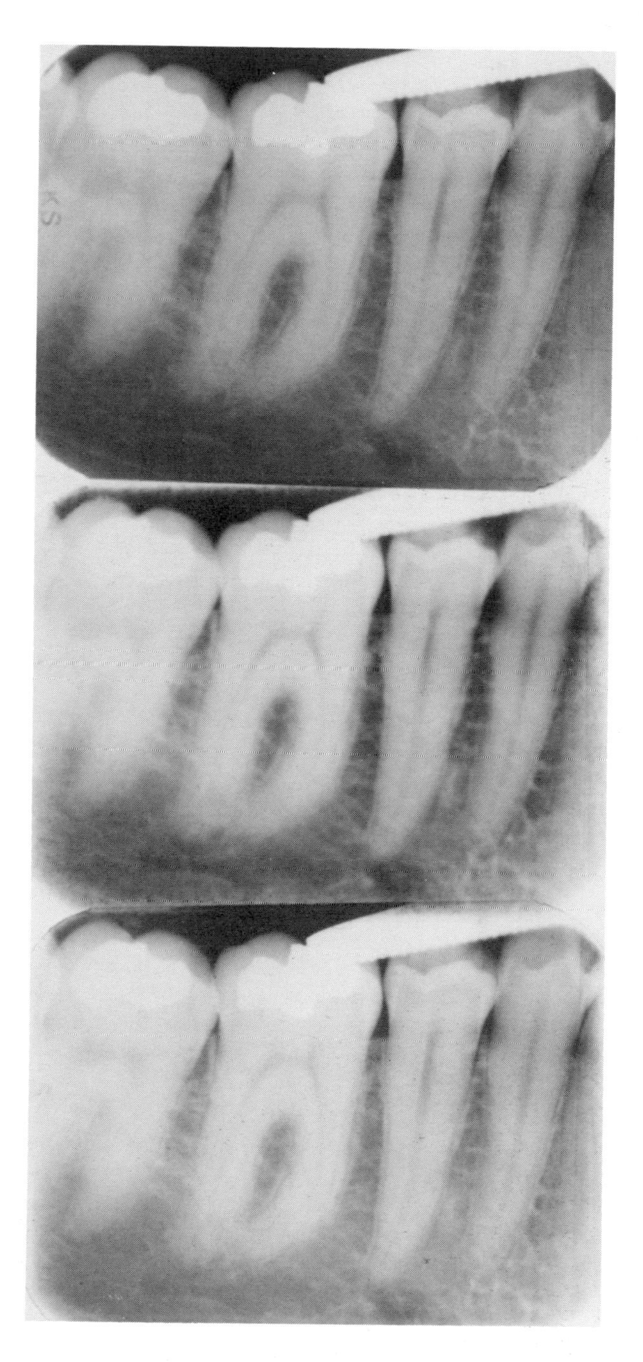

Figure 2–39. Original periapical radiograph (above) and duplicates made with periapical size duplicating film. The correctly exposed duplicate is shown in the middle. The bottom radiograph is a duplicate made with the incorrect side of the duplicating film in contact with the original radiograph and has the raised dot on the opposite side.

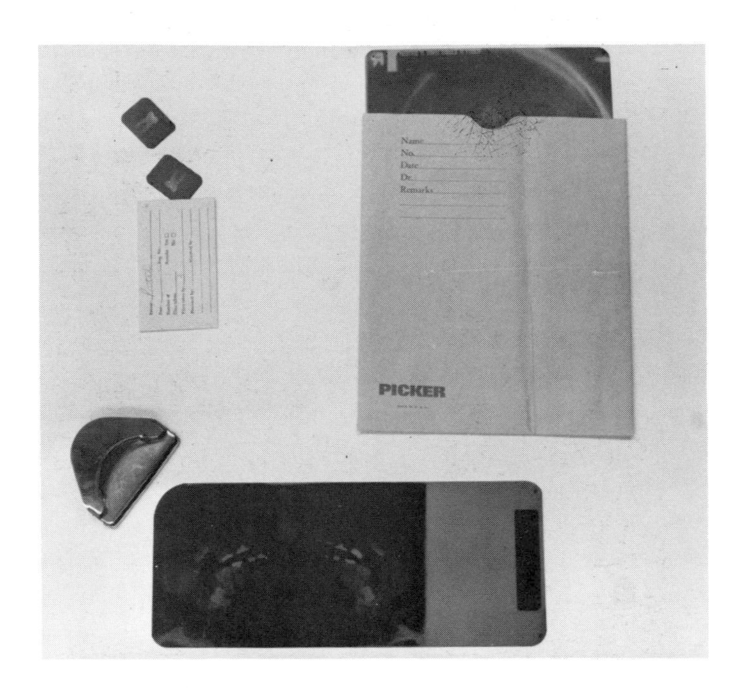

Figure 2–40. Labeled film envelopes and small hand-operated film cutter.

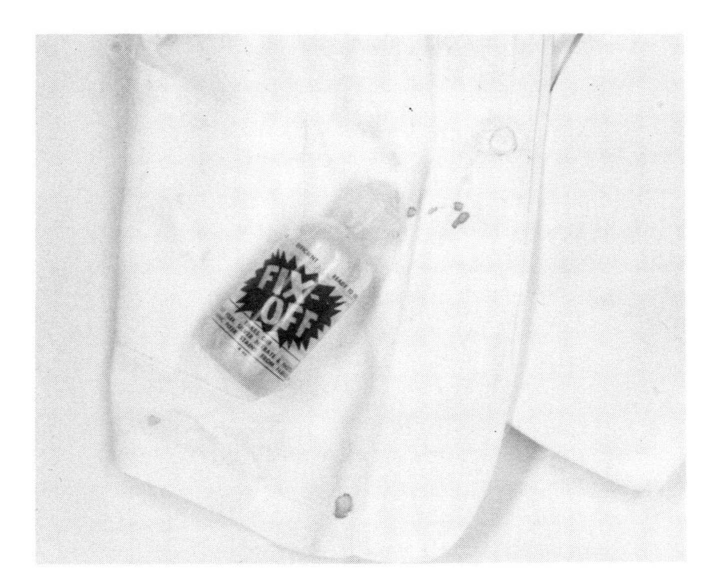

Figure 2–41. Stains created by splashed processing chemicals; commercially available stain remover.

ever, if a person is looking at only the duplicate, it is not possible to identify if it was incorrectly labeled. All duplicates should be checked clinically with the patient before being used for diagnostic purposes.

PREPARING RADIOGRAPHIC RECORDS

Intraoral periapical radiographs can be stored in envelopes in the patient's chart (Figure 2–40). Information about the patient and the date must be carefully recorded on envelopes and film mounts, since radiographs constitute an important part of the patient's record. When more than one radiograph is placed in the same envelope, all sharp corners or points created by film holder clips must be removed to prevent scratches on film emulsions. A variety of film cutters are available for this purpose.

REMOVING PROCESSING STAINS

Processing solutions spilled upon uniforms create unsightly stains. Wet spots should be immediately washed with a strong concentrated soap solution. Dried stains are best removed with a commercially available stain remover just prior to sending the uniform to the laundry (Figure 2–41). Home remedies include the use of a weak bleach solution and vinegar immediately prior to washing the uniform. Vinegar contains weak acetic acid similar to the fixer solution.

FILM STORAGE

Unexposed film must be protected from heat, humidity, chemicals, and x rays. Unopened boxes of film are best stored in a refrigerator or a cool place. The boxes should be stored so that the box with the earliest expiration date is used before the other boxes (Figure 2–42A). Because of stray radiation in the area of the x-ray machine, film is stored in lead-lined or steel containers or dispensers (Figure 2–42B).

B

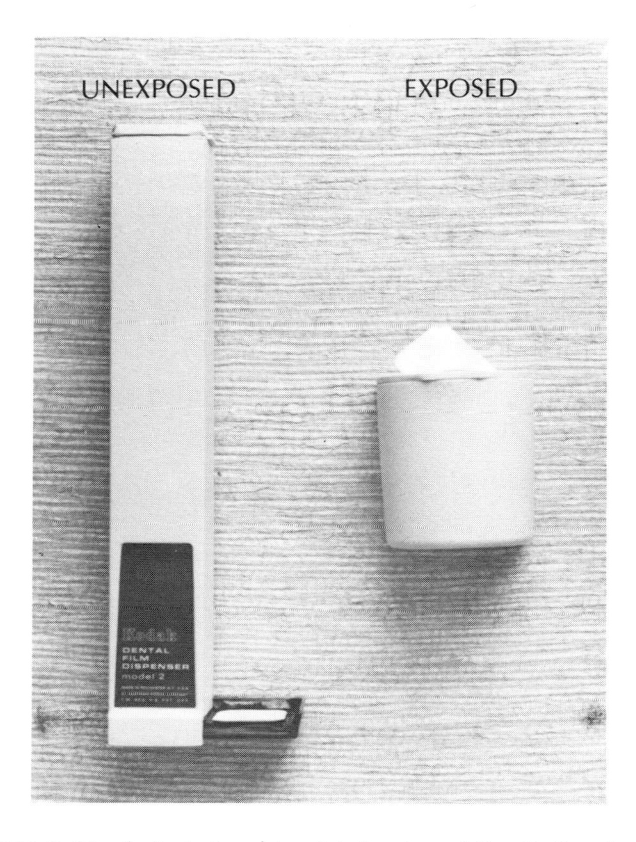

Figure 2–42. A, Expiration date printed on box of film. B, Containers for unexposed and exposed intraoral film.

Chapter 3

Radiographic Quality and Artifacts

Radiographs are made by producing x rays from electricity, exposing the patient's dental structures to the x rays to form an x-ray image, capturing the image in a film, and processing the film to make a visible image (Figure 3–1). Certain qualities are desirable in the diagnostic radiograph. The quality of a radiograph is determined by its density, contrast, image sharpness, image shape, and image dimensions. The images should have proper density and contrast to be identified, should be sharp to show object borders clearly, and should be of the same shape and size as the objects they represent.

DENSITY

Each spot on a radiograph has a certain blackness or density; however, the term *density* is usually used to denote the overall blackening of the film. Images of teeth and bone must have enough density to be seen on a viewbox in the dental office, but must not be overly black so that changes in the objects cannot be identified. Blackening of the film is affected by the amount of x-ray energy that reaches the film to produce a latent image and the subsequent processing of this image. When radiographic density is not satisfactory, knowledge of the factors affecting density is important in identifying which of the many factors affecting density is the cause. Basic factors affecting density are listed in Figure 3–2.

CONTRAST

The image of an object is seen as different densities on different areas of the radiograph. The variation of densities or "shades of gray" is referred to as radiographic contrast. Contrast is high when few density levels are shown between the black and clear areas; low contrast radiographs have many gradations and have less density difference between two adjacent density levels (Figure 3–3). A high contrast radiograph is sometimes said to have

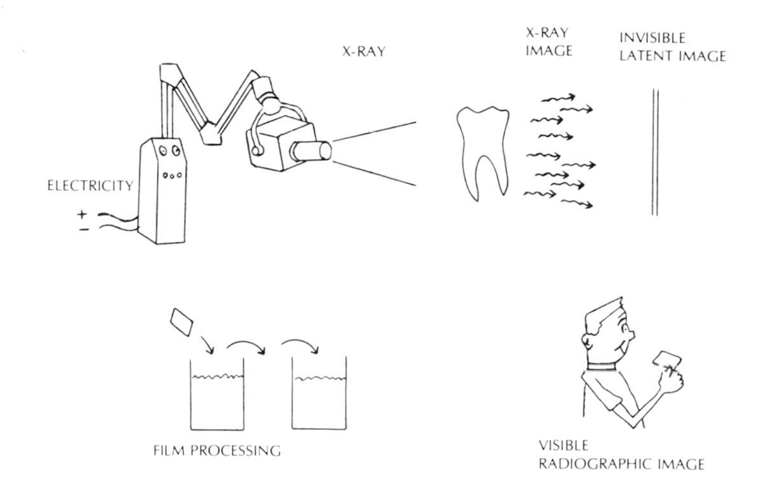

Figure 3–1. Factors in the production of a radiograph.

FACTOR	*DENSITY EFFECT*
Kilovoltage	Increases with kVp
Milliamperage	Increases with mA
Exposure time	Increases with time
Film	Increases with speed
Screens	Increases with speed
Developing time	Increases with time
Developer temperature	Increases with temp.
Fixing time	Decreases with overfixing
Object size	Decreases with thickness
Tube-film distance (TFD)	Decreases with TFD

Figure 3–2. List of basic factors affecting radiographic density.

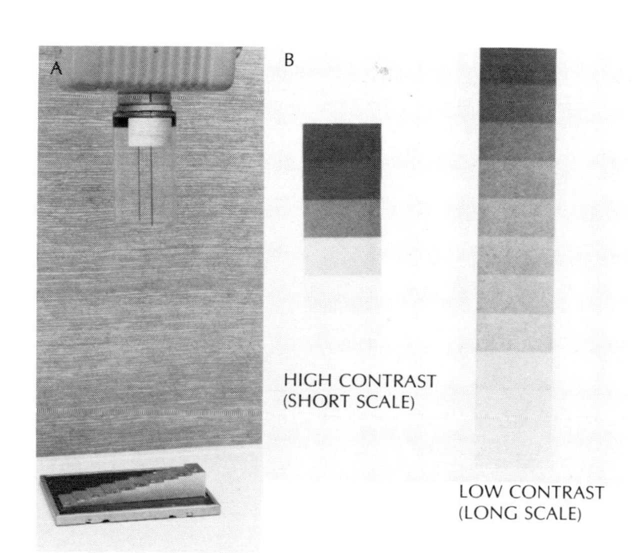

Figure 3–3. A, Exposure of step wedge made of 1 to 10 steps or thicknesses of aluminum producing varying exposure levels in film. B, Radiograph of step wedge made with different radiographic factors to show high and low contrast.

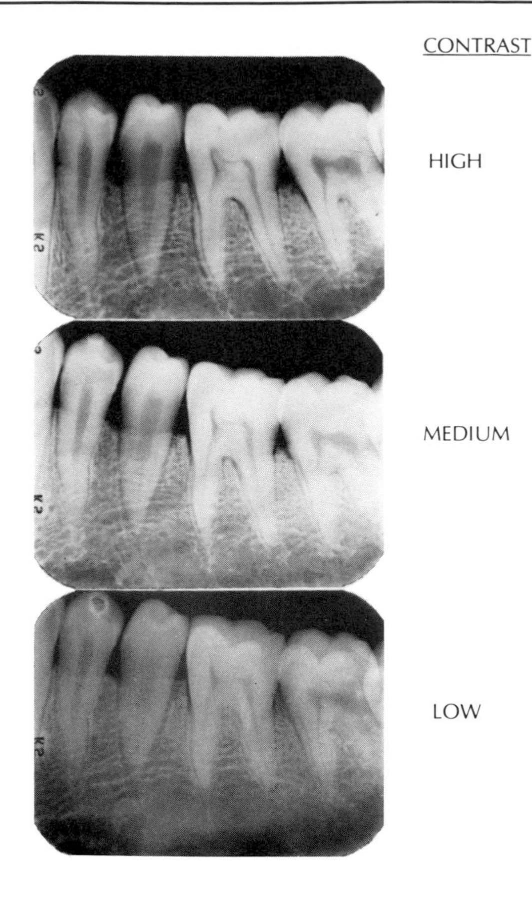

Figure 3–4. Clinically useful dental radiographs showing high, medium, and low radiographic contrast.

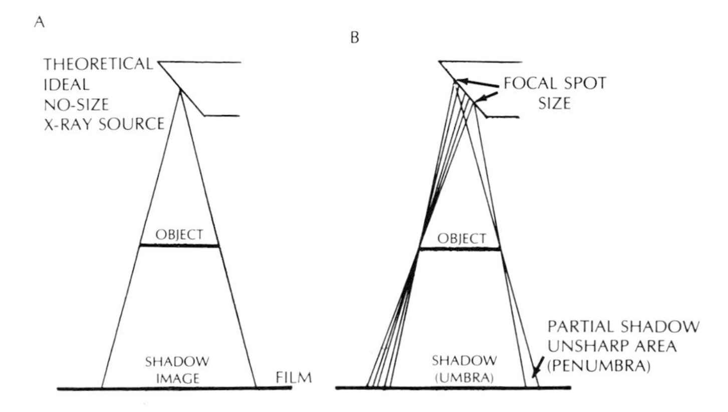

Figure 3–5. A, Sharp image produced by infinite size source of x rays. B, Edge or point of object represented on film by unsharp area due to size of focal spot.

short-scale contrast because there are fewer shades of gray or density levels; conversely, a low contrast radiograph has long-scale contrast.

The basic factors affecting contrast in a dental office are kVp and temperature of the developer solution. Higher kVp's produce more penetrating x rays and lower radiographic contrast. Higher film developing temperature produces higher contrast. Figure 3–4 shows varying contrast in three dental radiographs. A good understanding of high and low contrast can be obtained from a home television receiver. If a black-and-white picture is shown (color sets can suppress the color) and the control labeled "contrast" is increased and decreased, the picture will be produced with varying scales of contrast.

IMAGE SHARPNESS OR DEFINITION

The ideal image would have a point on the radiograph representing a point in the object. To achieve this all x rays would have to originate from the same point in the x-ray tube; since x rays originate from all points on the focal spot, the size of focal spot produces some unsharpness in the x-ray image (Figure 3–5). The greater the film area representing a point in the object, the greater is the image unsharpness. It is desirable to have as small a focal spot as possible in the dental x-ray machine.

Although the dentist has no control over the focal spot size, except when purchasing an x-ray machine, the effects of the focal spot upon unsharpness can be modified (Figure 3–6). When distance between the x-ray tube and the object is increased, a point on the object has its image cast upon a smaller film area, i.e., the image is sharper. If the film-to-object distance is reduced, the image is also made sharper. Note that if a film cannot be placed close to the object to obtain a sharp image, the image can be made sharp by increasing the tube-object distance.

Motion of the x-ray source, object, or film results in a less sharp image. If the x-ray tubehead moves during radiography, the effect is similar to using a large focal spot or source of radiation (Figure 3–5). Proper dental radiographic technic requires the patient to hold the film steady and the operator to control the patient's movement.

ARTIFACTS AND FILM FAULTS

The quality of a radiograph pertains to its ability to provide diagnostic information. In addition to the factors affecting radiographic quality discussed in shadow casting, many other film faults and artifacts that appear in radiographs reduce their diagnostic quality. The most common errors due to improper film exposure technic are shown in Chapter 4 following the discussion of intraoral radiographic technics; these are incorrect vertical angulation, incorrect horizontal angulation, cone cutting, and curved films.

Many artifacts are produced by improper film processing. The most common processing artifacts are shown in Figures 2–20 to 2–25 illustrating errors in film processing technic.

Fog is an artifact seen as a uniform darkening of the radiograph. Fog obscures the image and can have many sources. It can be produced by a darkroom or daylight processor that is not light tight, incorrect or cracked safelight filters, improper safelight bulb or position of the safelight, old or improperly stored film, excessive scattered or secondary radiation, improper processing solutions times or temperatures, weak developer solution and dirty processing tanks. Figure 3–9 shows two radiographs with and without fog.

Other common film faults are shown in Figures 3–10 to 3–19; the causes of these faults are described in the legends. Additional radiographic errors not shown in this or other chapters include chemical stains from a dirty darkroom, improper density due to individual factors affecting film density, improper contrast due to errors in kVp or developer temperature and distorted images due to many possible improper tube-object-film alignments.

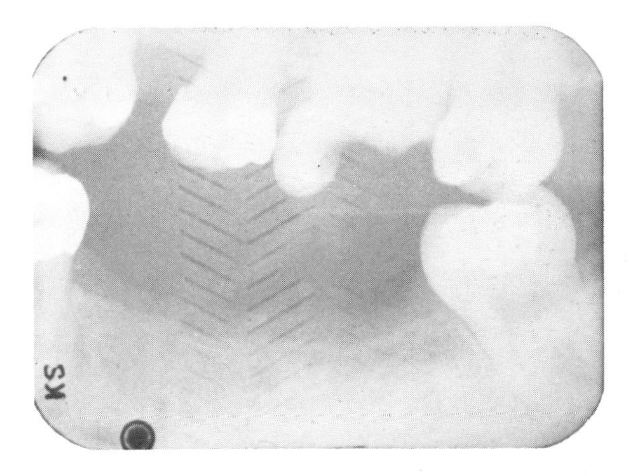

Figure 3–10. Film positioned backward in patient's mouth. X-ray beam passes through lead backing in film packet and prints pattern placed in lead backing into film; in this case film manufacturer uses a herringbone pattern.

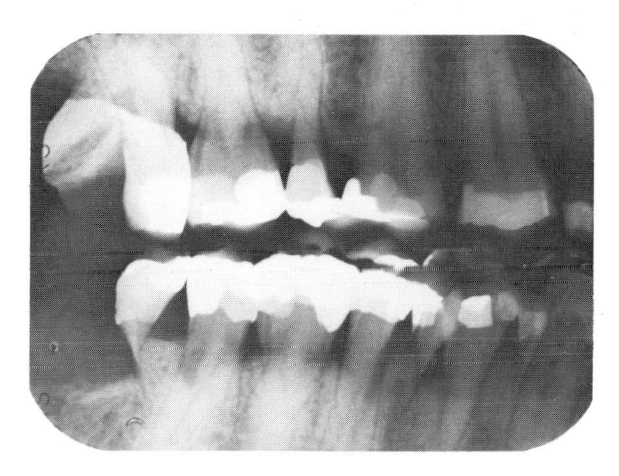

Figure 3–11. Double exposure. Film is exposed twice in patient's mouth, resulting in two images and dark or dense radiograph. This often occurs when operator keeps unexposed and exposed films in different pockets of uniform, instead of in proper film containers, and forgets which pocket contains unexposed film.

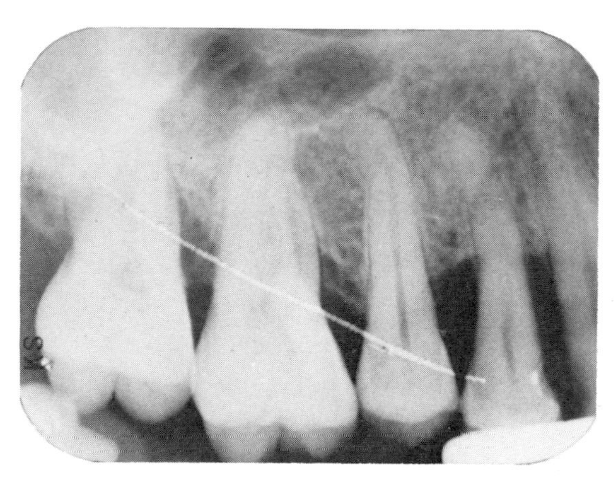

Figure 3–12. Scratches in emulsion appear as white lines. They can be differentiated from radiopaque images in emulsion by looking at film's surface in reflected light.

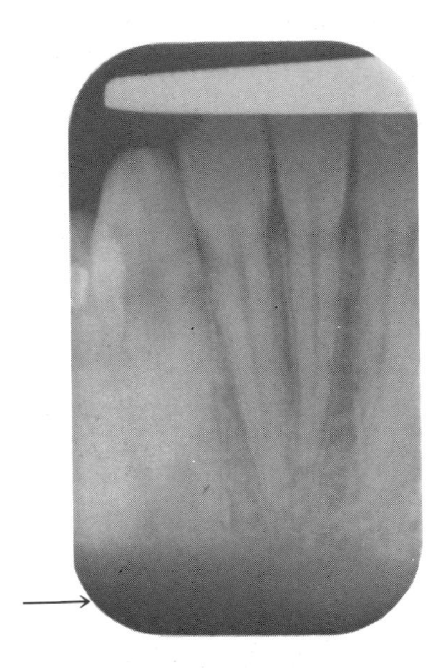

Figure 3–13. Wet or light-leaking film packets result in exposure of film around edges.

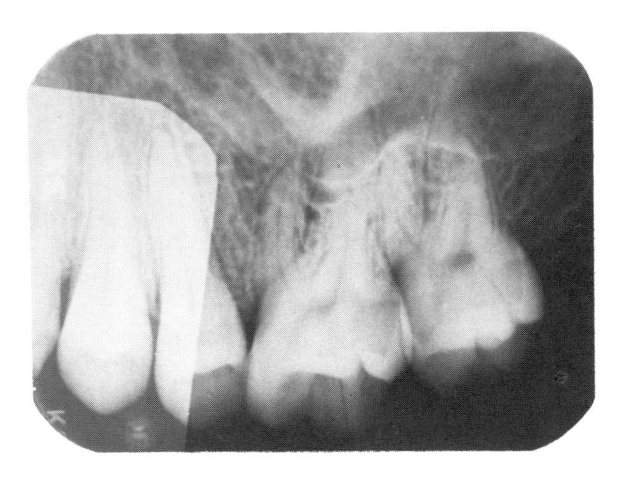

Figure 3–14. Overcrowding film in developer results in films on adjacent film holders overlapping each other. Developing solution cannot reach overlapped emulsions, and low density area results. Image is still observed in overlapped area because dental films have emulsions on both sides and only one emulsion is affected.

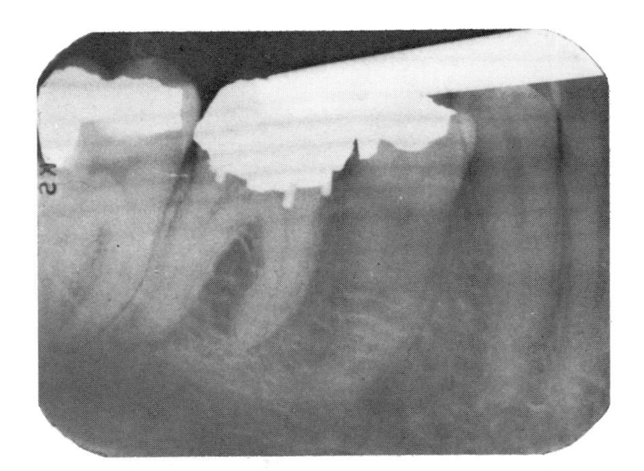

Figure 3–15. Light and dark streaks produced by unclean or worn rollers of automatic processor using roller type of film transport system or by faulty film manufacturing.

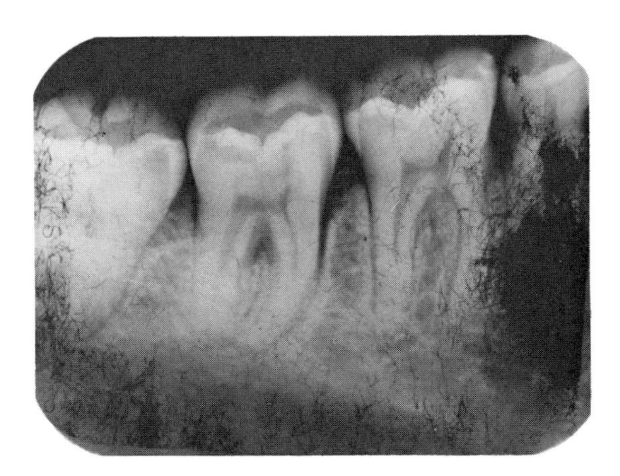

Figure 3–16. Paper of film packet sticking to emulsion due to water or saliva entering film packet.

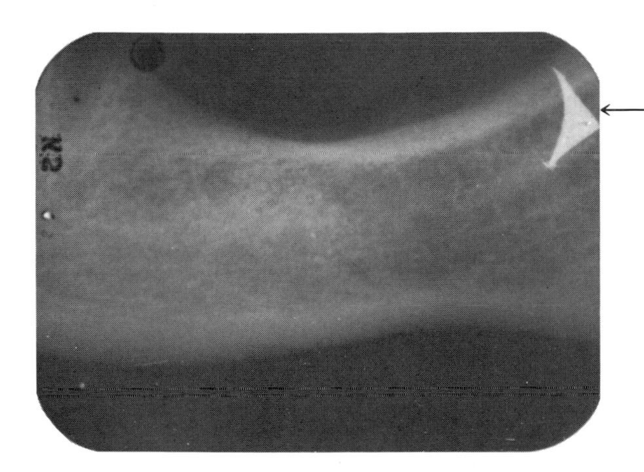

Figure 3–17. Metal foil in film packet between film and x-ray machine due to faulty film manufacturing.

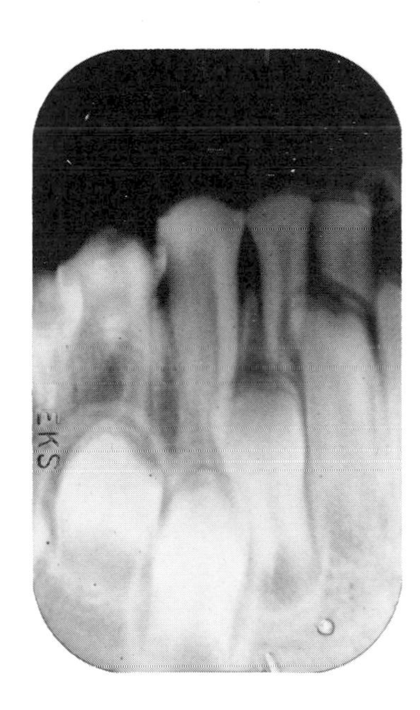

Figure 3–18. Blurred images owing to film movement during x-ray exposure of film in patient's mouth. Similar image blurring can also be caused by movement of patient or x-ray tube during film exposure.

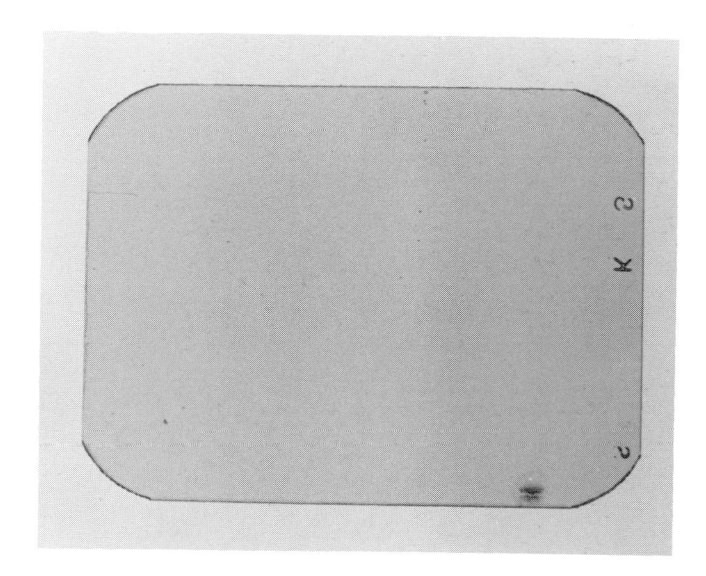

Figure 3–19. A blank clear film can be produced by non-exposure, exposed film placed in the fixer before the developer or processed radiograph left in strong fixer for 12 or more hours.

Chapter 4

Intraoral Radiography Prerequisites

Conventional intraoral radiography of teeth with film placed in the oral cavity is often called periapical radiography. Radiographs are made with the use of one of two basic technićs: the bisecting-the-angle or the paralleling technic. The two technics will be described in the following two chapters as they pertain to the adult patient. Modifications of technic applicable to children and edentulous patients will be discussed in Chapter 16.

Intraoral radiography requires the operator to possess some knowledge of the anatomy of the teeth and oral region, to know how to position the patient, and to be able to control film exposure. These basic conditions must be met before one begins to learn the actual placement of the film in the patient's mouth and subsequent exposure of the film by x rays.

TEETH AND X-RAY BEAM LOCATIONS

Intraoral radiography requires the operator to locate the long axes of the teeth and position the x-ray beam. Knowledge of the locations of these items is essential for accurate radiography. Accurate location of the long axis of a tooth is obtained by observing the crown of the tooth in the patient and using prior knowledge of the anatomy or shape of the tooth. Without prior knowledge of tooth anatomy, the long axes of teeth cannot be accurately located. However, approximate positions of the long axes of normally shaped and positioned teeth can be obtained from observing external landmarks on the patient's head. The long axes of maxillary incisor teeth point upward to the bregma (soft skull opening found in the top of a baby's head), located in the midline of the head slightly anterior to the center of the head (Figure 4–1A). The long axes of maxillary posterior teeth are midway between the buccal and palatal roots. Viewed from the front, the long axes of posterior teeth point to the middle of the top of the patient's head (Figure 4–1B). The maxillary cuspid is different; this tooth directs its long axis to the top of the nose.

The direction of the long axes of mandibular incisors varies from tilting slightly forward to slightly backward. These directions are easily observed. Long axes of mandibular bicuspids tend to be vertical (straight up and down) and mandibular molars have their crowns slightly tilting inward (Figure 4–2).

Knowledge of the location of teeth apices beneath the tissues of the patient's face is useful. The maxillary cuspid apex is located at the wing (ala) of the nose (Figure 4–3). Apices of maxillary posterior teeth are located along a line joining the nose wing with the ear opening (tragus). The molars lie beneath a line connecting the pupil of the eye and a point ½ inch posterior to the corner of the eye. The operator should be able to identify positions of mandibular teeth beneath their maxillary counterparts and the apices of mandibular teeth as being not much above the lower border of the mandible.

Location of the x-ray beam is aided by the standard open-end cone. The cone is sometimes called a PID (position indicating device). Some manufacturers indicate the location of the source of x rays with a mark on the tubehead (Figure 4–4). The edge and sides of the open-end cone are useful in positioning the x-ray beam. The side of the cone is parallel with the central ray and indicates the direction of the x-ray beam. The edge of the cone is a plane perpendicular to the central ray (i.e., any line on the plane of the edge of the cone is at right angles to the direction of the x-ray beam). Earlier machines were equipped with pointed cones. The point of the cone indicated the exit point of the central ray of the x-ray beam (Figure 1–18). Readers using a pointed cone should pay particular attention to the position and direction of the depicted central ray in the illustrations of this chapter.

PATIENT'S POSITION

The patient can be seated in an upright or reclining position during radiography. The upright position is preferred because, when the long axes of the patient and operator are similarly oriented to the horizontal floor, the operator more easily sees or identifies the

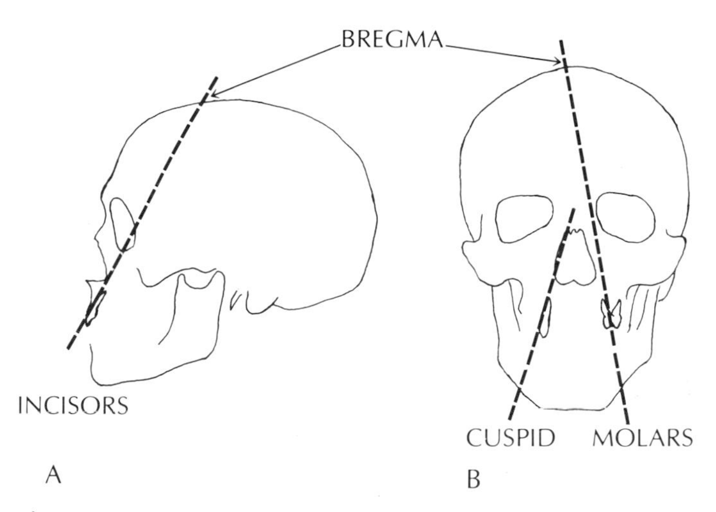

Figure 4–1. A, Approximate position of long axis of maxillary incisors seen from side of patient. B, Average long axis of maxillary cuspid and posterior teeth seen from front of patient.

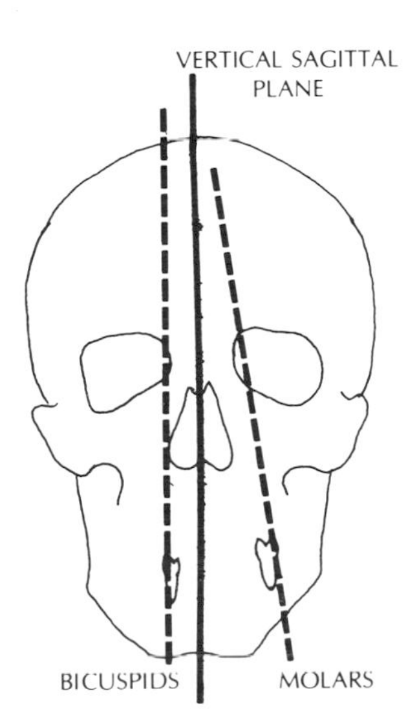

Figure 4–2. Long axes of mandibular bicuspid and molar teeth seen from front of patient.

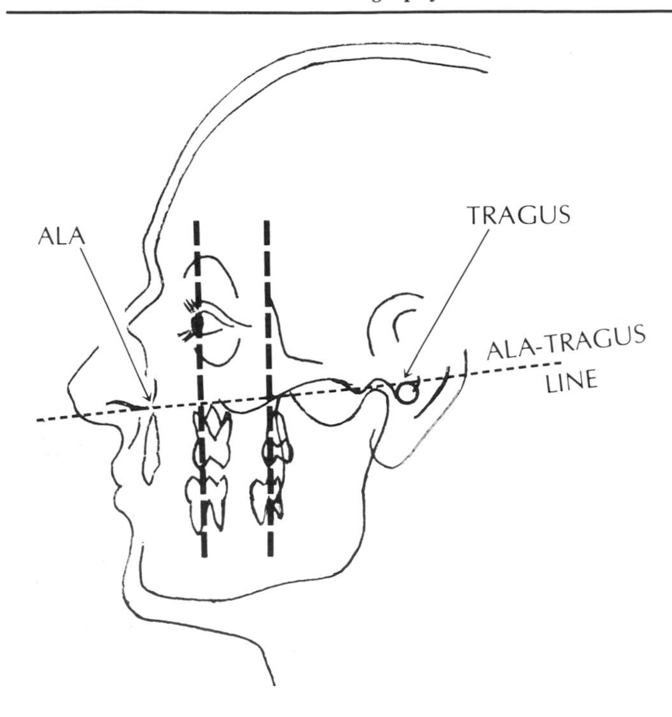

Figure 4–3. Location of apices of teeth as seen from side of patient.

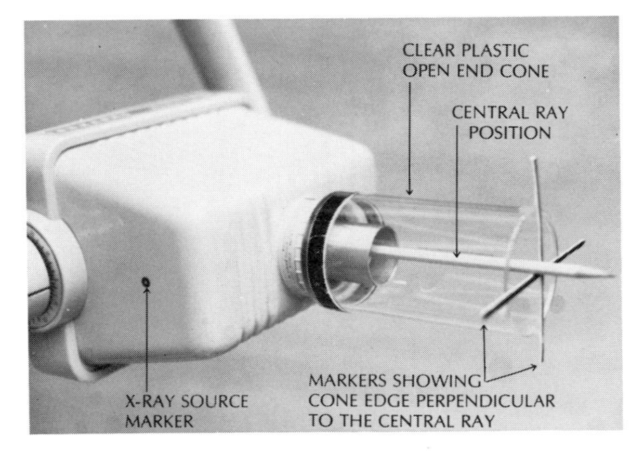

Figure 4–4. X-ray tubehead showing x-ray source location and beam-locating open-end cone. Note that any line on surface of end of cone is always perpendicular to central ray.

patient's teeth and film positions and the angles formed by the teeth, film, and x-ray beam (Figure 4–5). An upright patient position is strongly recommended for the new student of intraoral radiography. The occlusal plane of the jaw being examined is positioned as parallel to the floor as possible without making the patient uncomfortable.

ANGLES OF X-RAY BEAMS

The direction of the x-ray beam is related to the patient's teeth when the occlusal plane of the patient is parallel with the floor. Vertical angulation relates to movement of the x-ray tubehead in the vertical plane relative to the patient's occlusal plane (Figure 4–6A). When the x-ray beam is directed in the occlusal plane there is zero vertical angle. Movement of the x-ray source higher for the maxillary teeth and lower for the mandibular teeth increases the vertical angulation. Movement of the x-ray tubehead in the horizontal plane around the upright patient relates to horizontal angulation (Figure 4–6B). An x-ray beam can have correct horizontal angulation or have the beam directed too much from the mesial or too much from the distal of the area being examined. When the patient is not in the upright position, x-ray beam angulations remain related to the patient's occlusal plane and not to the horizontal floor or vertical walls of the room.

EXPOSURE TIME

The bisecting-the-angle technic is the most commonly used technic and the following radiographic factors usually are used with this technic: an 8-inch tube-patient distance, 65 kilovolts, 10 milliamperes, and varying exposure times. Each film needs a similar amount of energy to form a latent image regardless of the tooth area being examined. Various tooth areas have different thicknesses (Figure 4–7). The various tooth areas will absorb different amounts of x rays from the beam and more x-ray energy must be used in the thicker areas, such as with molar teeth. Tube-patient distance, kilovoltage, milliamperage, and exposure time affect the amount of energy the film is exposed to. Any of these factors can be changed to vary the energy delivered to the film. Exposure time is the most common factor varied; the other factors

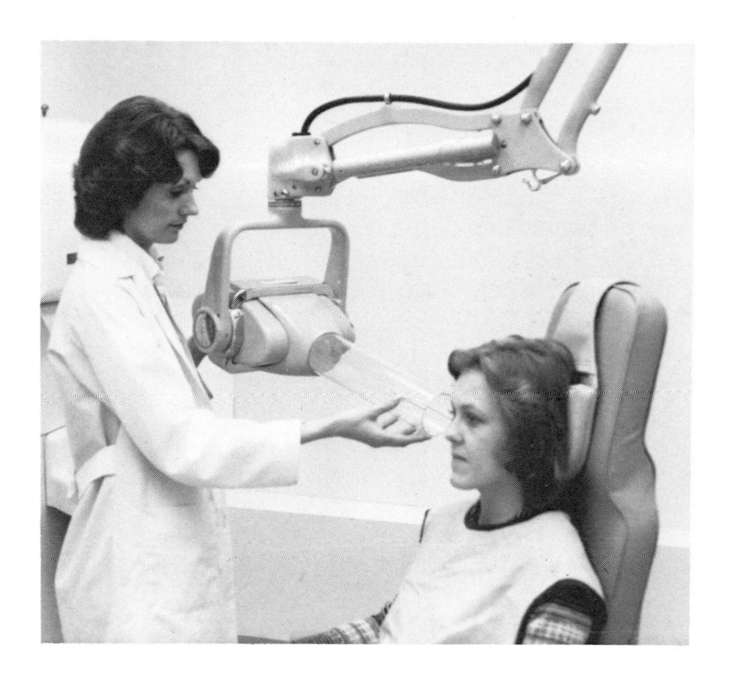

Figure 4–5. Recommended upright positions of patient and operator. Occlusal plane of the patient is positioned as nearly parallel to floor as is comfortable.

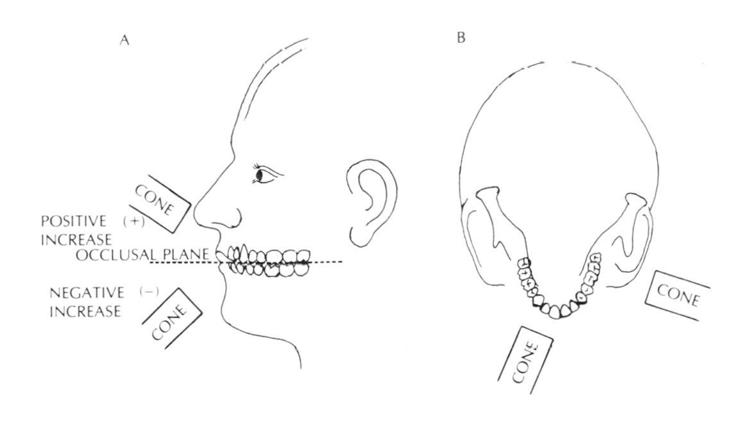

Figure 4–6. A, Changes in vertical x-ray beam angulations. B, Changes in horizontal x-ray beam angulation as seen from above patient's head.

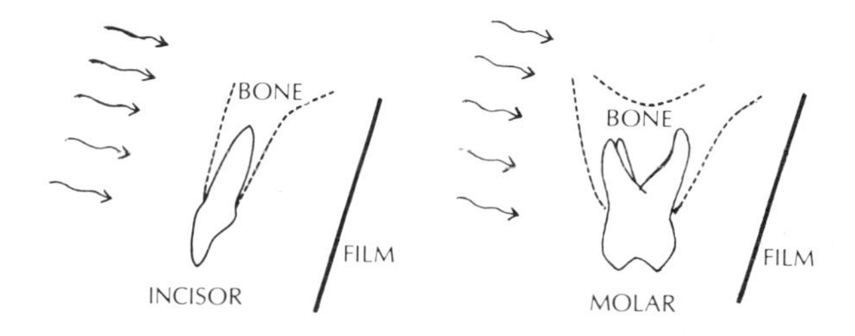

Figure 4–7. Example of different amounts of x-ray absorbing teeth and bone between x-ray beam and film in incisor and molar teeth areas.

Area	*Relative time*
Maxillary Incisors	1
Maxillary Bicuspids	1¼
Maxillary Molars	1¾
Mandibular Incisors	¾
Mandibular Bicuspids	1
Mandibular Molars	1¼

Figure 4–8. Exposure time relationships for different dental regions.

usually are kept constant. However, some clinicians tend to relate film exposure to milliampere seconds (MAS). This is because the total number of photons used is a product of milliamperes and seconds; thus 30 MAS could be 10 milliamperes for 3 seconds or 15 milliamperes for 2 seconds.

The exposure time of one tooth area is related to the exposure times of the other areas. Thus if the correct exposure time for one area is known, the approximate times for the other areas can be calculated. The relationship of the various tooth areas of an average patient is shown in Figure 4–8.

A fast film, for example, Kodak Ultraspeed or other ANSI speed group D film, is commonly used to reduce the patient's exposure to x rays. When such a film is used with the above-mentioned radiographic factors for the bisected-angle technic, the exposure time for the maxillary incisors is approximately 15 impulses (an exact time cannot be stated because machines have varying efficiencies in x-ray production). The exposure time of the other dental regions can be calculated. The operator must always remember that in establishing the correct exposure time, film processing must be standardized. When a radiograph has insufficient density, i.e., is underexposed, an increase of at least 50% in exposure time is usually needed to produce proper density. Conversely, a 50% reduction is usually needed for an obviously overexposed radiograph (Figure 4–9).

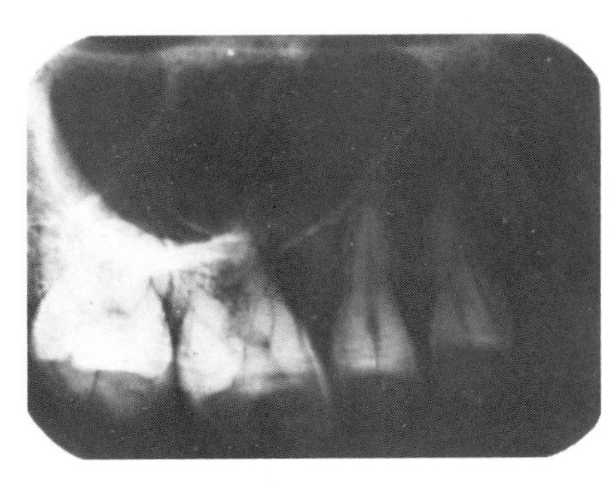
OVEREXPOSED
(decrease 50% time)

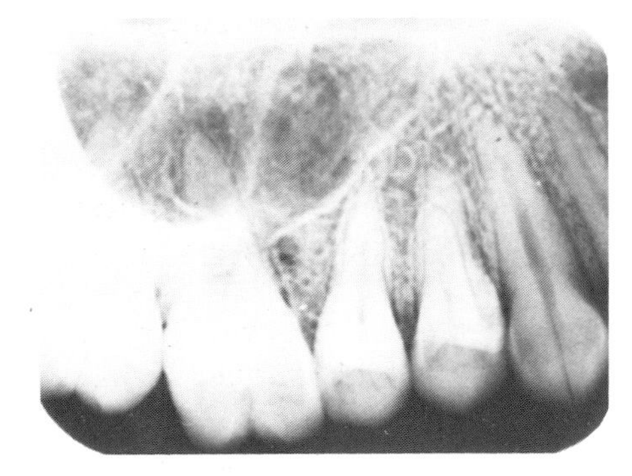
PROPER DENSITY

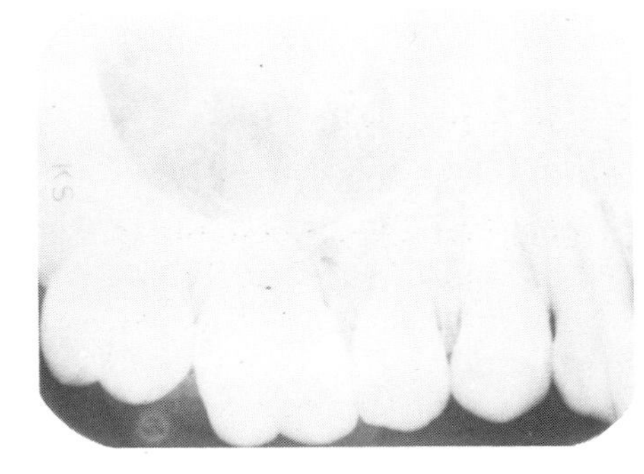
UNDEREXPOSED
(increase 50% time)

Figure 4–9. Examples of over- and underexposed radiographs.

FILM HOLDERS

The film must be held motionless in the patient's mouth. Many types of film holders are available; they are described in Chapter 9. The technic of placing a film in the patient's mouth with one type of film holder is quite different from many other types of film holders and individuals can have distinct preference for a particular film holder. However, the film position in the patient's mouth for a particular radiographic technic is the same regardless of the type of film holder. A film holding device is mandatory for the paralleling technic, while the patient's finger can be used with the bisecting-the-angle technic. However, all technics using a film holder are less difficult to perform than the patient finger method. In addition, film holders have the advantage of producing less bending of the film and keep the patient's hand out of the primary beam of x rays.

Chapter 5

The Paralleling Technic

Modern fast films and efficient x-ray machines can make intraoral radiographs with tube-film distances of 16 inches or more, with exposure times of approximately 1 second or less. The paralleling technic requires the use of a long tube-film distance, a film holding device and an ANSI 1.1 film size for the anterior teeth.

The paralleling technic positions the vertical plane of the film parallel to the long axes of the teeth. To maintain this position a film holder must be used and the film is attached to a bite block or some other type of film-holding device (Figure 5–1). The film is positioned far from the teeth and image magnification and blurring are increased. To counteract these undesirable effects and maintain proper image size and sharpness, an extended tube-film distance of 14 to 18 inches must be used. Thus the technic is sometimes called the long-cone technic. The x-ray beam is collimated to be no more than 2¾ inches in diameter at the end of the cone. A fast film is needed with this technic because the extended tube-film distance greatly reduces the x-ray intensity of the beam at the end of the cone and film exposure time must be below 2 or 3 seconds to keep unsharpness caused by the patient's movement at an acceptable level.

The paralleling technic conforms more closely to the principles of shadow casting described in Chapter 3. When the technic is used, teeth images closely resemble the teeth that form them.

THE MAXILLARY INCISOR RADIOGRAPH

The film is positioned parallel to the long axes of the teeth (Figure 5–1). The film used is ANSI size No. 1.1, which is much narrower in width that the commonly used No. 1.2 periapical film but is of similar length (Figure 5–2). The narrower width is needed to permit film placement high in the palate without bending or curving the film. One ra-

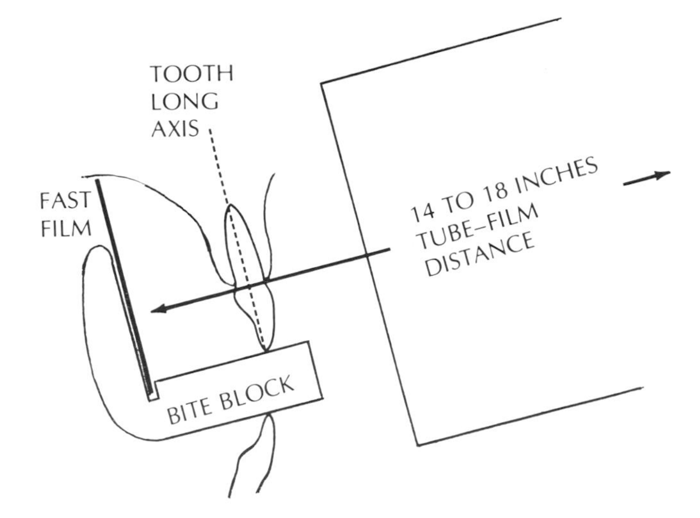

Figure 5–1. Basic positions of teeth, film, and x-ray tube in the paralleling technic. The film and tooth long axis are parallel. The central ray is perpendicular to the tooth and film. An extended tube film distance is mandatory.

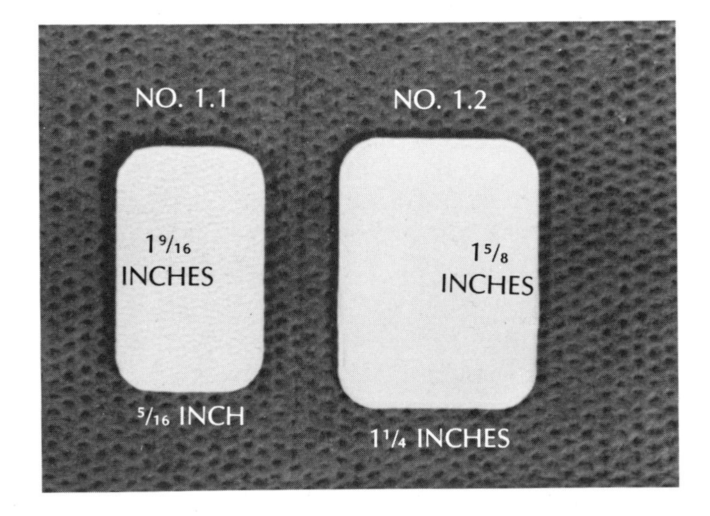

Figure 5–2. Comparison of dimensions of No. 1.1 and No. 1.2 dental films.

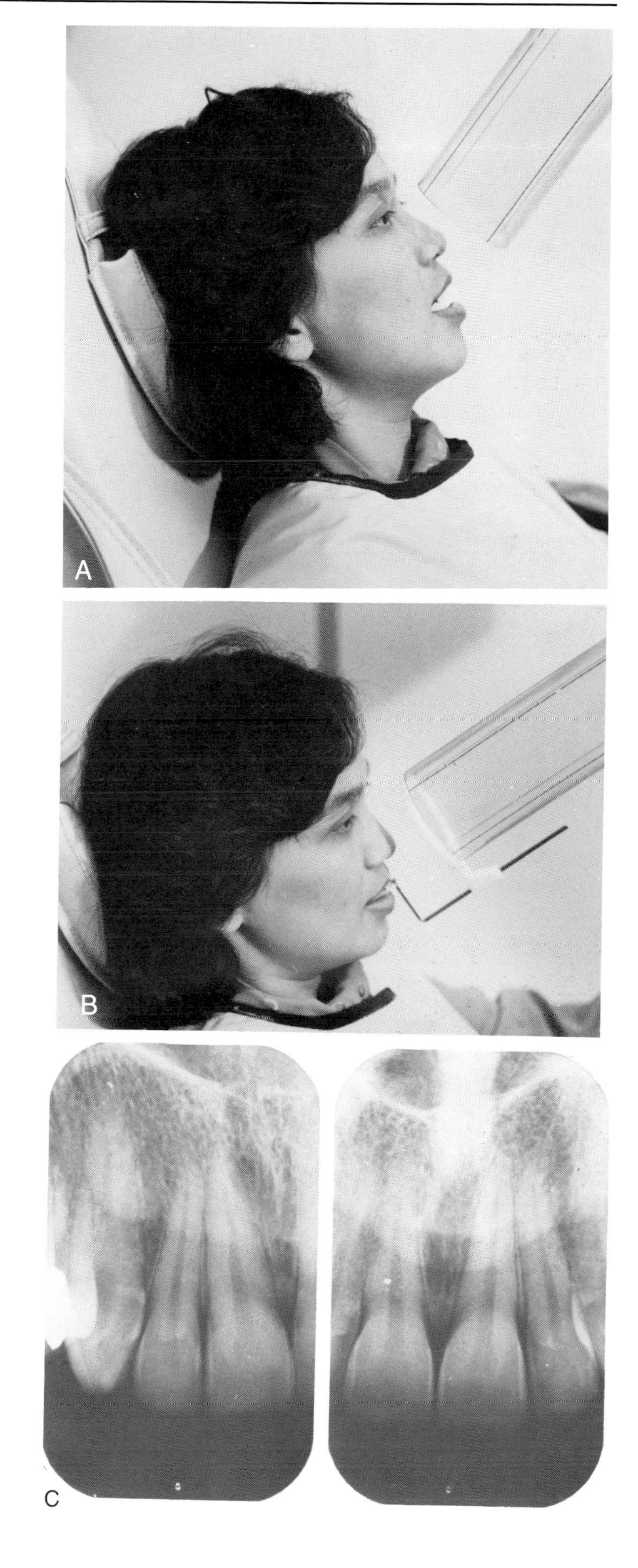

Figure 5–3. Radiographic technic for maxillary incisors. A, Using bite-block film holder. B, Using a film holder with attached cone positioning plastic ring and C, radiographs of maxillary midline and central-lateral incisors.

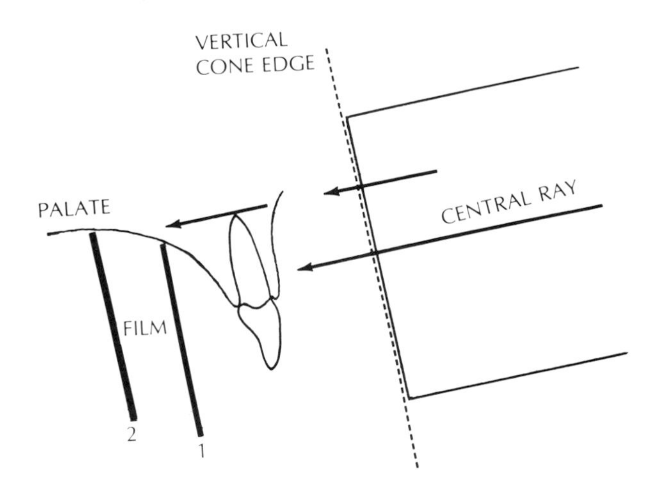

Figure 5–4. Films positioned parallel to long axis of maxillary incisors. Position 2 is farther in mouth and film is located higher to receive image of tooth's apex.

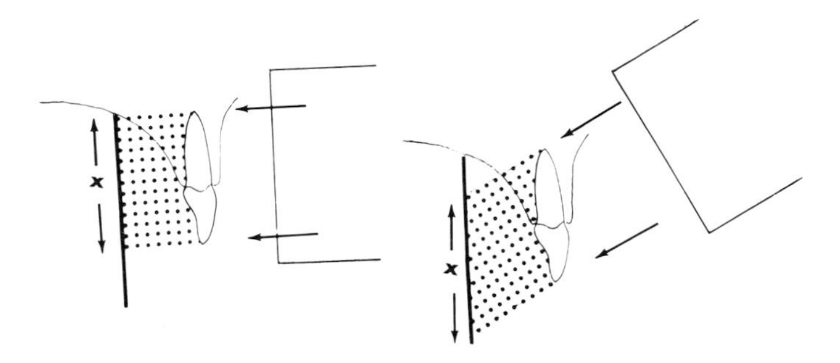

Figure 5–5. Effect of increasing vertical angulation (left to right) with film and tooth parallel is to lower entire tooth image. Vertical angulation does not appreciably change length of tooth's shadow (X).

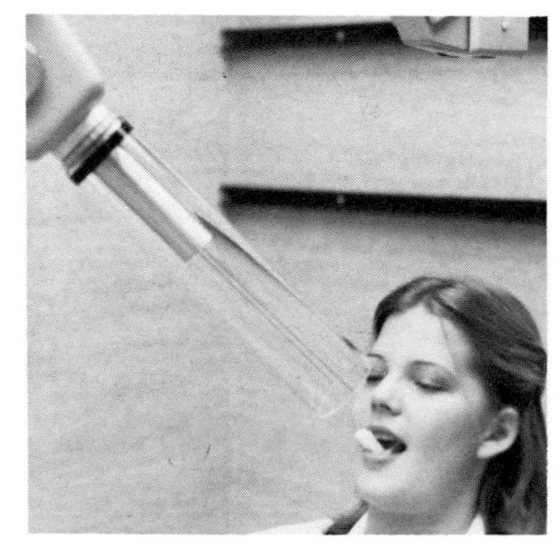

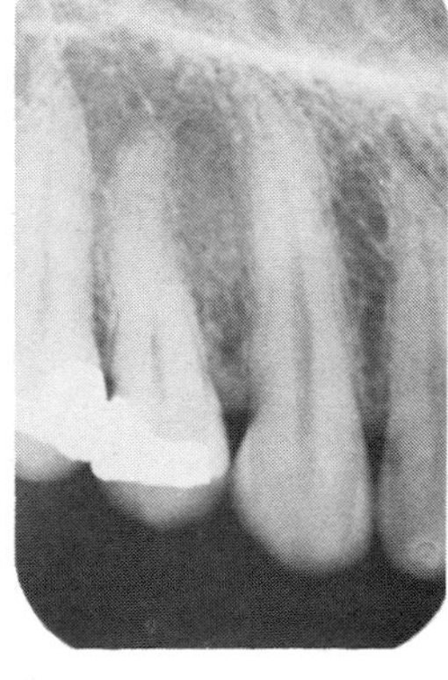

Figure 5–6. Technic for maxillary cuspid projection with paralleling technic and resultant radiograph.

diograph is made for the central and lateral incisors of each side. An additional midline projection is often useful. Figure 5–3 shows these radiographs and the exposure technic using two different types of film holders.

The film is positioned with its horizontal plane parallel to the labial surfaces of the teeth. It is placed as far as possible in the patient's mouth because it can be positioned higher in the palate when it is farther in the mouth (Figure 5–4). In most cases it is more efficient to introduce the film into the patient's mouth directly over the incisal edges of the teeth to be radiographed until approximately ¼ inch is not past the incisal edges of the teeth. The top of the film is then raised to touch the palate and the lower or outside border of the film pushed into the oral cavity until the film is parallel to the long axes of the teeth. The central ray is directed between the teeth of interest and perpendicular to the long axes of teeth and film. It is often easier for the operator to align the vertical edge of the cone parallel with the tooth and film.

In many cases the film may be close to but not quite reach the correct height in the mouth because of a shallow or narrow palate. To adjust for this problem the operator simply increases the vertical angulation until the shadows of the incisal edges of the teeth are cast on the film ⅛ inch above the lower border. With the film parallel to the long axes of the teeth the images of the apices of the teeth will automatically be lowered on to the film (Figure 5–5). When vertical angulation is changed, the tooth's shadow changes from a rectangle to a parallelogram. The length of the tooth's shadow does not change and thus the operator can concentrate on the visible incisal edge of the tooth and ignore the unseen apex. The horizontal position of the x-ray beam is adjusted to direct the central ray between the teeth being examined. This is best done when the operator directly sees the crowns of the teeth and is standing behind the x-ray tubehead.

THE MAXILLARY CUSPID RADIOGRAPH

The film is positioned behind the cuspid, parallel to the long axis of the cuspid and as high as possible in the palate. The vertical angle is adjusted to cast the shadow of the tip of the cusp to a point not more than 1/8 inch above the lower border of the film (Figure 5–6). The horizontal angle of the x-ray beam is adjusted by moving the tubehead distally until the shadow of the cuspid is close to the mesial border of the film. In this position the x-ray beam will be directed as close as possible through the contact area between the cuspid and first bicuspid, and any resulting overlapping of the images of these teeth will be minimized.

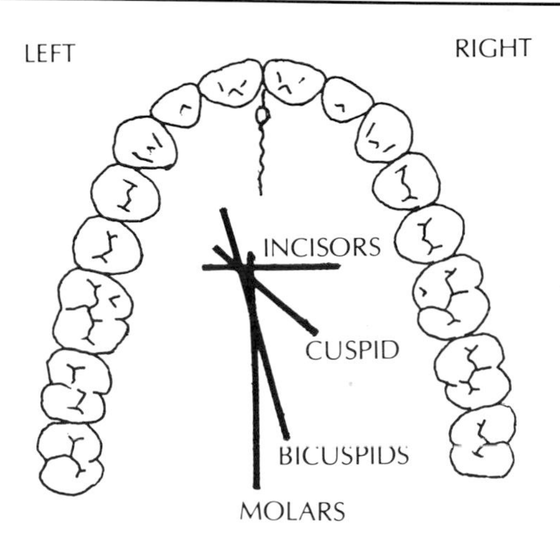

Figure 5–7. Locations of upper border of maxillary films on palate for paralleling technic radiographs of right side of patient.

THE MAXILLARY BICUSPID RADIOGRAPH

The standard No. 1.2 periapical film is used with the long dimension in the horizontal plane. It is placed parallel to the long axes of the bicuspid teeth in the vertical plane and parallel to the buccal surfaces of the bicuspid teeth in the horizontal plane. The upper border of the film is across the midline of the palate away from the teeth being examined (Figure 5–7). The anterior border should be placed behind the middle of the cuspid tooth.

While standing behind the tubehead and looking directly at the space between the teeth, the operator moves the x-ray tubehead in a horizontal direction to direct the x-ray beam between the bicuspid teeth. If the operator cannot see the teeth, the patient's cheek should be retracted. The horizontal direction of the beam can also be accomplished with the operator standing in front of the patient, looking at the line formed by the buccal surfaces of the bicuspid teeth, and positioning the horizontal edge of the open-end cone parallel to this line (Figure 5–8A). In this position the x-ray beam is also directed between the bicuspid teeth. The patient, film and x-ray beam positions are shown in Figures 5–8B and 5–8C using two types of film holders.

The vertical angulation is increased until the shadow of the tips of the cusps of the bicuspids are not more than 1/8 inch above the lower border of the film. The maxillary bicuspid radiograph is shown in Figure 5–8D.

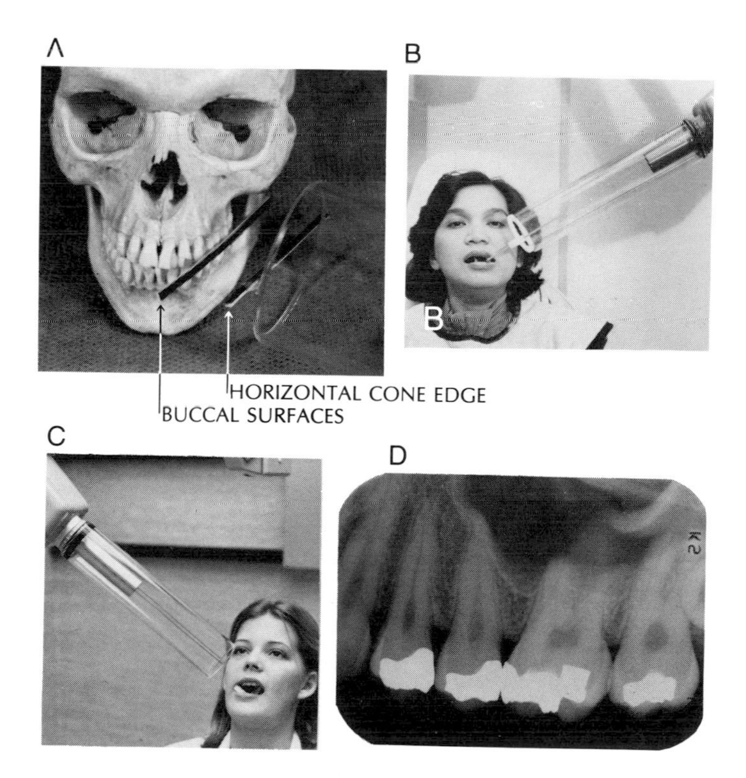

Figure 5–8. Paralleling film exposure technic for maxillary bicuspid teeth. A, Horizontal angulation of x-ray beam, placing horizontal edge of cone parallel to buccal surfaces of teeth. B, Using a film holder with attached cone positioning ring. C, Using a bite-block film holder. D, Maxillary bicuspid radiograph.

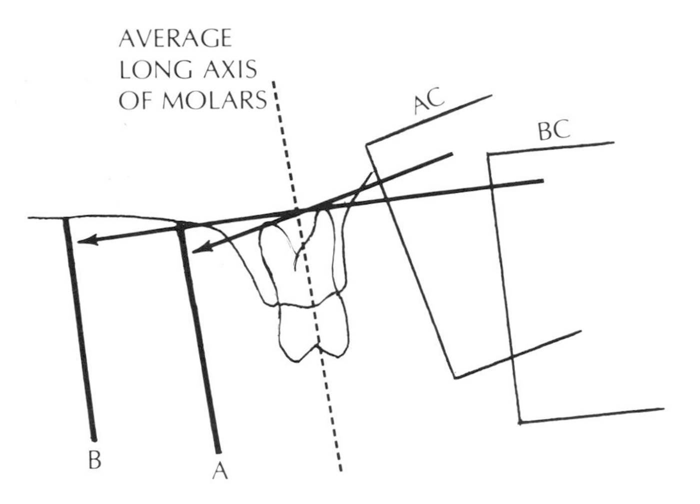

Figure 5–9. Diagram showing that when molar film is moved away from teeth (A to B) vertical angle needed to cast the shadow of tooth onto film is reduced (AC to BC).

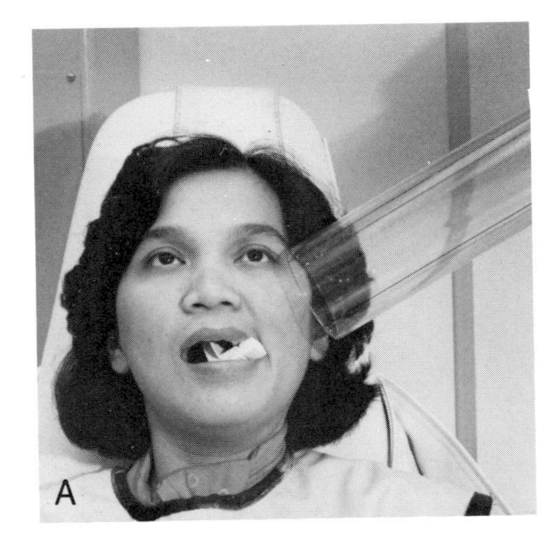

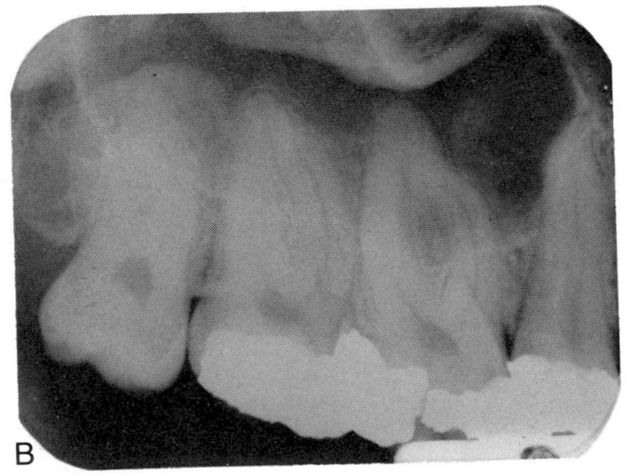

Figure 5–10. A, X-ray beam, patient and film positions for the maxillary molar projection. B, Maxillary molar radiograph.

THE MAXILLARY MOLAR RADIOGRAPH

The maxillary molar radiograph is similar to the bicuspid radiograph. The film is positioned more posteriorly to receive the image of the maxillary tuberosity. In the average adult patient the anterior border will be at the middle of the second bicuspid tooth. The upper border of the film is slightly across the midline of the palate (Figure 5–7). The farther the film is away from teeth the less vertical angulation is needed because the teeth apices are tilted medially (Figure 5–9). The vertical angle is adjusted to cast the shadow of the cusps of the molar teeth just above the lower border of the film. The horizontal angulation of the x-ray beam is achieved by directing the central ray between the molar teeth or by aligning the horizontal edge of the cone parallel to the buccal surfaces of the molars. Since the molar teeth cannot be easily seen by the operator, it should be observed that, in most cases, the correct horizontal angulation places the central ray in a slight mesiodistal direction from perpendicular to the sagittal plane of the patient's head. The molar projection and radiograph are shown in Figure 5–10.

THE DISTAL OBLIQUE MOLAR RADIOGRAPH

In some patients, when the film cannot be placed posteriorly enough into the mouth (e.g., a gagging patient), the film can be placed in the bicuspid region with the exposure side facing distally toward the molars (Figure 5–11A). The tubehead is placed in a more distal position and the shadows of the molars are cast anteriorly into the palate onto the film. The radiograph will not show the contact areas of the molars; however, these areas can be viewed on bitewing radiographs. The distal oblique projection is useful for viewing impacted maxillary third molars. In such cases the vertical angle is increased to direct the impacted tooth's shadow downward. An example of this projection is shown in Figure 5–11B.

THE MANDIBULAR INCISOR RADIOGRAPH

The No. 1.1 film is used with the long dimension positioned vertically. The film is

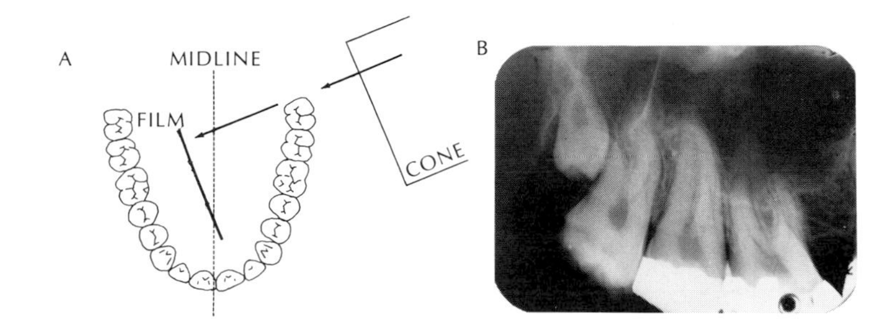

Figure 5–11. A, Distal oblique projection for maxillary molars with film in bicuspid region facing backward toward molars and x-ray tube positioned distally. B, Radiograph of impacted maxillary fourth molar.

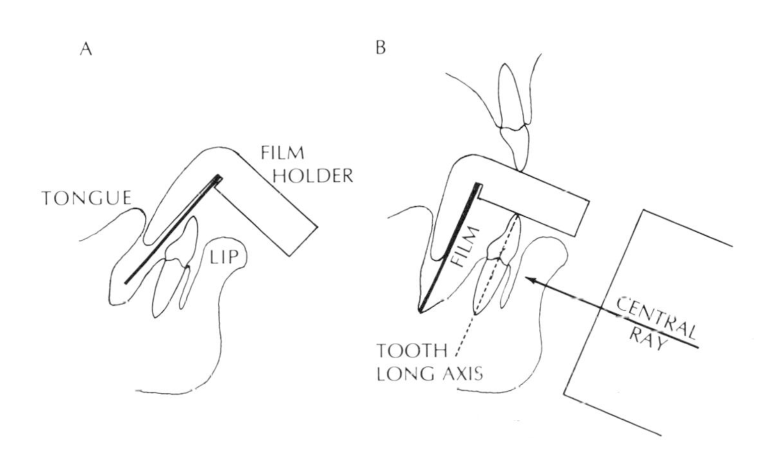

Figure 5–12. A, Initial placement of mandibular incisor film under tongue. B, Final position of incisor film.

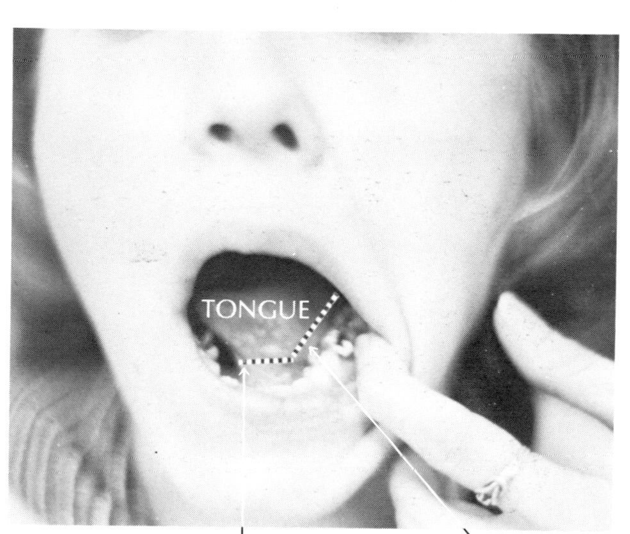

Figure 5–13. Location of the lower border of mandibular films.

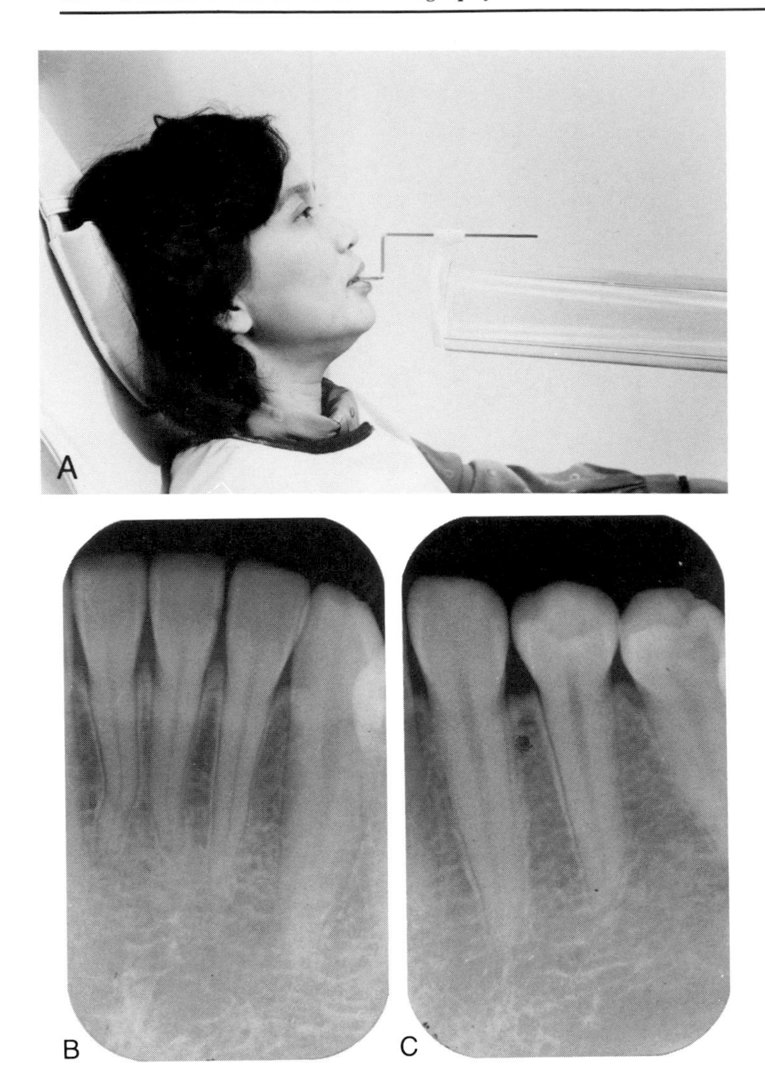

Figure 5–14. Radiography of mandibular incisor teeth. A, Using a film holder with beam locating ring. B, Mandibular incisor radiograph. C, Mandibular cuspid, first bicuspid radiograph.

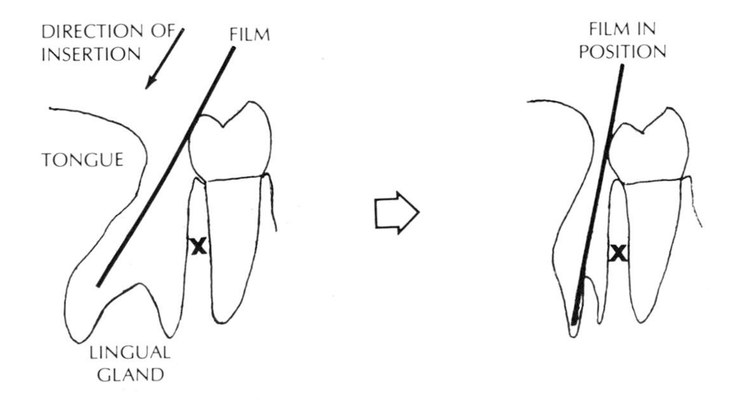

Figure 5–15. Film kept away from sensitive lingual gingiva (X) by placing lower border at base of tongue.

slipped over the central and lateral teeth of one side and under the tongue as far as possible; the operator sometimes has to ask the patient to lift the tongue (Figure 5–12A). The top edge of the film is then pushed into the patient's mouth until the film is parallel to the long axes of the teeth, and the patient is asked to close on the bite block (Figure 5–12B). It is important that the lower border of the film not move anteriorly when the upper edge is pushed into the patient's mouth. *The lower border of all mandibular films must be positioned away from the thin sensitive lingual gingiva covering the bone.* The lower border must be located at the base of the tongue where the tongue is attached to the floor of the mouth (Figure 5–13). The x-ray beam is positioned to direct the central ray between the teeth and to be perpendicular to the film and long axes of the teeth. The incisor radiograph is shown in Figure 5–14B.

THE MANDIBULAR CUSPID-FIRST BICUSPID RADIOGRAPH

The technic for this projection is identical to that for the incisor radiograph with the film positioned over the cuspid and first bicuspid. Unlike the maxillary cuspid radiograph, the mandibular first bicuspid can be radiographed clearly with the cuspid tooth since it is not greatly different in length or long axis position from the cuspid. An example of this projection is shown in Figure 5–14C.

THE MANDIBULAR BICUSPID RADIOGRAPH

Number 1.2 film is used with the long dimension positioned horizontally. The lower border of the film is placed under the tongue away from the lingual gingiva of the mandible. It is first inserted downward in a medial direction and then placed in an upright vertical position (Figure 5–15). The lingual gland tissue acts as a cushion to keep the lower border of the film away from the sensitive lingual gingiva covering the bone of the mandible. The film is moved as far anteriorly as comfortable for the patient. Note that when the film is parallel to the buccal surfaces of the bicuspid teeth, the anterior bor-

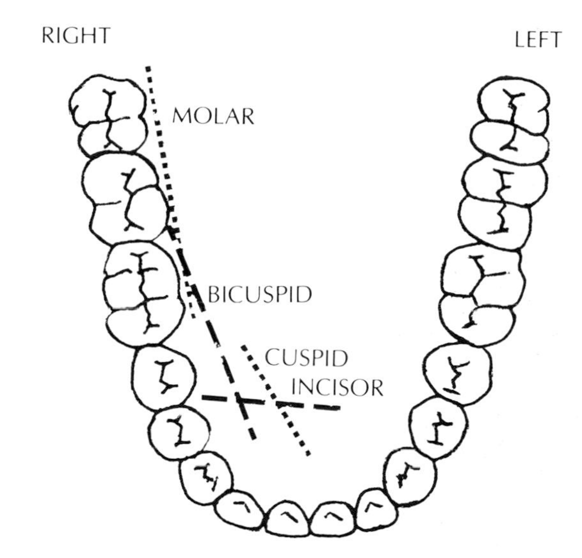

Figure 5–16. Location of lower border of films for different mandibular areas on the floor of the mouth for paralleling technic radiographs of the right side of the patient.

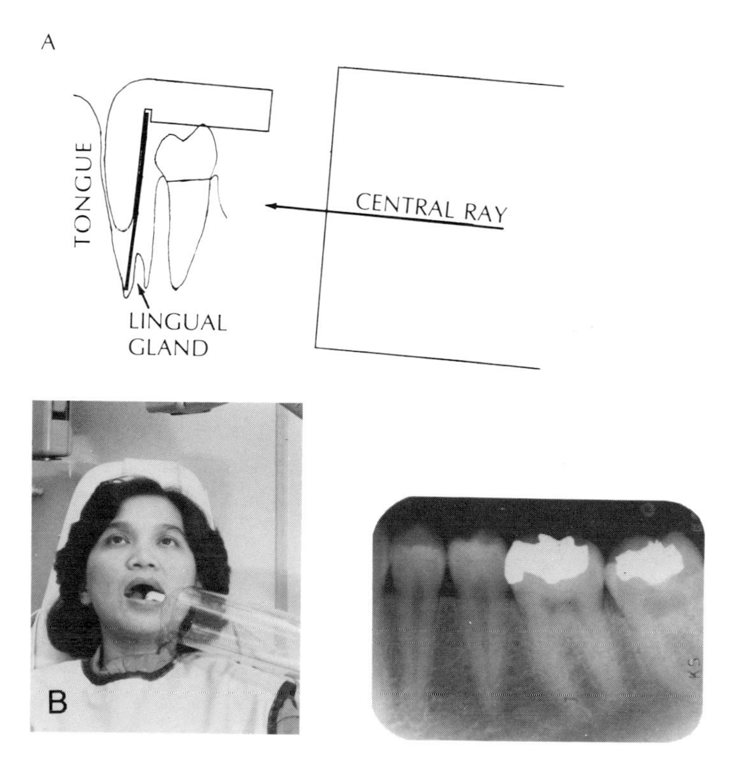

Figure 5–17. The mandibular bicuspid projection. A, X-ray beam and film positions. B, Using a bite-block film holder. C, The bicuspid radiograph.

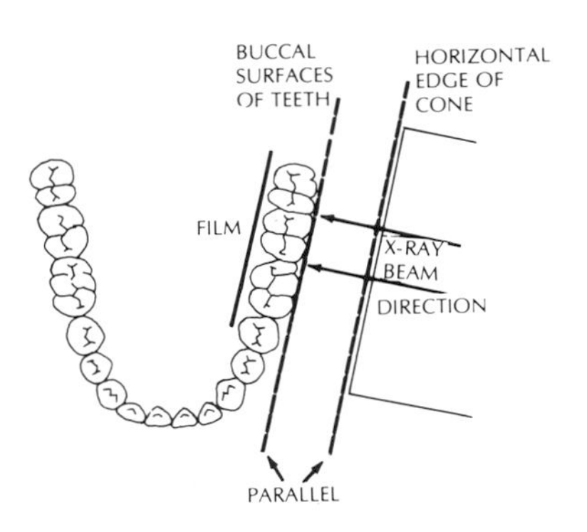

Figure 5–18. Horizontal beam angulation obtained by positioning horizontal edge of cone parallel to buccal surfaces of teeth.

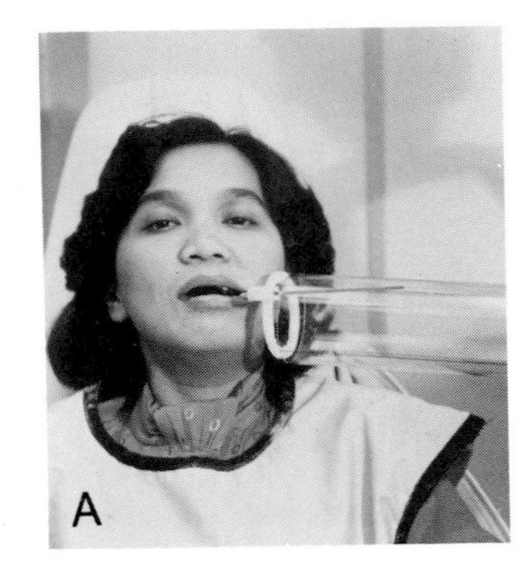

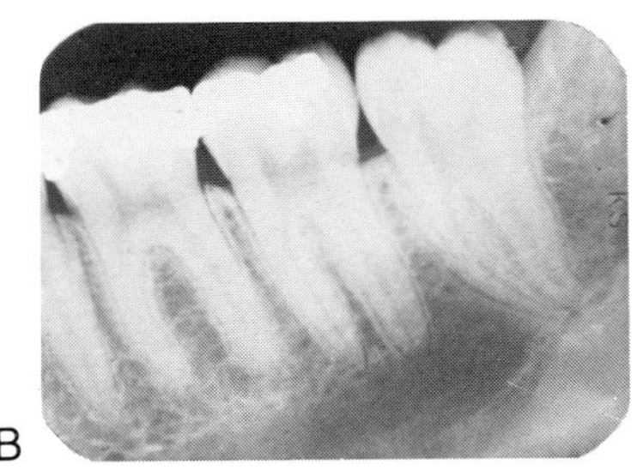

Figure 5–19. A, Mandibular molar technic and B, radiograph.

der is positioned medially. This is fortunate as it allows the film to be brought forward anteriorly into the curvature of the mandible in the incisor region without rising. The film position in the mandible for the bicuspid and other projections are shown in Figure 5–16.

With the patient's teeth closed upon the bite block the central ray is directed between the bicuspids and perpendicular to the film (Figure 5–17 A and B). The mandibular bicuspid radiograph is shown in Figure 5–17C.

THE MANDIBULAR MOLAR RADIOGRAPH

The molar radiographic technic is similar to the bicuspid projection. The same film size is used and the film is initially introduced into the patient's mouth in the same manner with the lower border under the tongue. The film is positioned posteriorly to examine the third molar. The anterior border in most adult patients will be at the middle of the second bicuspid tooth. In patients with large molar teeth or impacted third molars it is sometimes necessary to make a separate radiograph for the third molar. The x-ray beam is directed horizontally to pass between the teeth; as with other cheek covered teeth, the horizontal edge of the open-end cone can be positioned parallel to the buccal surfaces of the molar teeth to achieve the same result (Figure 5–18). The molar projection using a beam locating film holder and the molar radiograph are shown in Figure 5–19.

Chapter 6

The Bisecting-the-Angle Technic

The bisecting-the-angle technic was first used by dentists because it can be accomplished with a short tube-film distance. The early dental x-ray machines had poor x-ray production and films were of slow speed; thus tube-film distances of 8 inches or less had to be used to obtain exposure times of 3 seconds or less. If exposure time was greater than 3 seconds, the patient's movement often produced a blurred radiographic image. The bisecting-the-angle technic is sometimes called "the short-cone technic"; however, the bisecting-the-angle technic can be used with either a short-cone or a long-cone tube-film distance.

BISECTING-THE-ANGLE THEORY

The geometry of the bisecting-the-angle technic is isometric (same measurements) triangles. Figure 6–1 shows the type of triangles used in this technic in which the distance X to A is the same as X to B. During radiography the long axis of the tooth is in position X A and the film in X B, with the film touching the incisal edge of the tooth at X (Figure 6–2). The operator must visually bisect the angle formed by tooth and film and direct the x-ray beam perpendicular to the identified bisector. When this is done, the shadow of the tooth's apex (A) is cast upon the film at a point located the same distance from X as the tooth's apex. The radiographic image of the tooth will have the same length as the tooth.

THE FILM POSITIONER

Many useful types of film holders are available: they are described in Chapter 9. Unlike the paralleling technic a film holding device is not mandatory with the bisecting-the-angle technic. The patient's hand holding the film in position will be used in describing the bisecting technic in this chapter. This is done because there are situations where a film holder may not be available or the operator is not familiar with the available film holder.

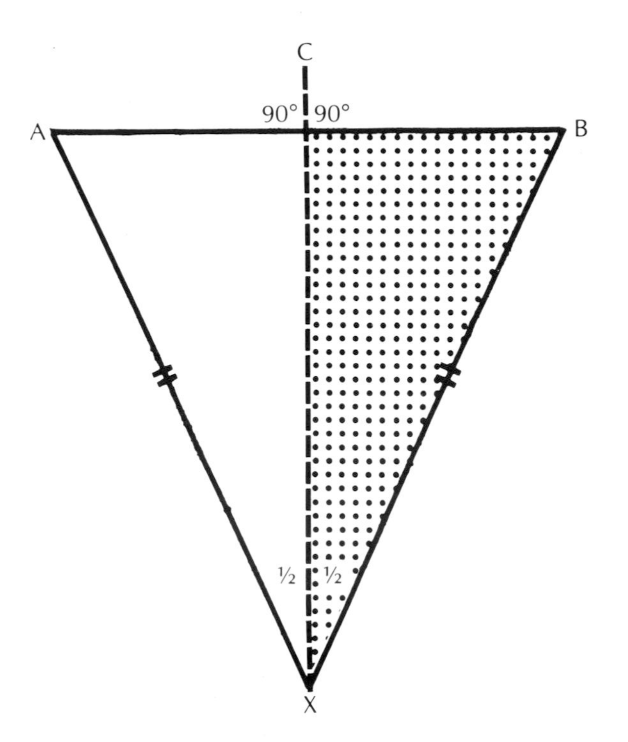

Figure 6–1. Geometry of isometric triangles. When angle formed by lines X A and X B is bisected (divided into 2 equal angles) by X C, and line A B is drawn perpendicular (90 degrees) to bisector X C, two triangles (one in dots) with same angles and dimensions are formed.

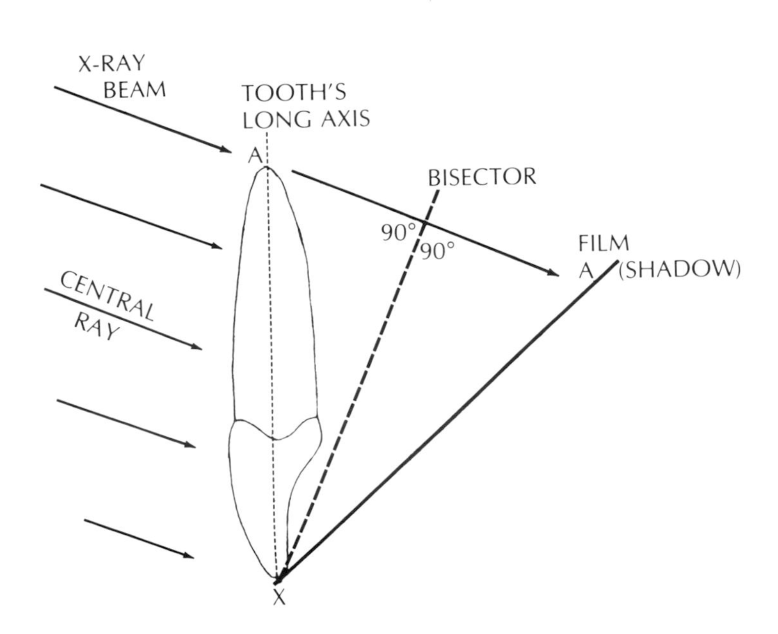

Figure 6–2. X-ray beam, tooth and film relationships in bisecting-angle technic.

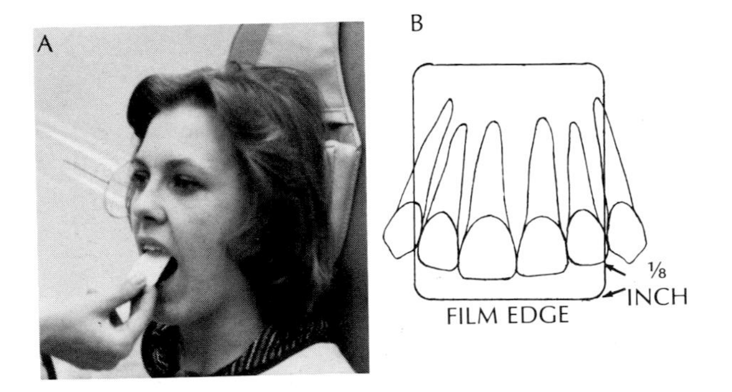

Figure 6–3. A, Film held by operator's thumb and forefinger with film exposure side facing upward. B, Film position in patient's mouth behind maxillary incisors.

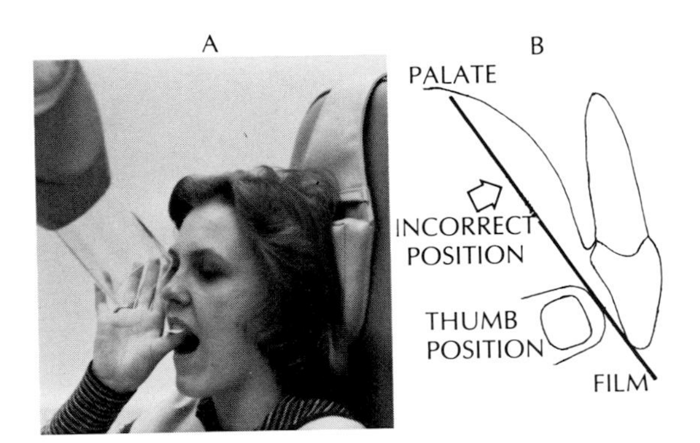

Figure 6–4. A, Film held by patient's thumb against palatal surfaces of crowns of teeth. B, Correct film position of thumb and incorrect thumb position area that will produce curved film.

The finger holding method is less preferred because it places the patient's hand in the primary x-ray beam. While all film positioning systems are designed to place the film in the same position, holding the film flat and in position is much easier to accomplish when a film holding device is used. In learning the various ways of retaining a film in the patient's mouth, information is most needed when the patient finger system of film holding is being studied.

THE MAXILLARY INCISOR RADIOGRAPH

The film is held with the long dimension vertically positioned by the thumb and forefinger (Figure 6–3A). The film is inserted into the patient's mouth and the operator's thumb is used as a "stop" to feel the incisal edges of the central teeth and indicate when the proper amount of film is in the oral cavity (Figure 6–3B). Approximately ⅛ inch of the film will extend below the incisal edges of the teeth when the proper amount of film is in the patient's mouth.

The film is held in place by the patient's thumb (Figure 6–4A). The objective is to keep the film in place without excessively bending the film. The flat part of the thumb is used to gently press the film against the palatal surface of the teeth (Figure 6–4B). Great force must not be used or the film will bend. If the thumb is placed on the upper part of the film, the film will be curved like the palate and a distorted tooth image will be produced.

The x-ray tubehead is moved to position the end of the cone over the film. The tubehead is positioned directly in front of the patient, and the horizontal direction of the x-ray beam is adjusted to direct the central ray between the central incisors (Figure 6–5A). The central ray is aimed at the center of the film. The operator visualizes the long axis of the central incisors, the film plane, and the angle formed by teeth and film (Figure 6–5B). The bisector of the angle is now identified and the central ray is positioned perpendicular to the bisector (Figure 6–6A). An easier way to position the central ray perpendicular to the bisector is to place the vertical edge of the open end of the cone parallel to the bisector. This method achieves the

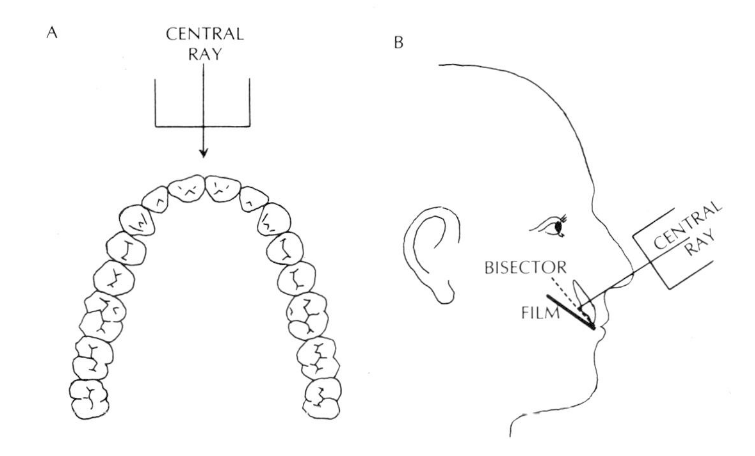

Figure 6–5. A, Horizontal angulation of x-ray beam for maxillary incisor teeth. B, View from side of patient for locating long axes of teeth, bisector of teeth-film angle and position of central ray perpendicular to bisector.

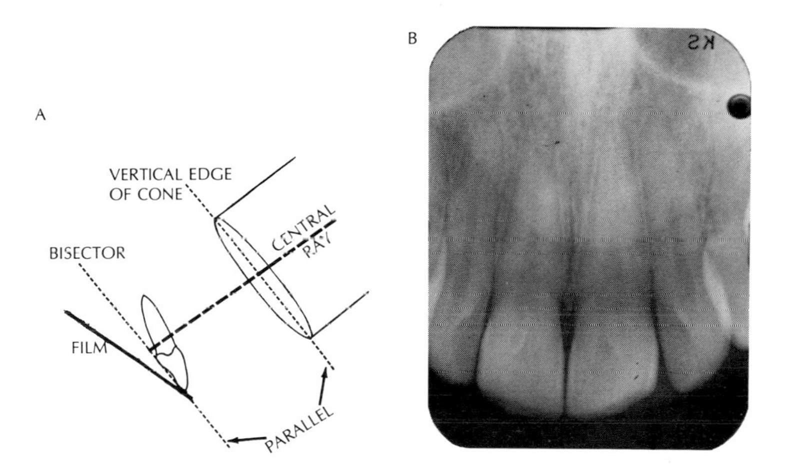

Figure 6–6. A, Placing vertical edge of cone parallel to bisector to position central ray perpendicular to bisector. B, Radiograph of maxillary central incisors.

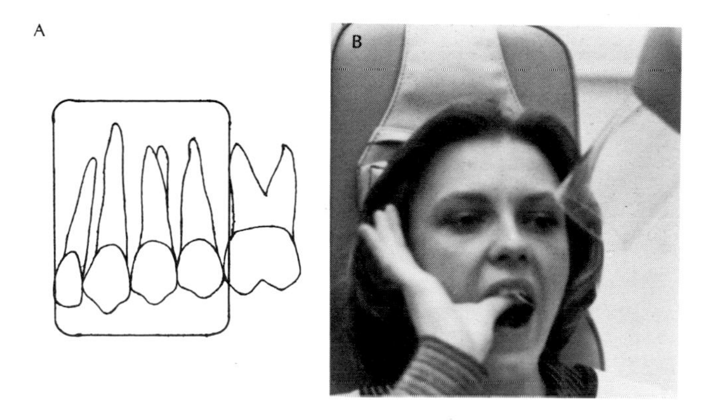

Figure 6–7. A, Position of film for radiograph of maxillary cuspid. B, Film held by opposite thumb of patient and position of patient and x-ray tubehead for radiograph of maxillary cuspid.

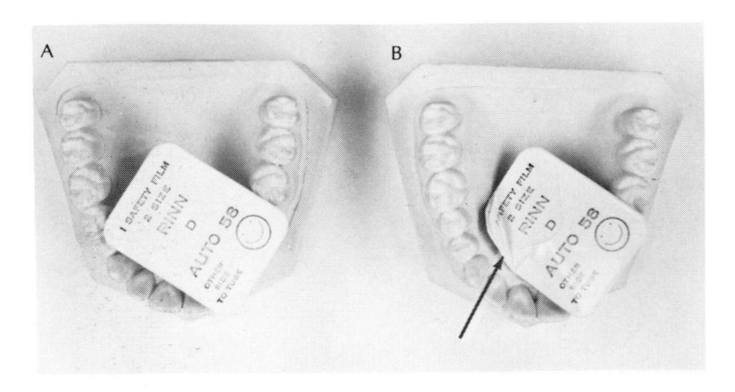

Figure 6–8. A, Cuspid film unable to be placed on palate because of interference of opposite teeth in patient with narrow maxillary arch. B, Film in correct position touching palate obtained by bending obstructing part away from opposite teeth.

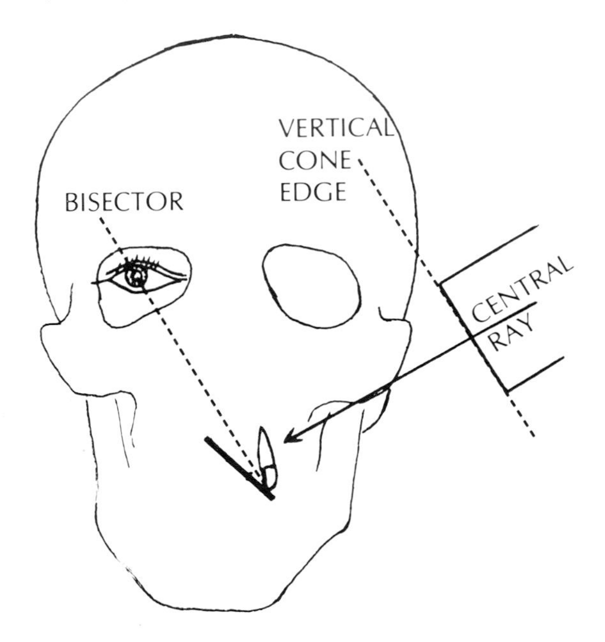

Figure 6–9. Approximate location of bisector of average person's film-cuspid angle.

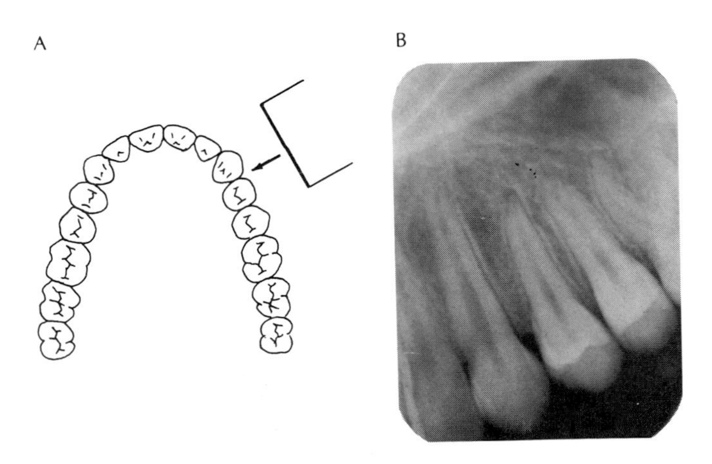

Figure 6–10. A, Horizontal angulation to direct central ray between maxillary cuspid and first bicuspid teeth. B, Maxillary cuspid radiograph.

same objective, since the central ray is always perpendicular to the edge of the cone. The first method uses an unseen central ray and an unseen bisector; the second method uses a visually observed cone edge and only one unseen factor, the bisector. The film is then exposed and processed. A radiograph of the maxillary central incisors is shown in Figure 6–6B.

THE MAXILLARY CUSPID RADIOGRAPH

The film is positioned in the patient's mouth behind the cuspid tooth in a manner similar to that for the maxillary incisor radiograph, but with less than ⅛ inch of the film extending below the cusp of the cuspid (Figure 6–7A). The film is held in position by the patient with the thumb of the hand opposite the cuspid being examined (Figure 6–7B). If the patient's maxillary arch is wide, the film can be placed in this position; however, many arches are of a size that do not permit this placement and the size of the film must be reduced to fit a narrow arch by bending part of the film (Figure 6–8). The film must not be curved. The unwanted part must be bent completely out of the way.

With the film positioned, the operator visualizes the long axis of the cuspid, the film plane, and the bisector of the angle formed by tooth and film. The x-ray tubehead is adjusted to place the central ray perpendicular to the bisector (Figures 6–6A and 6–7B). In this position the vertical edge of the cone is parallel to the bisector. If the operator has difficulty in locating the bisector, an external landmark on the patient can be of assistance; the bisector will be close to a line drawn from the cusp of the cuspid to the pupil of the opposite eye of the patient (Figure 6–9). To position the x-ray beam over the tooth the operator should recall that the cuspid's apex is located at the wing of the nose. The tubehead is moved horizontally to direct the central ray as close as possible through the interproximal space between the cuspid and first bicuspid (Figure 6–10A). The tubehead must not be moved so far distally that the image of the cuspid will not appear in the radiograph; this is particularly important in patients with narrow arches. The operator should note that the cuspid-first bicuspid contact surface is in a direction not greatly different from the contact direction of the first and second bicuspids. A cuspid radiograph is shown in Figure 6–10B.

THE MAXILLARY BICUSPID RADIOGRAPH

The film is positioned in the patient's mouth with the long dimension in the horizontal plane. The anterior border should be placed at the middle of the cuspid tooth (Figure 6–11A). The lower border of the film must be parallel to the cusps of the teeth and must not extend more than ⅛ inch below the cusps. The operator may find it useful to grasp the lower anterior corner of the film with the thumb and forefinger (Figure 6–11B). The thumb is then placed on the buccal surfaces of the teeth between the cuspid and first bicuspid. The film can be held by the operator's right or left hand, depending on whether the operator is standing in front of, or behind the patient. This film placement technic permits quick and accurate positioning of the film with a minimum amount of film movement in the patient's mouth. The relationship of the film to the palate is shown in Figure 6–12A. The film is held in place with the thumb of the opposite hand of the patient. Care is taken not to curve the film excessively by pressing it too firmly to the palate.

The operator observes the film plane, bicuspid axis, and bisector of the angle formed. The central ray is positioned perpendicular to the bisector, or the vertical edge of the cone parallel to the bisector (Figure 6–12B). A rough estimate of the location of the bisector is obtained by visualizing a line connecting the buccal cusp of the bicuspid and the top of the nose between the eyes of the patient. The nose point is located approximately midway between the top of the palate (to which the film plane is directed) and the top of the head (to which the tooth's long axis is directed). While standing behind the tubehead and looking directly at the space between the teeth, the operator moves the x-ray tubehead in a horizontal direction to direct the x-ray beam between the bicuspid teeth. If the operator cannot see the teeth, the patient's cheek should be retracted. The horizontal direction of the beam can also be accomplished

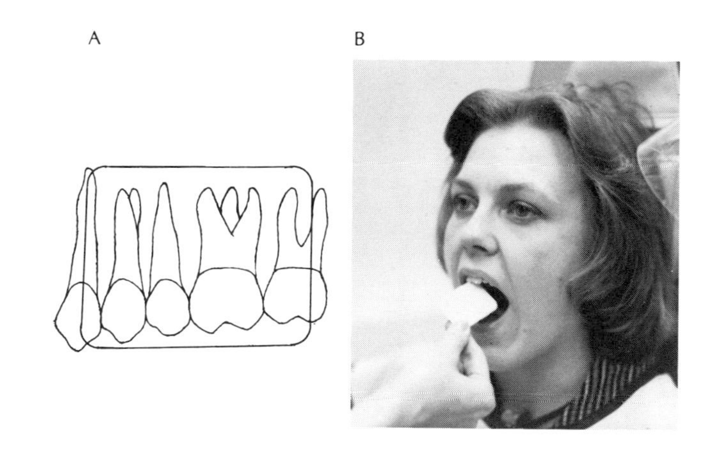

Figure 6–11. A, Area covered by maxillary bicuspid film. B, Operator placement of film for bicuspid radiograph when operator is in front of patient and holds the film with right hand.

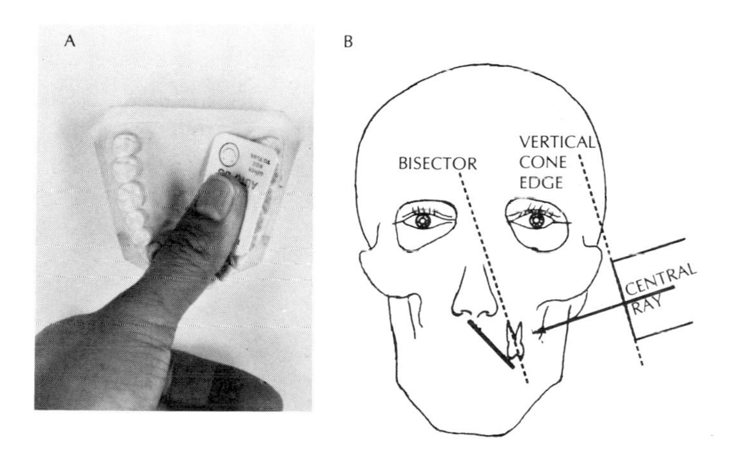

Figure 6–12. A, Position of bicuspid film on palate. B, Relationship of film, teeth, and cone for maxillary bicuspid radiograph. Note that bisector is directed close to point midway between eyes.

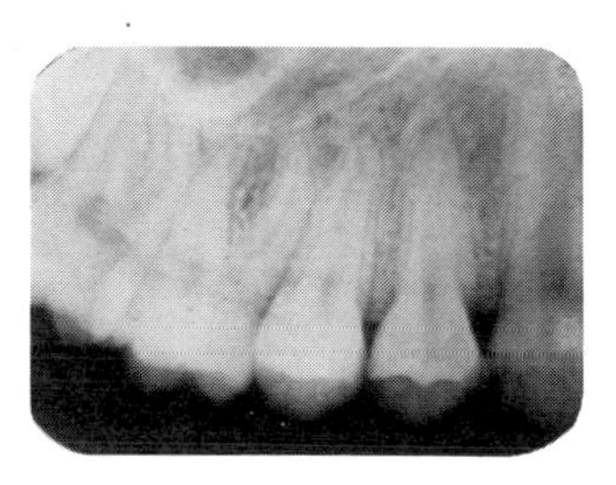

Figure 6–13. Maxillary bicuspid radiograph.

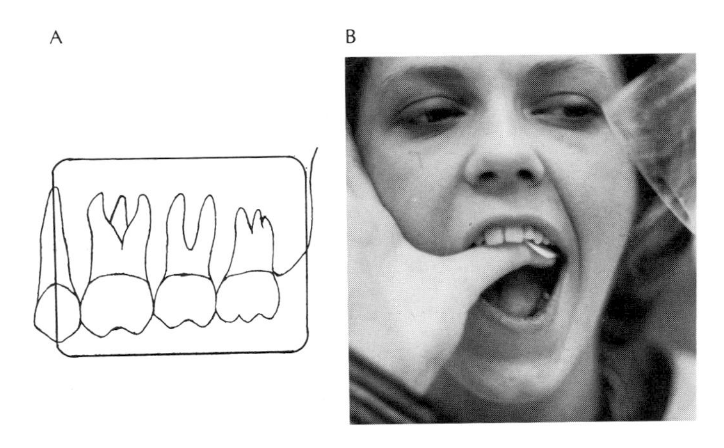

Figure 6–14. A, Area examined by maxillary molar film. B, Position of molar film.

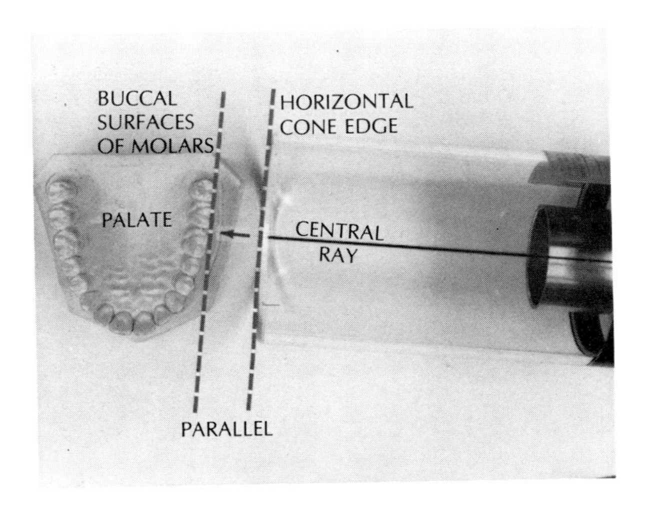

Figure 6–15. Horizontal beam angulation with horizontal edge of open-end cone parallel to buccal surfaces of molar teeth.

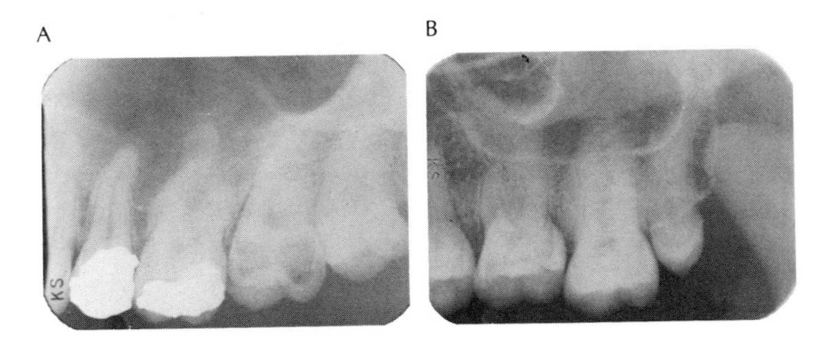

Figure 6–16. A, Radiograph of maxillary molar. B, Radiograph of maxillary third molar.

with the operator standing in front of the patient, looking at the line formed by the buccal surfaces of the bicuspid teeth, and positioning the horizontal edge of the open-end cone parallel to this line. In this position the x-ray beam is also directed between the bicuspid teeth. The bicuspid radiograph is shown in Figure 6–13.

THE MAXILLARY MOLAR RADIOGRAPH

The film is positioned and held in the mouth like the film for the bicuspid radiograph but is placed distally until the posterior film border is slightly past the tuberosity of the maxilla (Figure 6–14). The operator sometimes has difficulty in seeing the posterior border of the film and can use a slightly less accurate method by placing the anterior film border at the middle of the second bicuspid tooth. The second method is most useful when the patient has average-sized teeth. The vertical angulation of the x-ray beam is slightly greater than that for the bicuspid region because the molar film tends to lie in a slightly more horizontal or less upright position. The horizontal angulation of the x-ray beam is adjusted to direct the beam between the molars. Since the patient's cheek prevents the operator from looking directly into the interproximal spaces between the molars, an alternative method of horizontal beam angulation using the horizontal edge of the cone will be found useful (Figure 6–15). In many patients the beam will not pass directly through all molar contact points because the molars are often shaped to position the contact points in slightly different buccolingual directions. However, since the first molar appears in both bicuspid and molar radiographs, all contact points are usually seen when both radiographs are made. A molar radiograph is shown in Figure 6–16A.

When the third molar is the single tooth of interest, the film is positioned slightly more posteriorly and in most cases slightly higher in the oral cavity. The vertical angle used is slightly greater than that for the normal molar radiograph and the x-ray tubehead is placed in a slightly more distal location. These modifications are designed to place the film behind the area of interest and cast the shadow of the apex of the third molar slightly more forward and downward than is done in the normal molar radiograph (Figure 6–16B).

THE MANDIBULAR INCISOR RADIOGRAPH

The patient is positioned with the occlusal plane of the mandible parallel to the floor when the patient's mouth is open. The film is positioned with the long dimension in the vertical plane and held by thumb and forefinger of the operator as shown in Figure 6–17A. The film is gently placed under the patient's tongue until the operator's thumb encounters the incisal edges of the teeth to indicate that enough film is in the mouth to receive the images of the teeth. Approximately ¼ inch of film will extend above the incisal edges of the teeth. The film is held in place by the anterior or palm surface of the index finger of either hand of the patient (Figure 6–18A). Note that to accomplish this the patient's elbow must be elevated. The finger presses the film against the lingual surfaces of the crowns of the incisors with enough pressure to stabilize the film (Figure 6–18B). Too much pressure will curve the film to the shape of the arch. Positioning the finger too low in the mouth will curve the film in the vertical plane. Excessively curved film produces distorted images.

The x-ray tubehead is moved horizontally until it is directly in front of the patient and the horizontal beam angulation directs the central ray between the central incisors. The operator must identify the tooth axis, vertical film plane, and the bisector of the tooth-film angle (Figure 6–19A). The central ray is directed to the center of the film perpendicular to the bisector. An alternative procedure is to note that the open end of the cone covers the film and that the vertical edge of the cone is parallel to the bisector. The mandibular incisor radiograph is shown in Figure 6–19B.

THE MANDIBULAR CUSPID RADIOGRAPH

The film is placed and held in the patient's mouth in a manner similar to that for the incisor radiograph. The patient uses the index finger of the opposite hand and the film is positioned with the cuspid in the middle of the film (Figure 6–20A). The horizontal

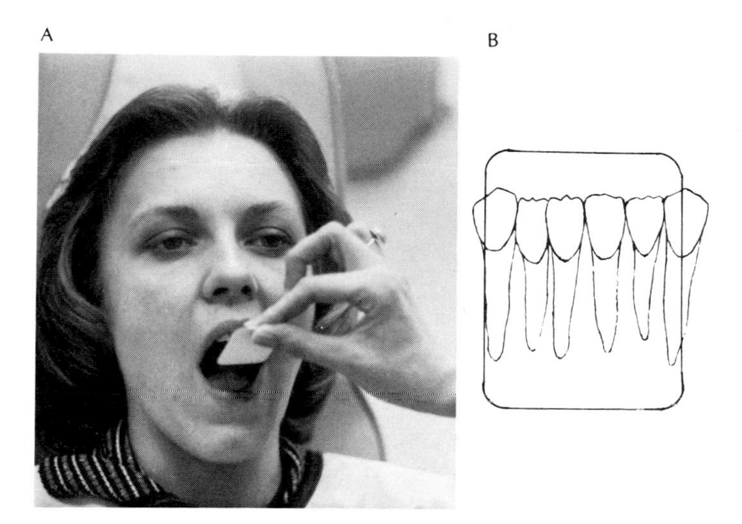

Figure 6–17. A, Film held by operator's thumb and forefinger with film exposure side facing downward. B, Area covered by film for mandibular incisor.

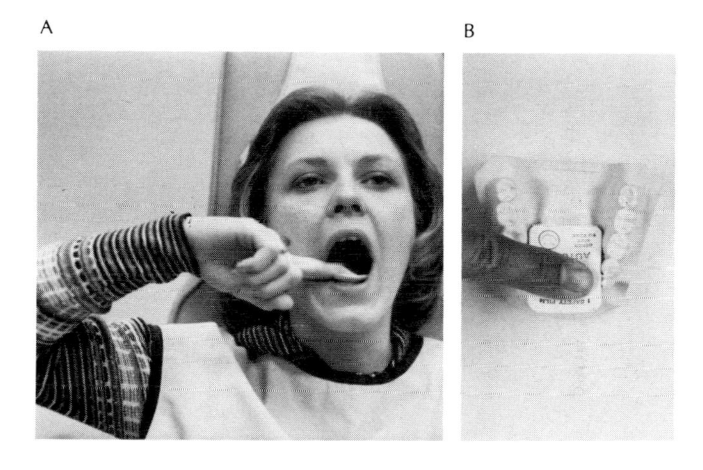

Figure 6–18. A, Patient holding film with index finger. B, Index finger position on film.

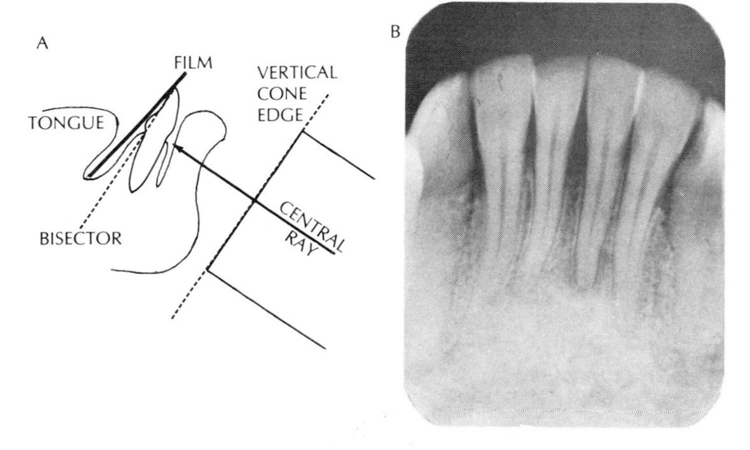

Figure 6–19. A, Relationship of central ray and open-end of cone to film, long axis of tooth, and bisector of tooth-film angle. B, Radiograph of a mandibular incisor.

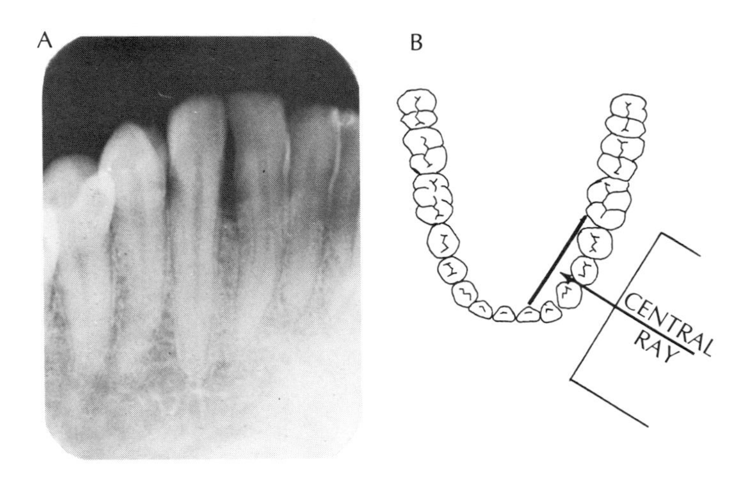

Figure 6–20. A, Radiograph of mandibular cuspid. B, Central ray directed between cuspid and first bicuspid teeth.

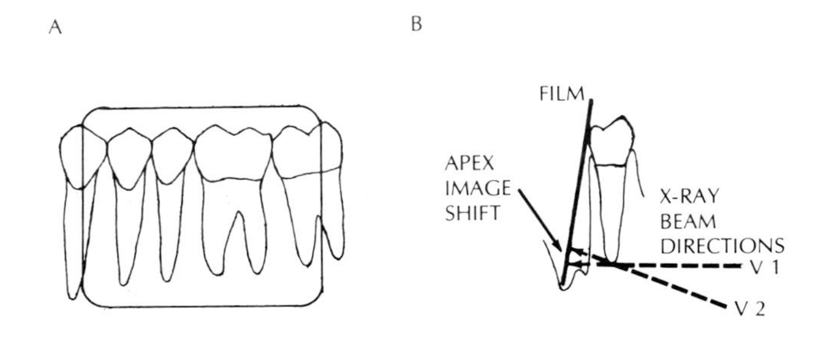

Figure 6–21. A, Area covered by mandibular bicuspid radiograph. B, Film positioned close to apex of bicuspid with little vertical shift of apex image when relatively large changes are made in vertical angulation of x-ray beam (V1 to V2).

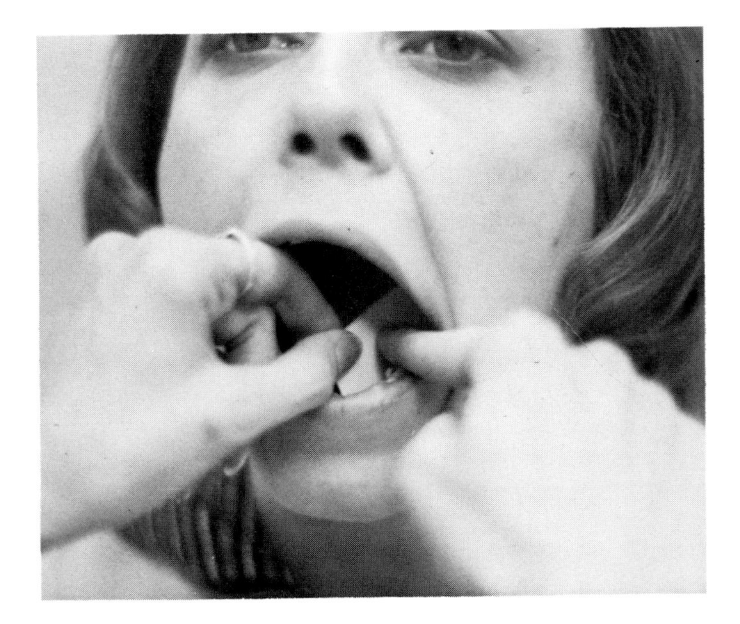

Figure 6–22. Placement of film for mandibular bicuspid while pushing tongue medially to keep film away from lingual gingiva.

angle of the x-ray beam is adjusted to direct the central ray between the cuspid and first bicuspid (Figure 6–20B). The beam's vertical angulation is established like that of the incisor radiograph (Figure 6–19A).

THE MANDIBULAR BICUSPID RADIOGRAPH

The film is placed in the patient's mouth with the long dimension in the horizontal plane. The anterior border of the film should be at the middle of the cuspid (Figure 6–21A). The upper border of the film should be parallel to the cusps of the teeth and should not protrude above the cusps more than ⅛ inch. The operator should note that the short dimension of the film is only slightly greater than the lengths of the bicuspids; if the film extends more than ⅛ inch above the teeth, the lower border will be above the apices of the teeth in many patients. The operator should also observe that the film is quite close to the crowns and apices of the posterior mandibular teeth (Figure 6–21B). With this relationship, large changes in x-ray beam vertical angulation produce relatively small changes in the position of the images of the apices of teeth on the film. These two observations indicate that the placement of the bicuspid film deep in the patient's mouth is of utmost importance.

The lower border of the film must always be at the base of the tongue between the fold of the lingual gland (the rise in the tissue of the floor of the mouth between the tongue and the inner surface of the mandible) and the base of the tongue (Figure 5–15). The lower edge of the film must not press on the lingual gingiva; pressure here is painful to the patient because the gingiva in this area is thin and there is hard unyielding bone underneath it. To achieve deep placement of the film with little discomfort to the patient the film can be positioned slightly posteriorly and pushed downward while the other hand of the operator is used to push the tongue medially and keep the lower border of the film away from the sensitive lingual gingiva (Figure 6–22).

After the film is positioned deep in the mouth, it is brought forward until the anterior border is at the middle of the cuspid. The film is held in place by the patient with the index finger of the opposite hand (Figure 6–23). The patient must elevate the arm used so that well-controlled pressure can be applied to the film to press it against the lingual surfaces of the teeth. If the elbow is close to the patient's chest, the side of the index finger will be touching the film and the patient has less control over elevation of the film by the tissues of the floor of the mouth.

As with the other projections, the tooth-film angle is bisected and the central ray is positioned perpendicular to the bisector. The angle is usually so small that the bisector can usually be easily found close to the vertical plane of the film (Figure 6–24A). Another point to observe is that the long axis of the bicuspid is close to perpendicular to the occlusal plane; thus the central ray will have a slight upward direction or minus vertical angulation. The x-ray beam is also directed horizontally to pass between the bicuspids. A bicuspid radiograph is shown in Figure 6–24B.

THE MANDIBULAR MOLAR RADIOGRAPH

This projection is similar to the bicuspid radiograph. The film is placed deep in the mouth in the same way. It is then moved posteriorly until the posterior border is past the distal surface of the third molar (Figure 6–25A). The vertical angle of the x-ray beam is approximately the same as that for the bicuspid radiograph. Although this angle is the same relative to the occlusal plane, it is actually increased relative to the molars because the crowns of the molars tend to be tilted lingually (Figure 6–25B). The tubehead is positioned horizontally to direct the x-ray beam between the teeth; as with other cheek-covered teeth, the horizontal edge of the open-end cone can be positioned parallel to the buccal surfaces of the molar teeth to achieve the same result.

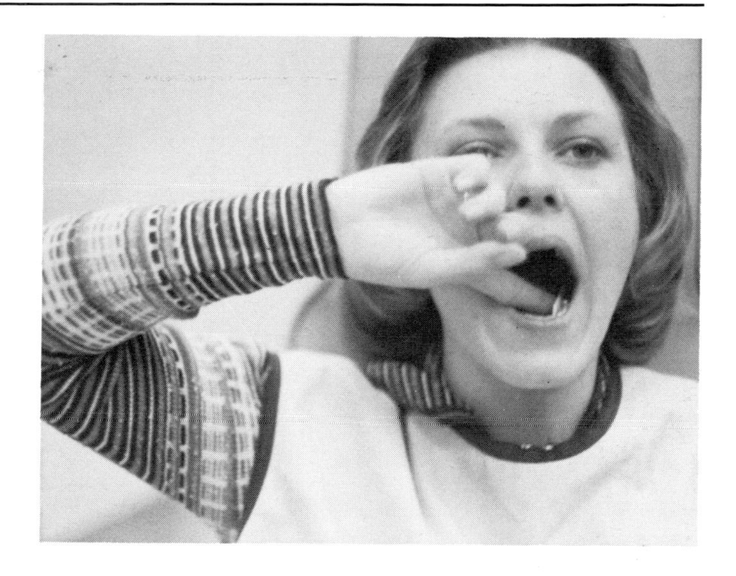

Figure 6–23. Patient holding film for mandibular bicuspid in position with anterior (palm) surface of index finger against lingual surfaces of teeth. Note that patient has to elevate elbow.

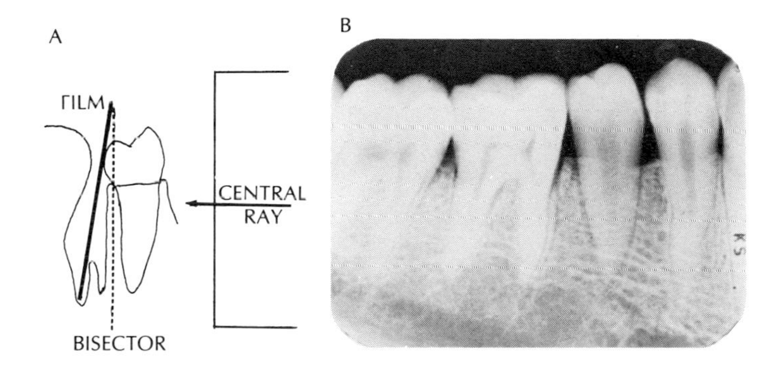

Figure 6–24. A, Positions of tooth, film, and x-ray beam for mandibular bicuspid radiograph. B, Radiograph of a mandibular bicuspid.

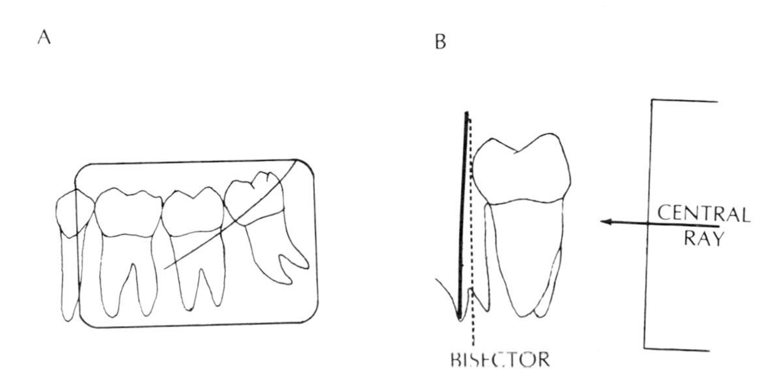

Figure 6–25. A, Area covered by mandibular molar radiograph. B, Position of molar film in relation to teeth. Vertical angle of beam is similar to angle used for bicuspid radiograph.

Chapter 7

The Bitewing Radiograph

The bitewing radiograph is made to show the proximal surfaces of the teeth and the crest of the alveolar bone of both the maxilla and mandible on the same film. Two films of the standard periapical No. 2 size, one bicuspid and one molar bitewing, are usually needed for each side of the adult patient. Two films are needed because all bicuspid and molar contact surfaces do not lie in the same buccolingual direction.

The bitewing film has a film tab projecting from the exposure surface of the film packet (Figure 7–1A). The film is manufactured in this form or can be constructed by placing a standard periapical film in a bitewing loop (Figure 7–1B). It can also be placed in some film holders.

The film for the bicuspid bitewing radiograph is positioned in the patient's mouth by placing the lower half between the tongue and mandibular teeth, with the anterior border at the middle of the cuspid (Fig. 7–2A). It is held in place by the operator's forefinger pressing the tab on the occlusal surface of the mandibular teeth. The patient is asked to close slowly; the operator removes the finger and the patient occludes the upper and lower teeth, holding the film tab firmly between the teeth (Figure 7–2B).

A common problem is one in which more than half of the film is positioned below the occlusal plane. This occurs when the upper border contacts the palatal cusp of the maxillary teeth or the palatal gingiva at the necks of teeth and is pushed downward when the patient closes (Figure 7–3A). This problem can be avoided by using a throat stick or thin instrument to keep the upper edge of the film away from any obstructions when the patient closes the mouth on the film tab (Figure 7–3B). The stick is removed just before the patient bites on the tab.

The operator must instruct the patient to keep the teeth in contact or the film will be pushed out of position by the tissues of the floor of the mouth. The patient will often

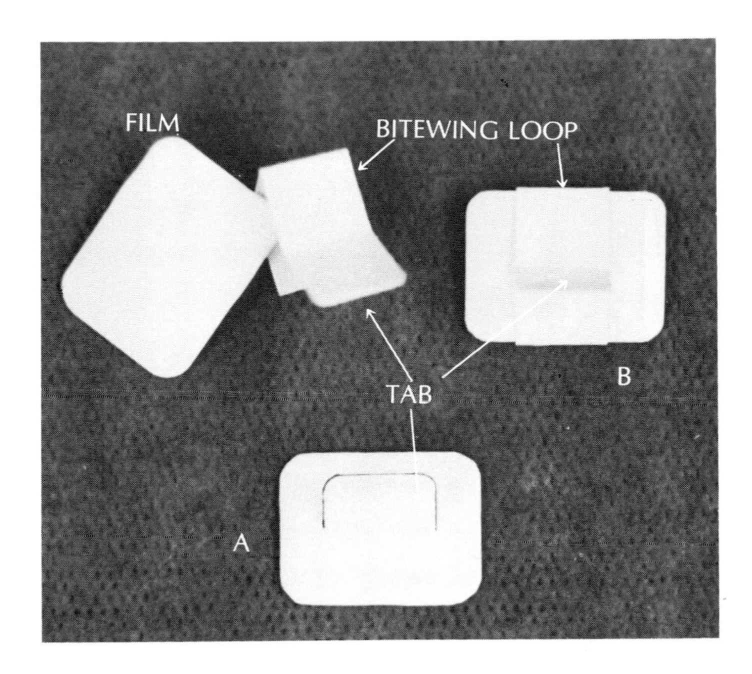

Figure 7–1. A, Bitewing film manufactured with attached film tab. B, Bitewing loop and standard periapical film used to construct bitewing film.

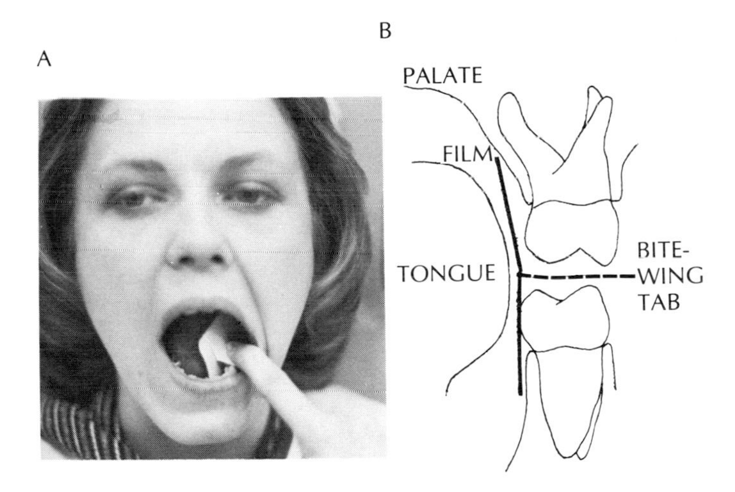

Figure 7–2. A, Placement of mandibular half of bitewing film in patient's mouth. B, Position of bitewing film in oral cavity.

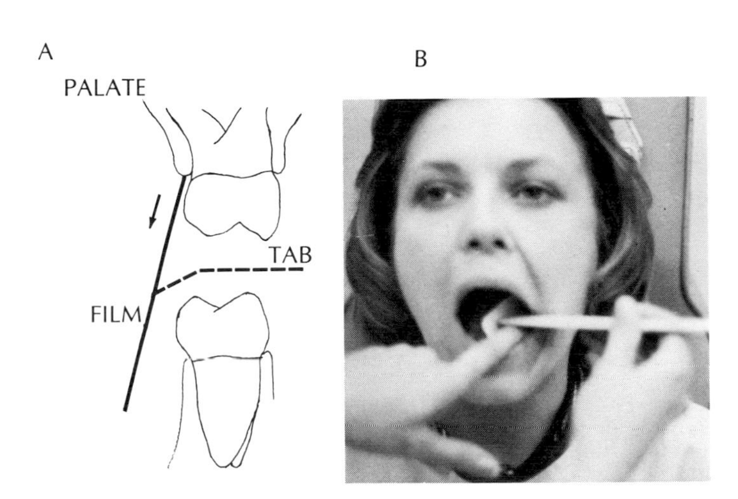

Figure 7–3. A, Film contacting free palatal gingiva before patient closes mouth. B, Top of film kept away from palatal obstructions with throat stick during closure of the mouth. Throat stick or tongue blade is removed just before patient bites on bitewing tab.

A

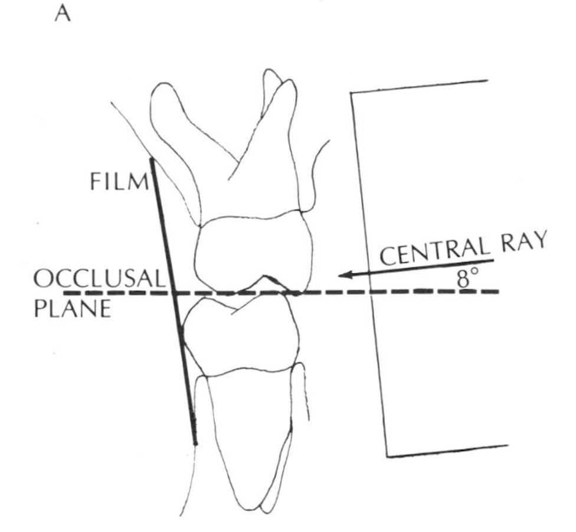

B

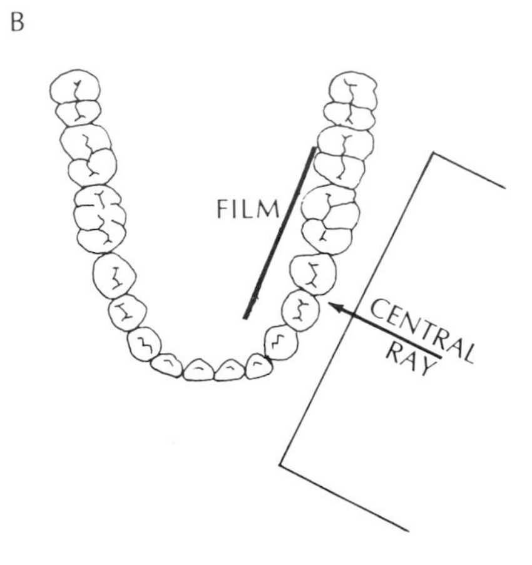

Figure 7–4. A, Vertical beam angulation for bitewing radiography. B, Horizontal angulation of x-ray beam for bicuspid bitewing radiograph.

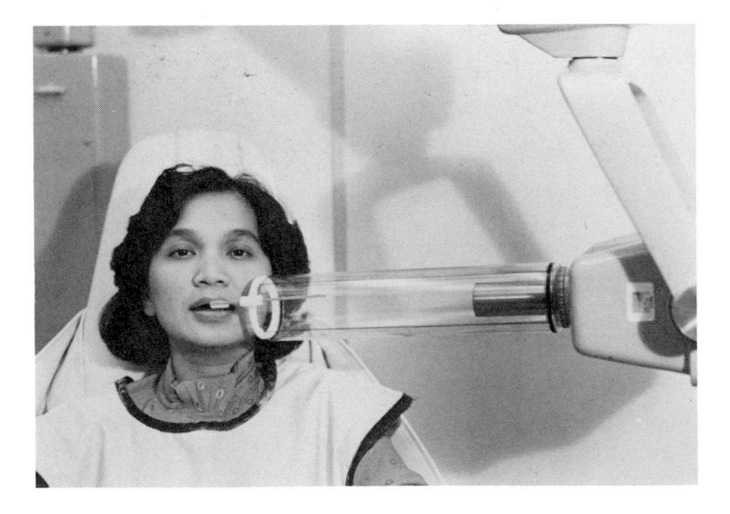

Figure 7–5. Bitewing radiography using a film holder with attached beam positioning ring.

A

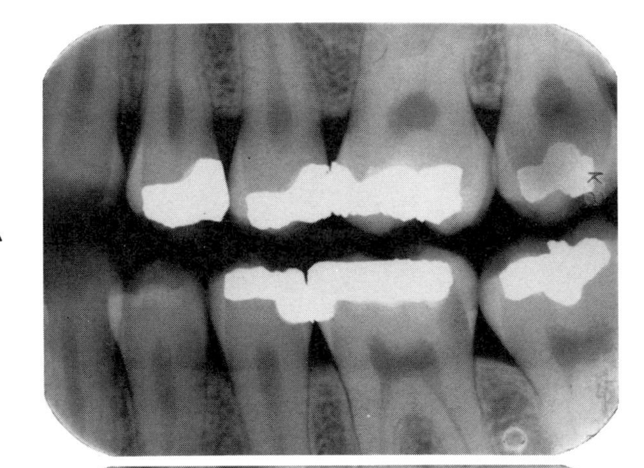

B

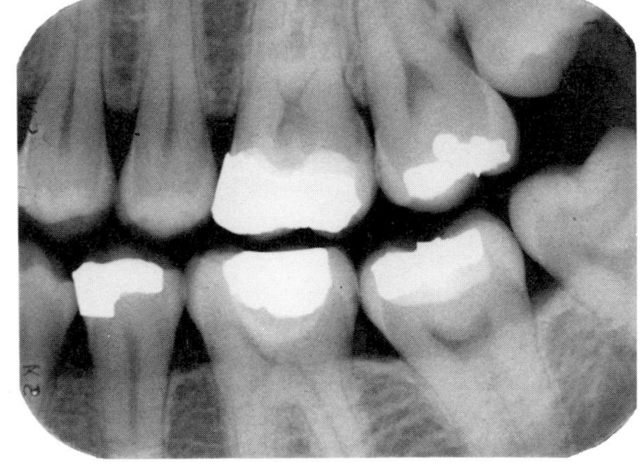

Figure 7–6. A, Bicuspid bitewing radiograph. B, Molar bitewing radiograph.

open and close the mouth unless instructed not to open the mouth.

With the film in position the x-ray beam is directed with a vertical angle of plus 8 degrees, or the central ray is directed slightly downward to the occlusal plane (Figure 7–4A). The horizontal angle is obtained by directing the central ray between the bicuspids or by placing the horizontal edge of the cone parallel to the buccal surfaces of the bicuspids (Figure 7–4B). Figure 7–5 shows patient and x-ray tube positions for bitewing radiography using a film holder with a cone positioning ring. Examples of bicuspid and molar bitewing radiographs are shown in Figure 7–6.

The molar bitewing is positioned similar to the bicuspid film but with the posterior border slightly distal to the third molar. The vertical angulation of the x-ray beam is the same as for the bicuspids and the central ray is directed between the molars. When the film can extend from the cuspid to the last molar, only one bitewing radiograph is usually needed on each side of the patient.

Patients with missing teeth can present a problem for proper closure of teeth on the bitewing film tab resulting in the film being malpositioned. The crowns of missing teeth can be replaced with cotton rolls or the patient's denture, if the patient has a denture made without metal materials (Figure 7–7A). If a bitewing loop is used and some properly occluding teeth are in the area, the loop can be moved along the film until it is in the area of the opposing teeth and these teeth can be used to hold the tab and film in the correct position (Figure 7–7B).

An anterior bitewing is used by some dentists. The technic is the same as for posterior teeth; however, a smaller film is usually used and the long dimension is placed vertically (Figure 7–8).

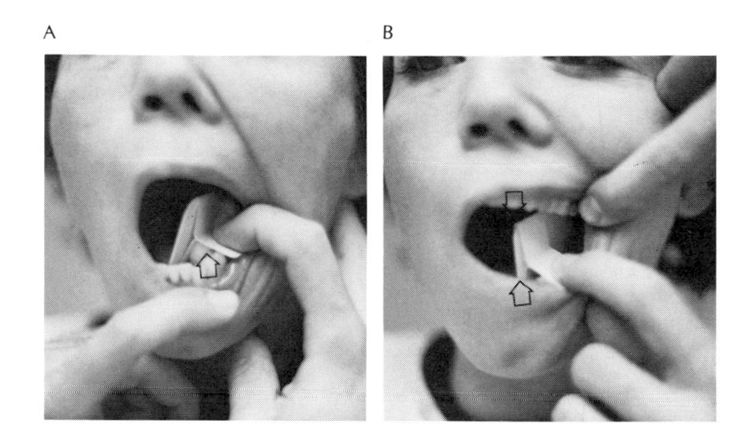

Figure 7–7. A, Missing mandibular molar teeth replaced by cotton roll to support molar bitewing film. B, Bitewing loop moved forward on film to position tab between existing upper and lower bicuspid teeth for molar bitewing radiograph.

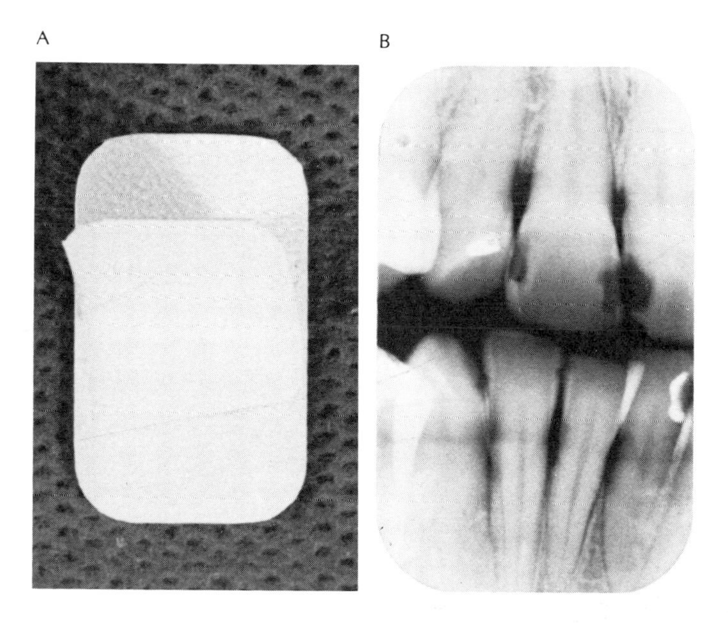

Figure 7–8. A, Anterior bitewing film with attached tab. B, Anterior bitewing radiograph.

Chapter 8

Comparing Technics and Evaluating Technical Errors

Two intraoral radiographic technics have been described in Chapters 5 and 6. It is useful for clinicians to understand the basic advantages and disadvantages of the two technics that are relevant to clinical problems. This chapter presents some important differences between the bisecting-angle and paralleling technics, and the four most common film exposure technical errors: incorrect vertical angulation, incorrect horizontal angulation, cone-cutting, and curved films. Other less common technical errors and artifacts are shown in Chapter 3 which discusses the quality of radiographs.

The paralleling technic conforms more closely to the principles of shadow casting described in Chapter 3. When the technic is used, teeth images more closely resemble the teeth that form them.

The paralleling technic positions the film parallel to the long axes of the teeth and thus produces images that have minimal distortion and are more representative of the teeth. The technic uses less vertical angulation than the bisecting-angle technic and thus similar buccal and lingual parts of teeth appear close to each other in the radiograph (Figure 8–1). When less vertical angulation is used, more tooth area underneath restorations is revealed. When good paralleling technic radiographs are available, bitewing views are seldom needed. Less vertical angulation in the maxillary molar region is desirable to avoid superimposing the shadow of the zygomatic arch on the teeth (Figure 8–2). Teeth apices and the maxillary sinus are better visualized with the paralleling technic.

The short cone is preferred by many dentists because it is easier to maneuver in a small room and in situations where the x-ray tubehead is close to obstructions such as the dental chair and unit. Only the bisecting-angle technic can be used with a short cone.

The paralleling technic must be used with the long cone to counteract the loss of image sharpness produced when the film is moved away from the crowns of the teeth. Compared to the bisecting-angle technic using the short cone, the paralleling long-cone technic has similar image sharpness in the crown areas of the teeth and improved sharpness in the apical areas. The apical sharpness is improved because the apex-to-film distance is similar in both technics and the increased tube-object distance in the paralleling technic improves image sharpness. When the bisecting-angle and paralleling technics both utilize the long cone, the bisecting-angle technic produces sharper images because most of the film is closer to the teeth.

The lengths of teeth can be more easily measured with the paralleling technic. When the film is positioned parallel to a tooth's long axis, variation in vertical angulation does not appreciably change the radiographic length of the tooth (Figure 5–5). In the bisecting-angle technic, when the x-ray beam is not perpendicular to the bisector, overangulation produces a radiographic tooth image that is shorter than the tooth; underangulation produces a longer radiographic image (Figure 8–3). These technical errors are called *foreshortening* and *elongation*.

The technical error of incorrect horizontal angulation produces the same result in the bisecting, paralleling, or bitewing technics. The radiograph shows superimposition or overlapping of the proximal images of adjacent teeth (Figure 8–4).

The paralleling technic cannot be effectively used when the film cannot be placed parallel to the long axis of the tooth and also high enough in the maxilla or low enough in the mandible to receive the image of the tooth apex; for example, in children who have adult size permanent teeth located in underdeveloped jaws and many teeth apices above the palate or below the floor of the mouth (Figure 8–5).

In rare cases when the teeth are longer than the film, only the bisecting technic can produce an image of the entire tooth on the film. This is accomplished by overangulating the vertical direction of the x-ray beam and deliberately foreshortening the tooth's image to a length shorter than the film's vertical dimension. The bisecting-the-angle technic can be accomplished without size ANSI 1.1 film, without a film holding device, and without a long cone.

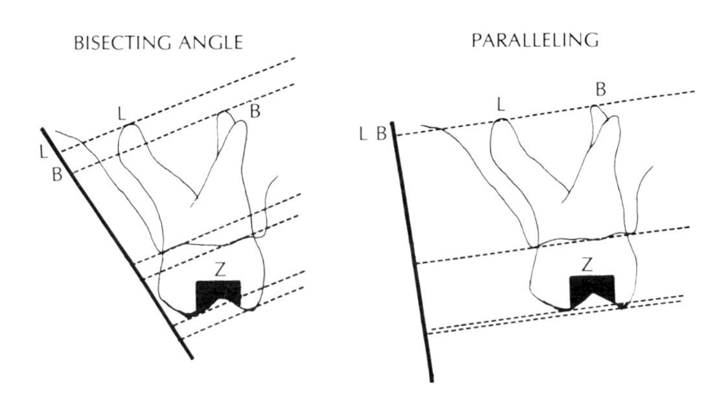

Figure 8–1. Diagrams showing vertical angulations of bisecting-angle and paralleling technics placing buccal and lingual tooth parts at different levels on radiograph. Less vertical angulation shows more of area underneath dental restorations (Z).

A

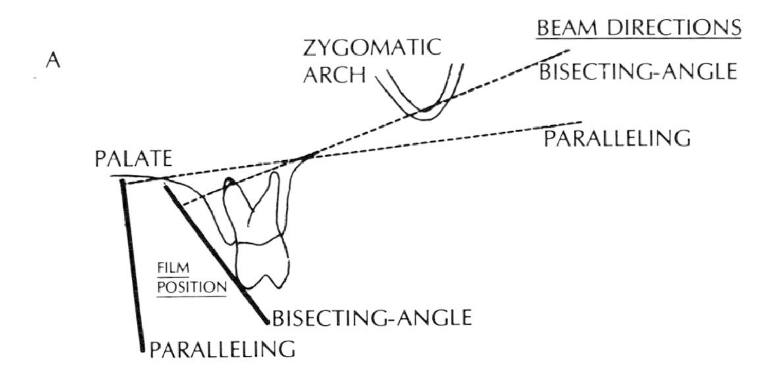

B

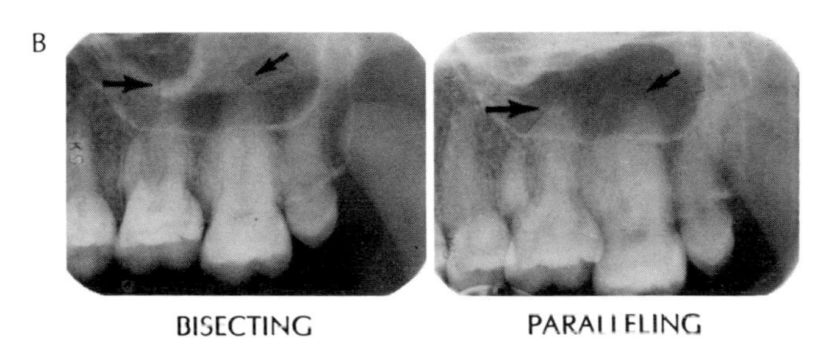

Figure 8–2. A, Vertical x-ray beam directions and film positions in bisecting-angle and paralleling technics for maxillary molar region. B, Radiographs made with two technics.

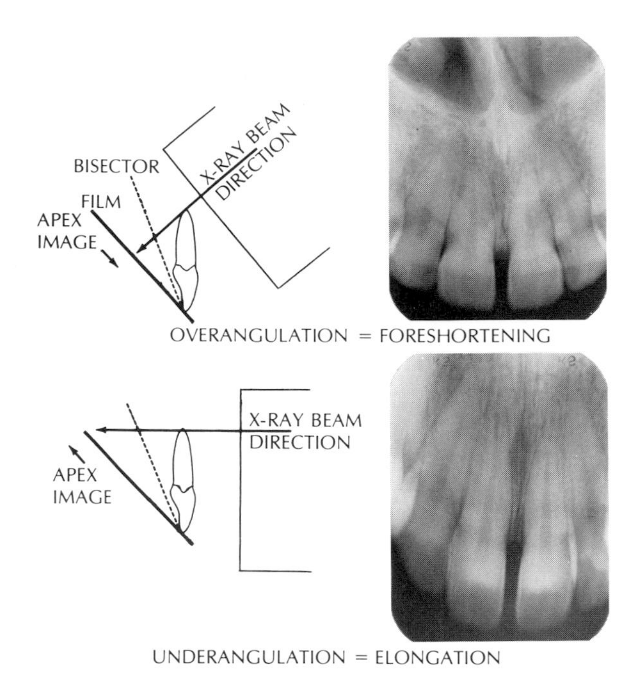

Figure 8–3. Effect of over and under vertical angulation in bisecting-the-angle technic.

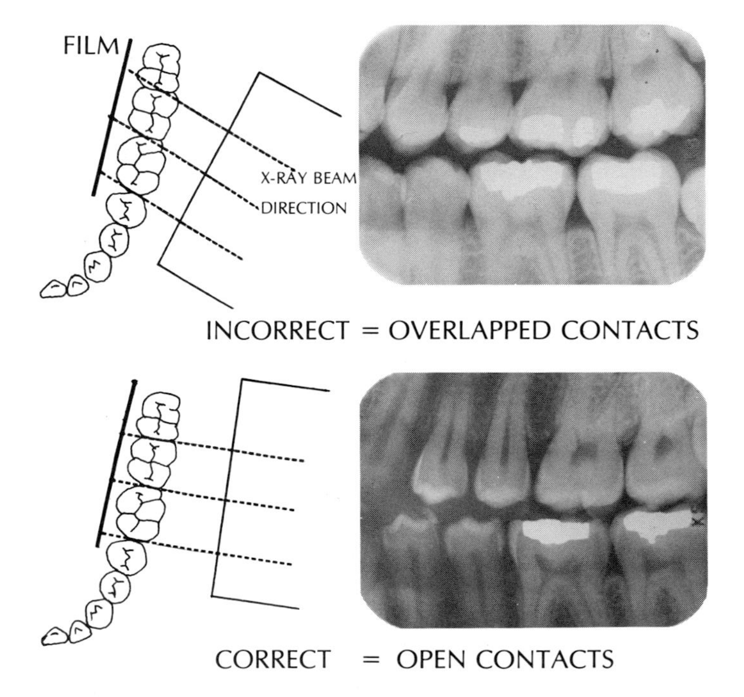

Figure 8–4. Incorrect and correct horizontal angulations and resultant radiographs.

Occasionally a patient cannot keep perfectly still and a very short exposure time is needed. In such cases a short tube-film distance is indicated and this necessitates the use of the bisecting-the-angle technic.

Cone-cut is the term commonly used to describe a radiograph made with the beam of x rays not completely covering the film (Figure 8–6). Cone-cutting often occurs when the operator aims the x-ray beam toward the occlusal plane or incisal edges of the teeth instead of toward the center of the tooth. The operator must remember that the x rays are traveling downward in the maxilla (upward in the mandible) as they move away from the end of the cone and thus the end of the cone will not be located at the same horizontal level as the teeth.

A common area of cone-cutting is the anterior border of posterior radiographs Figure 8–7). In this example, the cone is positioned too far posteriorly. To correct this error the operator must remember that the third molar teeth are no farther distally than a point just posterior to the corner of the eye (see Figure 4–3) and that the posterior border of the open-end cone must not be near the external opening of the ear; in other words, there are no teeth near the ear opening.

Curved film is another common technical error. The images on the resultant radiograph are unequally magnified, distorted, or streaked (Figure 8–8). The operator must see that the film is not bent. When there is no film holder note that the patient uses the palmar surface of the finger or thumb to press the film against the teeth, that the finger is placed opposite the lingual surface of the teeth, and that excessive pressure is not applied to curve the film to the shape of the inner surface of the mandible or palate.

When a radiograph is made it is evaluated for its quality before it is used. Basic criteria for a good quality radiograph include a density acceptable for viewing on a viewbox; contrast capable of showing changes in enamel, dentin and bone; film extending at least 1 mm beyond the apices of teeth being examined; undistorted teeth images; demonstration of the proximal surfaces of the teeth being examined; the absence of a cone cut; no fog present and no artifacts. Aside from the multitude of errors that can occur when handling sensitive film emulsions, the

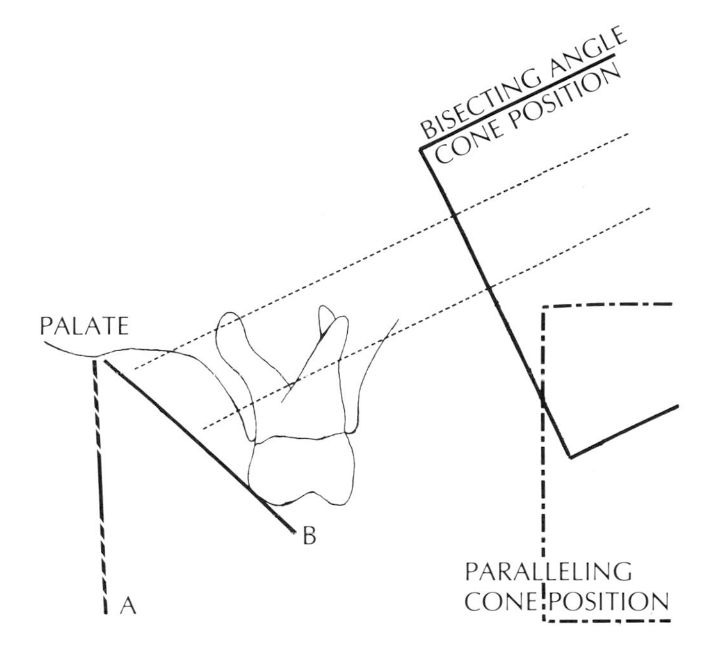

Figure 8–5. Shallow palate vault. Film in paralleling position (A) cannot achieve sufficient height. Bisecting-angle technic (B) can provide satisfactory radiographic image.

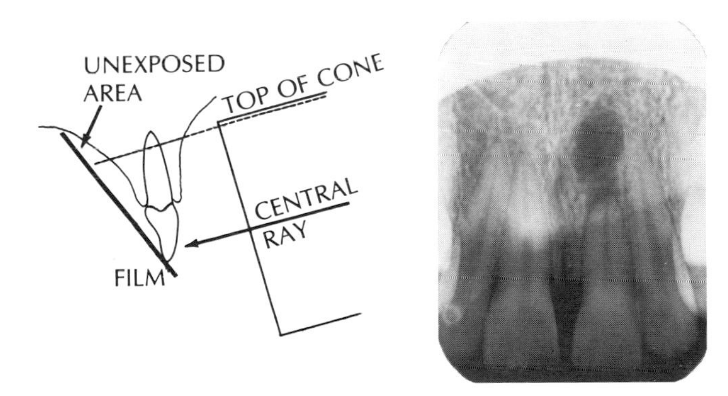

Figure 8–6. Cone-cutting of upper part of maxillary anterior radiograph due to central ray being directed to incisal edge of tooth instead of center of tooth.

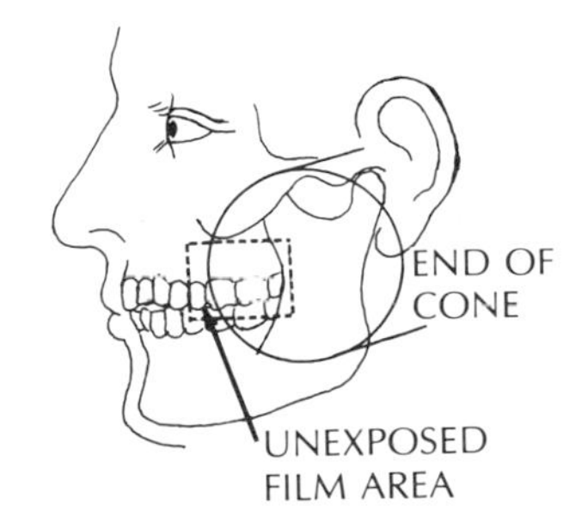

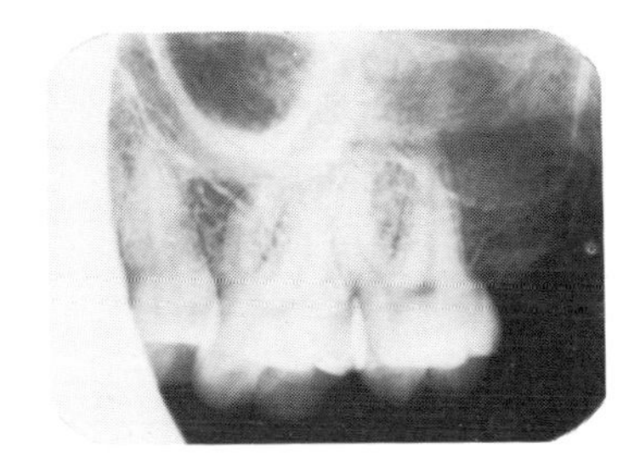

Figure 8–7. Cone-cutting of mesial portion of maxillary molar radiograph.

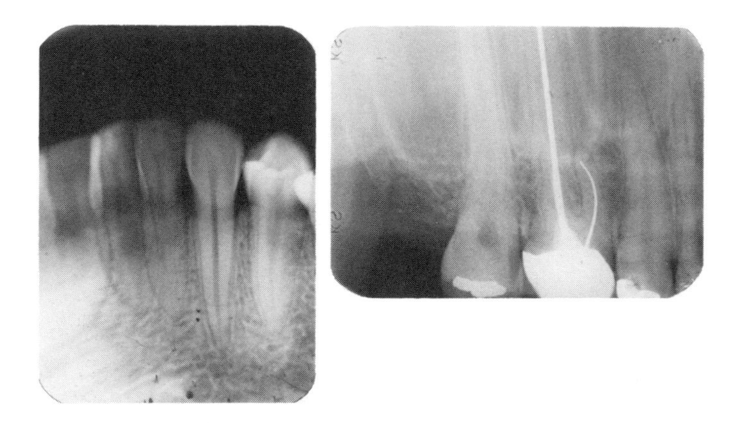

Figure 8–8. Streaked and distorted teeth images caused by curved films.

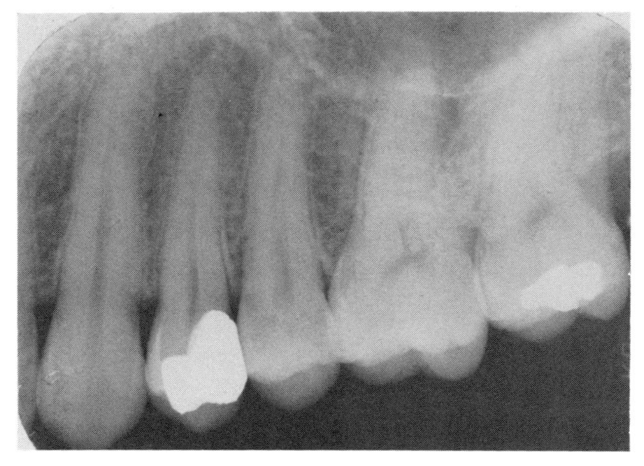

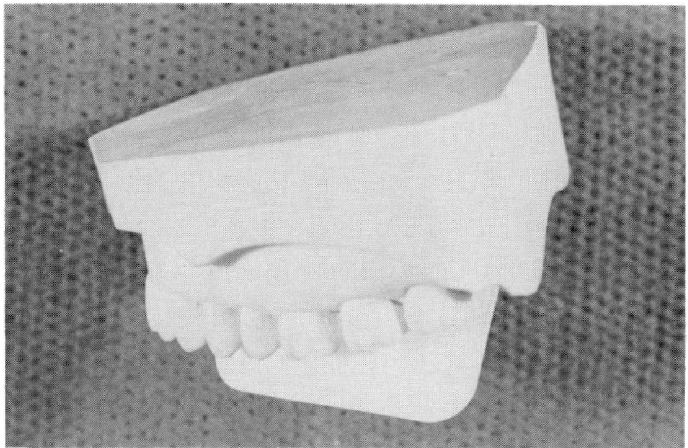

Figure 8–9. Observation of the position of the cusps of teeth on the film (above) indicates that the film packet was placed in the patient's mouth as indicated on the model (below).

greatest need is to identify the cause of film exposure technic errors. The following is presented to assist in this evaluation.

The student radiographer often has difficulty in identifying the specific cause of an exposure technic error observed in a radiograph. There is a tendency to confuse one error with different technic factors. When the bisecting-the-angle technic is used, a simple step-by-step analysis is useful in identifying specific causes of common exposure technic errors. There are four steps that begin in the form of questions:

(1) Was the film position correct? The answer is obtained by observing the position of the incisal edges or teeth cusps on the radiograph (Figure 8–9). Note that when the objects touch the film their images cannot be moved from that position by changes in beam angulation. Thus the position of the tooth cusps on the film indicates where the film was placed in the patient's mouth.

(2) Was the cone position correct? The answer is obtained by observing if there is a cone-cut error in the radiograph. The actual position of the end of the cone that locates the beam position can be observed from the position and curve of the cone-cut (Figures 8–6 and 8–7).

(3) Was the horizontal angulation correct? The answer is obtained by observing the overlapped and non-overlapped proximal teeth surfaces in the radiograph (Figure 8–10). In this case, if the radiograph was made to examine the cuspid tooth, the horizontal angle was correct. If the radiograph was made to examine the bicuspid teeth, the horizontal angle is incorrect and it is known that the x-ray tubehead must be placed more distally to be in the correct position since the beam is directed between the cuspid and first bicuspid teeth instead of between the bicuspid teeth. Note that in severe cases of malocclusion non-overlapped proximal surfaces are not to be expected in radiographs.

(4) Was the vertical angulation correct? The answer is obtained by observing the lengths of the teeth images. If the teeth images are longer than normal the x-ray beam was under-angulated (Figure 8–3) and the vertical angle must be increased to shorten the images. If the teeth images are shorter than normal, the x-ray beam was overangulated and the vertical angle must be de-

creased to lengthen the images. Note that a curved or bent film may simulate elongation but the image will have a great amount of uneven distortion (Figure 8–8).

Basic technic evaluation is useful for the beginning student. A structured evaluation of the quality of the radiograph is obtained when criteria for evaluation are presented. In addition, a formal analysis of film exposure technic is beneficial to a student radiographer as it enables the student to perform a self analysis of film exposure technic.

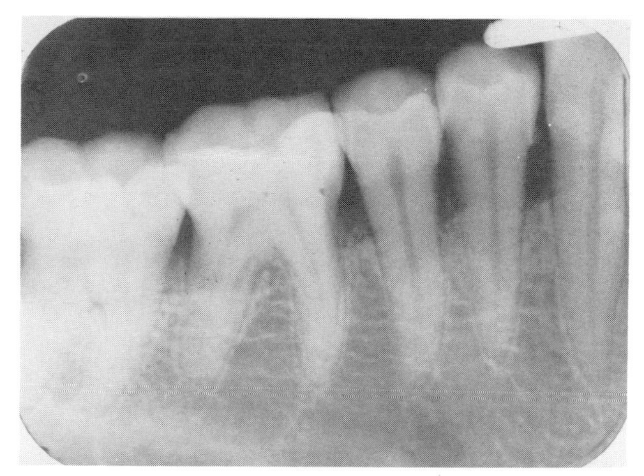

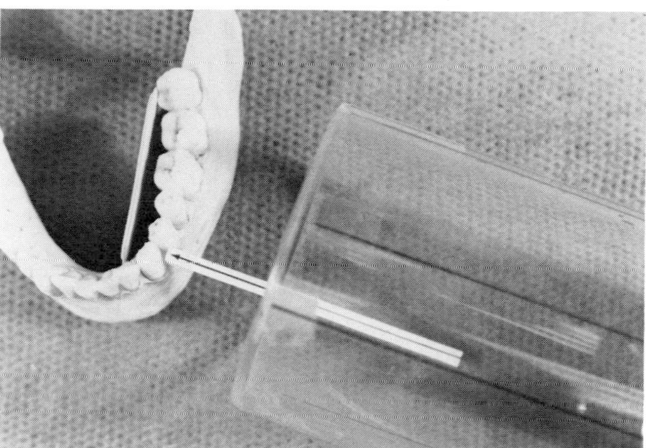

Figure 8–10. The radiograph shows separate adjacent proximal surfaces of the cuspid and first bicuspid teeth, with overlapped bicuspid and molar images. This information indicates that the x-ray beam was directed between the cuspid and first bicuspid teeth as indicated in the photograph.

Chapter 9

Film Holders

Film can be held in position during intraoral radiography by the patient's finger or by a film-holding device. The bisecting-angle technic can be accomplished with any method. The paralleling technic requires a film-holding device. When a film holder is used, the patient's hand is kept out of the primary x-ray beam. In addition, the film is easily kept flat and not curved. The ideal film holder is one that is simple, light in weight, usable on all types of patients, and sterilizable in an autoclave or disposable. Unfortunately, no single instrument has all these properties.

A great variety of film holders are commercially available; some are simple, others are complex. Some are light in weight, others relatively heavy. Some holders can be autoclaved, some need chemical sterilization, and some are of a disposable type. The dental radiographer should be able to assess the value of a film holder in order to select the device that best meets the needs of the patients being examined, the technical ability of the operator, and the sterilization requirements of the dental office or clinic. In the main, film holders made of plastic cannot be autoclaved and other nonmetallic holders or parts of holders may not withstand repeated autoclave sterilization. Information in this chapter is of great importance when the radiographer is an auxiliary person. Because dental offices do not have all types of holders or the same type of film holder, an auxiliary may be called upon to function with different film-holding devices.

A film holder is more practical or adaptable to more situations if it is disposable or can be autoclaved, can be held by the patient's teeth instead of the patient's hands, can be held by teeth not being radiographed, can place the film in any position in all parts of the dentition, holds the film firm without slipping, is not bulky and allows maximum closure of the patient's mouth to lower the floor of the mouth, is lightweight and needs little biting force, can be used with rubber

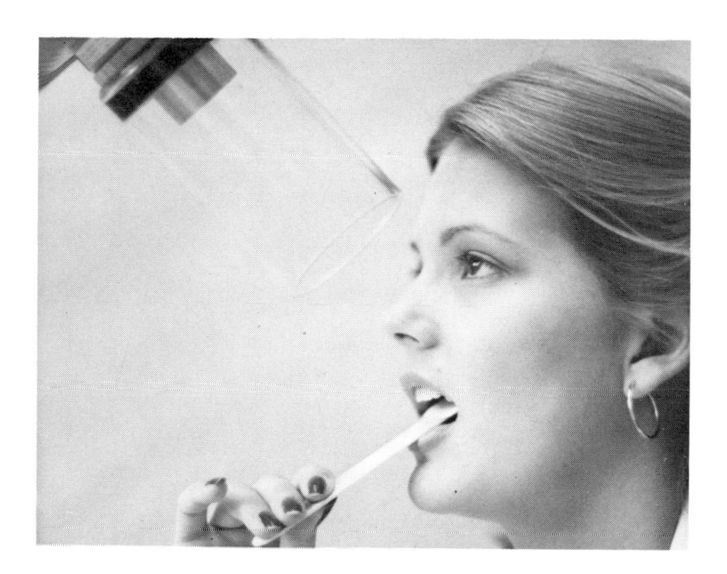

Figure 9–1. Use of blade-type film holder.

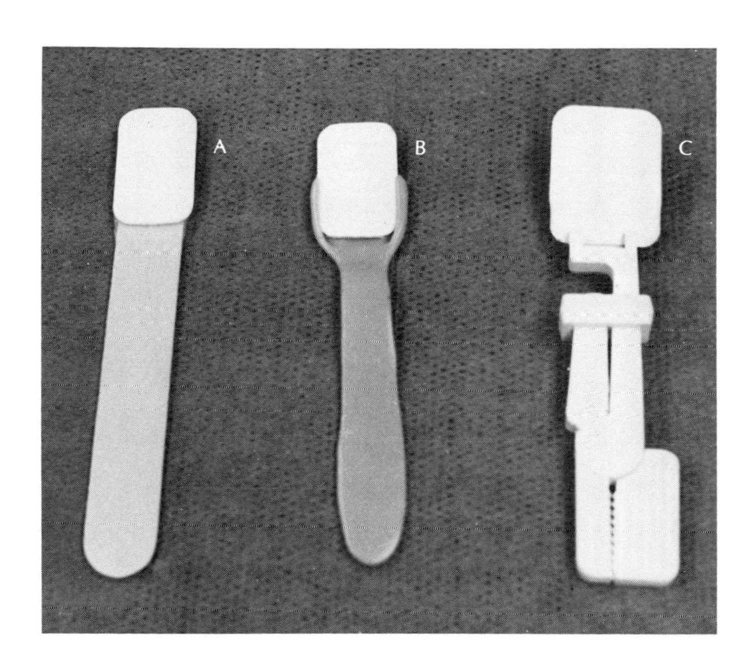

Figure 9–2. Examples of blade-type film holders. A, Disposable throat stick with film attached by cellophane tape. B, Acrylic blade with film inserted in a slot. C, Plastic Snap-A-Ray® film holder.

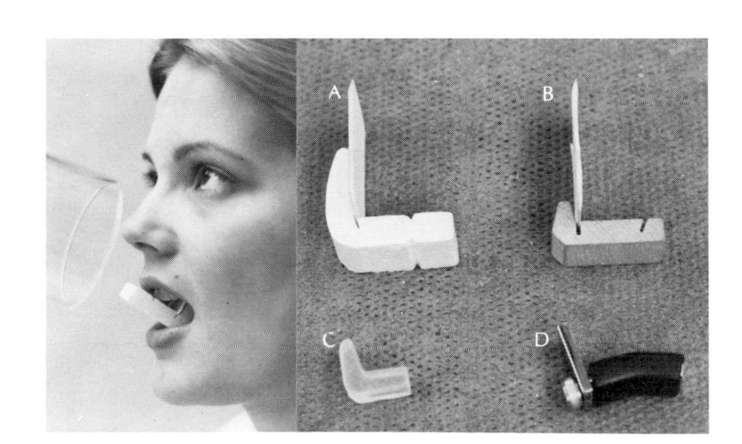

Figure 9–3. Patient using bite block and examples of bite blocks. A, Disposable Styrofoam block. B, Wood block. C, Plastic block. D, Sterilizable metal and rubber block with tightening screw to hold the film.

dams and clamps in the patient's mouth, and assists in x-ray beam positioning.

BLADE-TYPE HOLDERS

The film attached to a blade-like holder is useful in radiography of the maxillary anterior teeth. The film can be positioned in either the bisecting or paralleling positions with the blade held between thumb and forefinger by the patient and resting on the mandibular incisors (Figure 9–1). Some blade-type film holders are shown in Figure 9–2. Of great advantage is the fact that the operator can place the film in position without placing his hands in the patient's mouth. This minimizes any trauma of the oral tissues during radiography.

BITE BLOCKS

Bite blocks are the most common type of film holder. These devices can be used in any area of the mouth with the film in the bisecting-angle or paralleling positions. The film is held in position in a slot in the block. The patient holds the block in position by biting on the horizontal portion of the bite block. Figure 9–3 shows a bite block in use and blocks manufactured from different materials.

The great advantage of a bite block is the nonuse of the patient's hands. When the patient does not have the use of his hands or the hands cannot be kept steady, the bite block system is invaluable. However, this same advantage can be a disadvantage when there are no opposing teeth or the opposing teeth or the tooth being examined cannot be used in biting the block. For example, a tooth with an endodontic file in place cannot be examined with a simple bite block.

Modified bite blocks can avoid the problem of biting on the teeth being radiographed (Figure 9–4). The film holder is held in position by teeth that are not being radiographed. Additional stability, when required, can be obtained by having the patient hold the part of the film holder that extends out of the mouth.

The hemostat plus bite block is a versatile instrument because the film position can be adjusted at three different points. This flexibility permits the operator to place the film

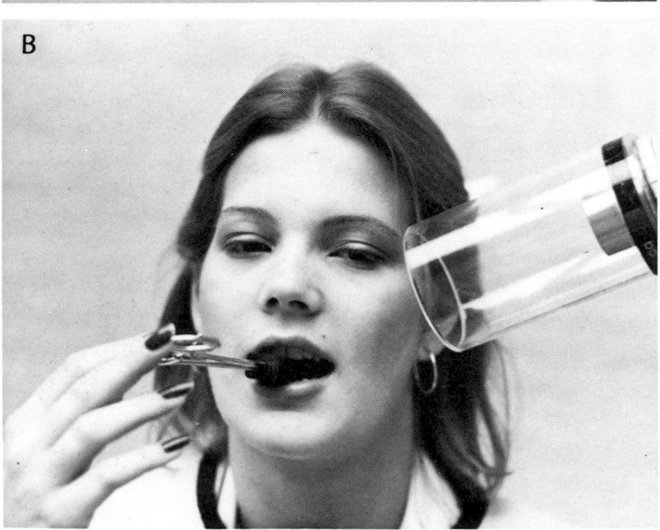

Figure 9–4. Modified bite blocks. Block is held between teeth that are not being radiographed. A, Prokem® rubber block with notch at incisal region of tooth being examined. B, Hemostat-rubber block holder.

in any position. Figure 9–5 shows the three points of adjusting the film's position and one end of the plastic Snap-A-Ray® film holder that is used in a similar but less versatile manner. The use of the hemostat and bite block is shown in Figure 9–6.

BEAM ALIGNING HOLDERS

Film holders sometimes have extensions used for directing the x-ray beam. The extensions, like the cone on the x-ray machine, are basically x-ray beam position indicating devices or PIDs. An aligning type of film holder may consist of a bite block with a rod extending out of the patient's mouth (Figure 9–7). The rod is positioned close to the side of the cone. In addition to the rod, a loop may be added to enable the operator to use the end of the cone instead of the side of the cone to locate the x-ray beam position (Figure 9–8). All beam aligning holders position the x-ray beam over the film and thus cone cutting is avoided whenever these devices are properly used.

Beam aligning holders are designed to establish a fixed angle (bisecting or paralleling) of the central ray to the film. These devices will thus produce the best possible x-ray beam to teeth relationship only when (1) the patient's teeth are in the ideal positions and (2) the film can be placed perfectly parallel to the long axes of the teeth when the paralleling technic aligning holder is used or the same ideal angle exists between film and teeth when the bisecting-angle holder is used. An illustration of the effect of having to use a less than ideal film position in the horizontal plane because of a lingual torus is shown in Figure 9–9. Part A of the figure shows the idealized situation in a patient without problems; part B shows the film not parallel to the buccal surfaces of the teeth in the horizontal plane. The result will be superimposition of the images of the proximal surfaces of adjacent teeth.

In dental diagnostic radiography it is important to see the contact areas of teeth; thus the x-ray beam should still be directed between teeth when films cannot be placed in the ideal location. A slightly distorted image is always preferable to an image that does not show the desired part of the object.

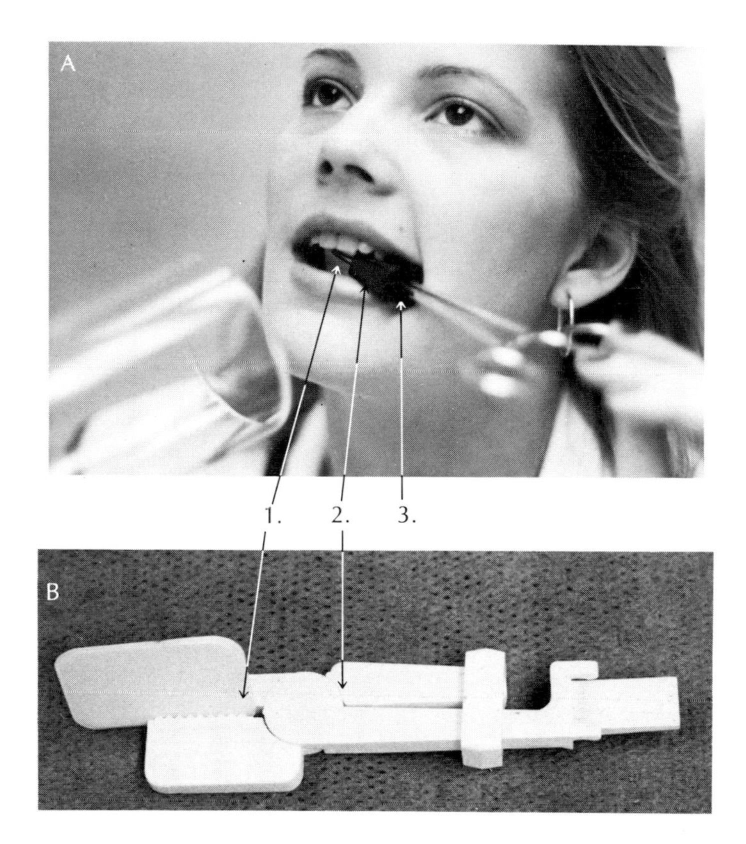

Figure 9–5. Hemostat-type bite block and adjusting points: (1) where film is positioned between beaks of hemostat, (2) where block contacts teeth, and (3) where hemostat passes through rubber block. A, Hemostat and rubber block. B, Snap-A-Ray® holder.

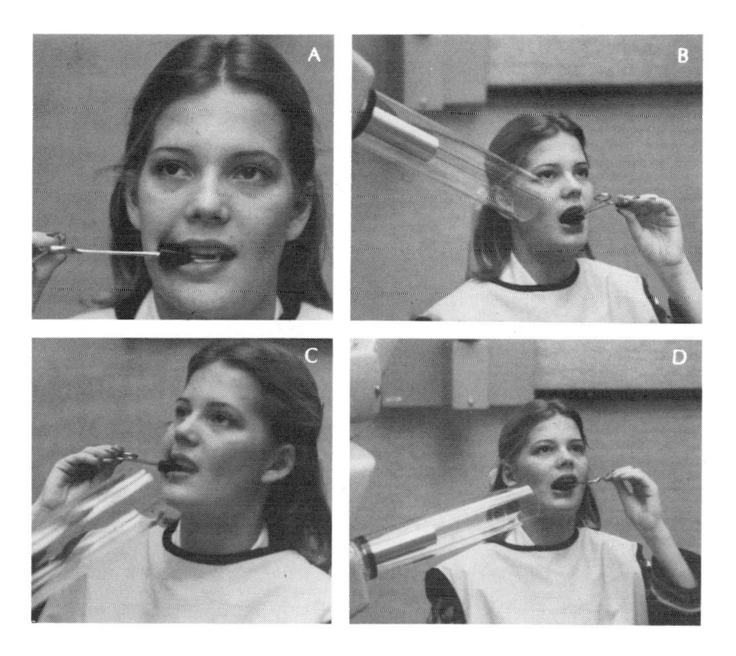

Figure 9–6. Intraoral radiography using hemostat plus bite block. A, Maxillary anteriors; B, Maxillary posteriors; C, Mandibular anteriors; D, Mandibular posteriors.

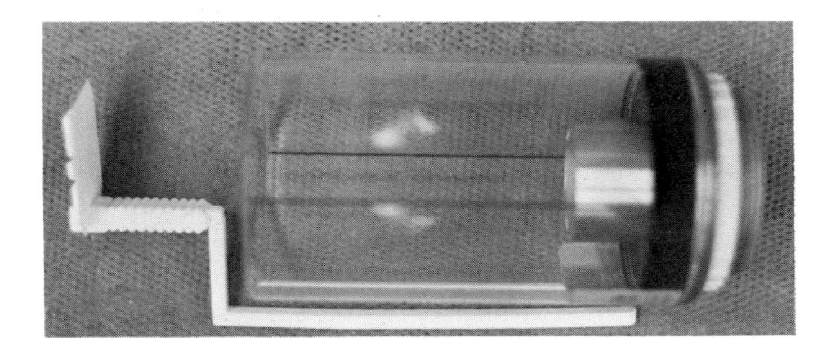

Figure 9–7. Bite block with beam aligning rod used with open-end cone. Rod is aligned with side of cone.

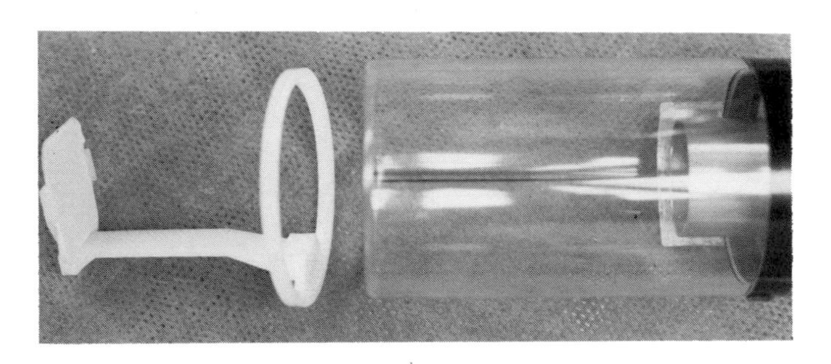

Figure 9–8. Margraf® beam aligning type of film holder using loop to position end of cone relative to film.

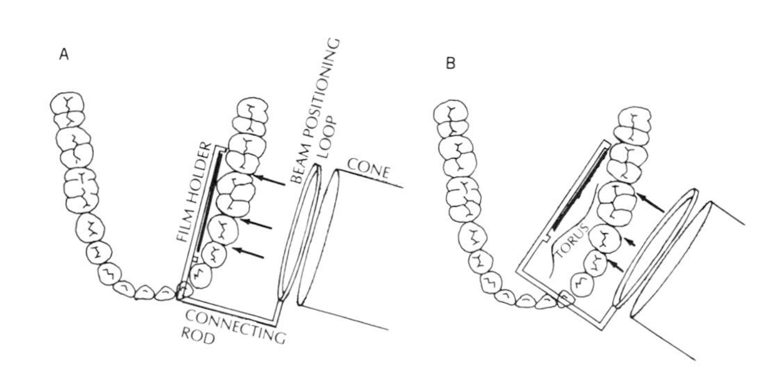

Figure 9–9. Beam aligning type of film holder. A, X-ray beam directed between teeth when film is in correct position. B, X-ray beam with incorrect horizontal angulation when lingual torus prevents film from being placed parallel to teeth in horizontal plane.

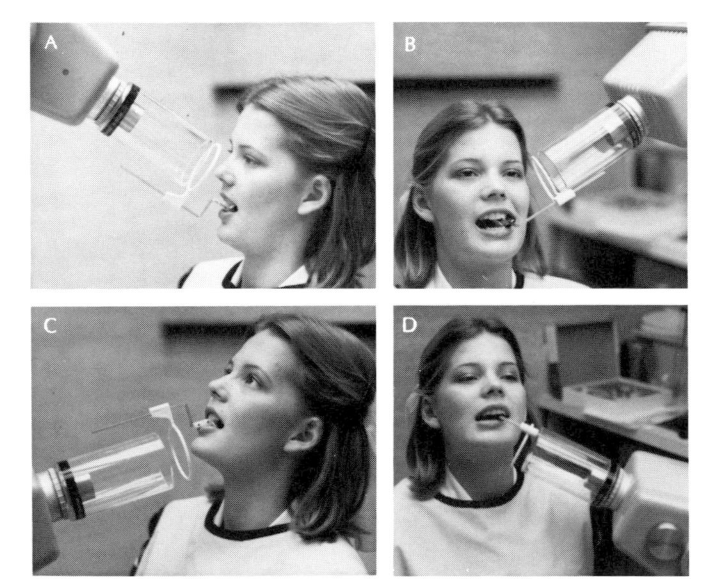

Figure 9–10. Intraoral radiography using the Rinn XCP® position indicating device. A, Upper anteriors; B, Upper posteriors; C, Lower anteriors; D, Lower posteriors.

Operators using a beam aligning type of film holder must keep in mind that the device positions the x-ray beam in an idealized relationship to the film (not the teeth) and that the device may not give the best relationship of the x-ray beam to the teeth after the film is placed in the patient's mouth. Slight deviations in the angles indicated by an aligning type of film holder may be desirable. The use of the Rinn XCP instrument is shown in Figure 9–10.

One beam aligning type of film holder incorporates a beam collimator (Figure 9–11). The beam locating loop is made of a sheet of stainless steel with a hole in the center the shape and size of the film used. The steel sheet acts as a collimator or diaphragm and restricts the x-ray beam to a size slightly larger than the film. The collimating ability of this film holder removes from the primary beam most of the patient's tissue around the film that is irradiated by circular-shaped x-ray beams.

Beam aligning holders also are available for rectangular shaped x-ray beams (Figure 9–12). This type of film holder locates the rectangular end of the cone with a similar rectangular shaped loop. Rectangular collimators must be used with a beam aligning film holder or cone cutting will be a common radiographic technical error. The long dimension of the rectangular x-ray beam must be positioned vertically for anterior teeth and horizontally for posterior teeth. The collimator has a moveable joint at its base that permits a rotary movement of the cylindrical extension of the device which turns the rectangular-shaped beam. When this beam aligning film holder system is used, the operator must make this additional x-ray beam adjustment along with the horizontal and vertical angulations.

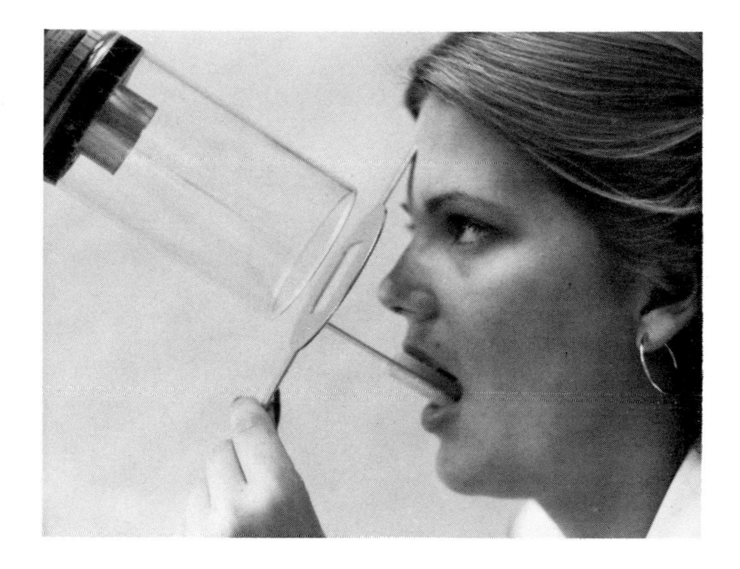

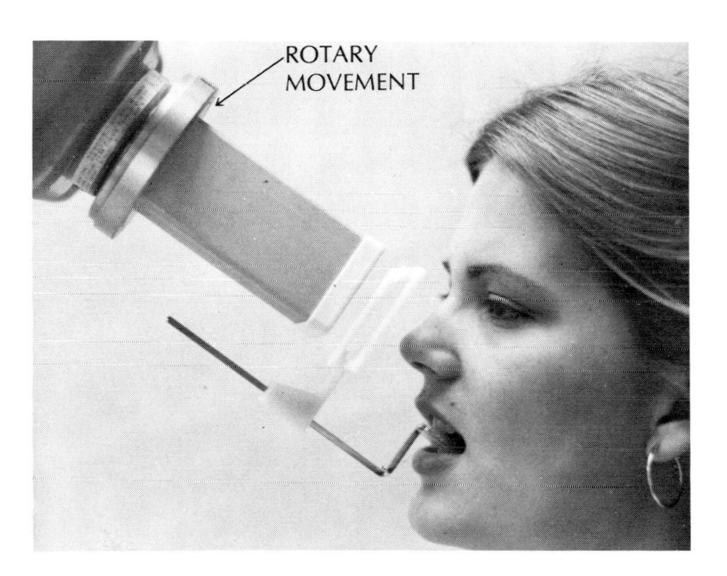

Figure 9–12. Rinn® film holder for rectangular collimated x-ray beams. Collimator on machine tubehead can be turned to position long dimension of x-ray beam in horizontal plane or vertical plane.

Chapter 10

Skull Anatomy

Radiographs show mainly the calcified tissues of the human head. In dentistry, knowledge of the shape and positions of the teeth and bones of the skull and face is important in recognizing and identifying the shadow images in dental radiographs. In addition, it is important to know the locations of calcified structures relative to recognizable external soft tissue structures of the head; this information helps the operator to best position a patient's head for the various intraoral and extraoral radiographic projections.

A detailed presentation of skull osteology is not possible in a book of this type devoted to radiographic fundamentals. Only the larger bone structures and important anatomic landmarks will be presented in this chapter. However, a more detailed description of the calcified structures of the teeth and osseous landmarks of the mandible and maxilla is useful for the dental radiographer; the details of the facial region will be presented in Chapter 11 where they are correlated with intraoral radiographic anatomy and film mounting.

The student radiographer should obtain an adult human skull when learning or reviewing skull osteology. The information presented in this chapter needs to be visualized in three dimensions, and a skull, or a good representative model, is useful for this purpose. Readers must remember that the illustrations relate to an adult human and that additional study of differences in skull size and form, due to growth and development, is needed if they are to achieve excellence in caring for all types of patients.

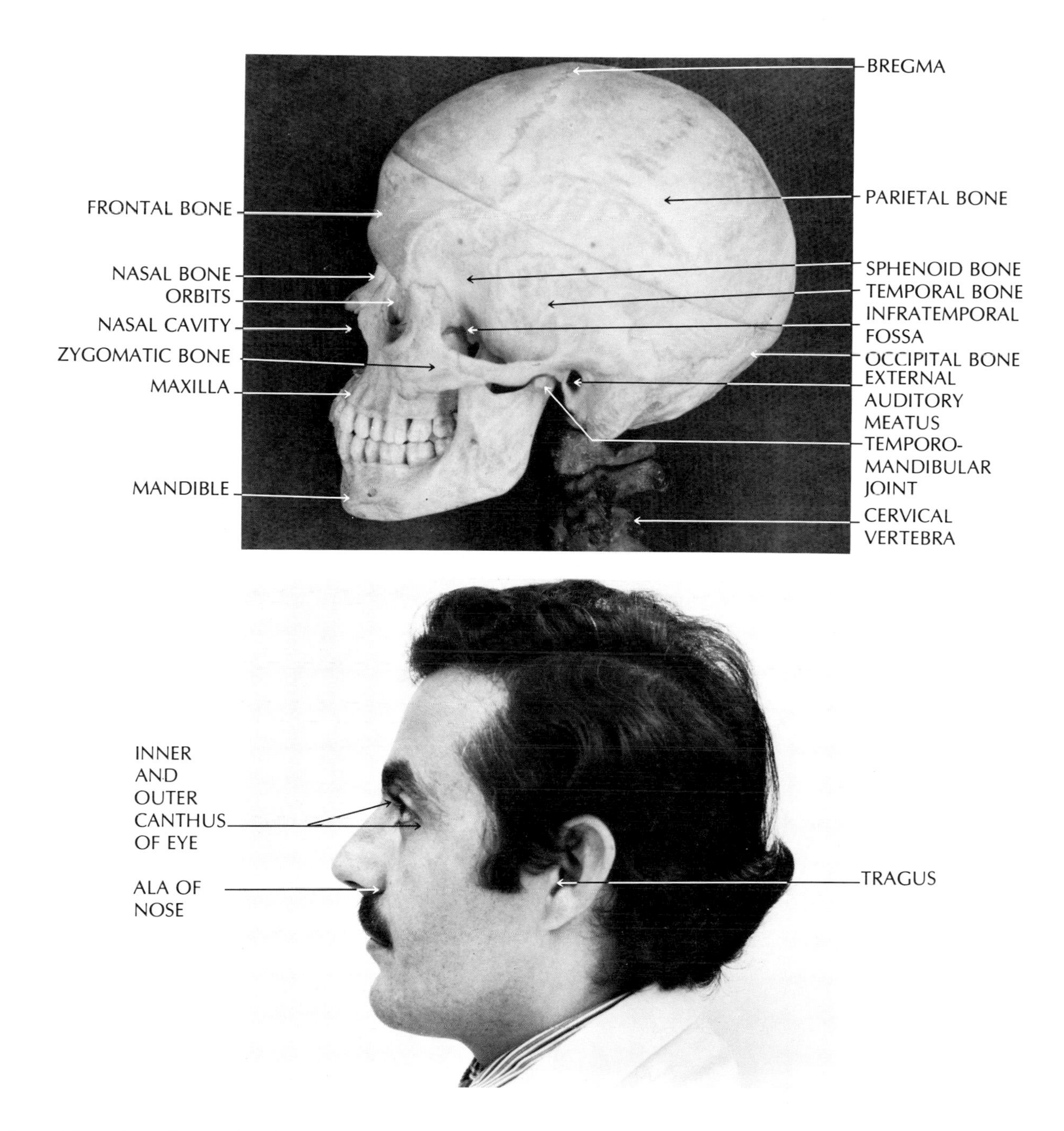

Figure 10–1. Lateral view of skull and patient's head.

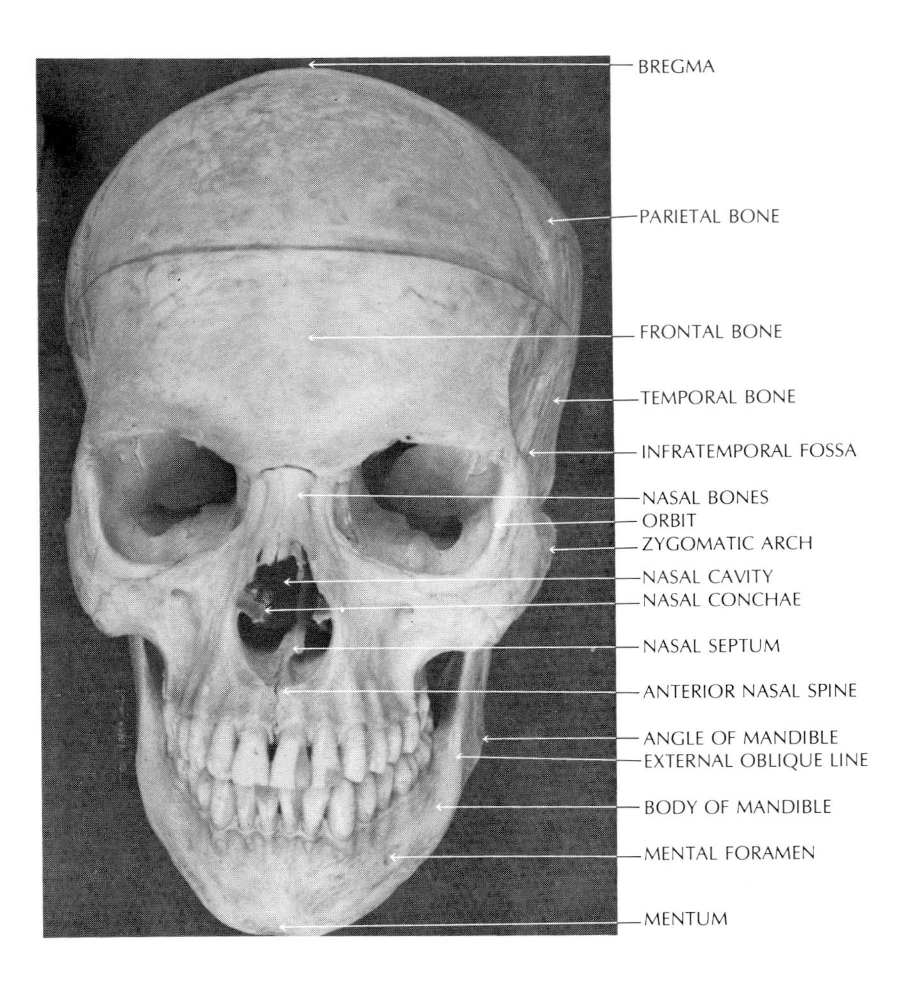

Figure 10–2. Frontal view of skull.

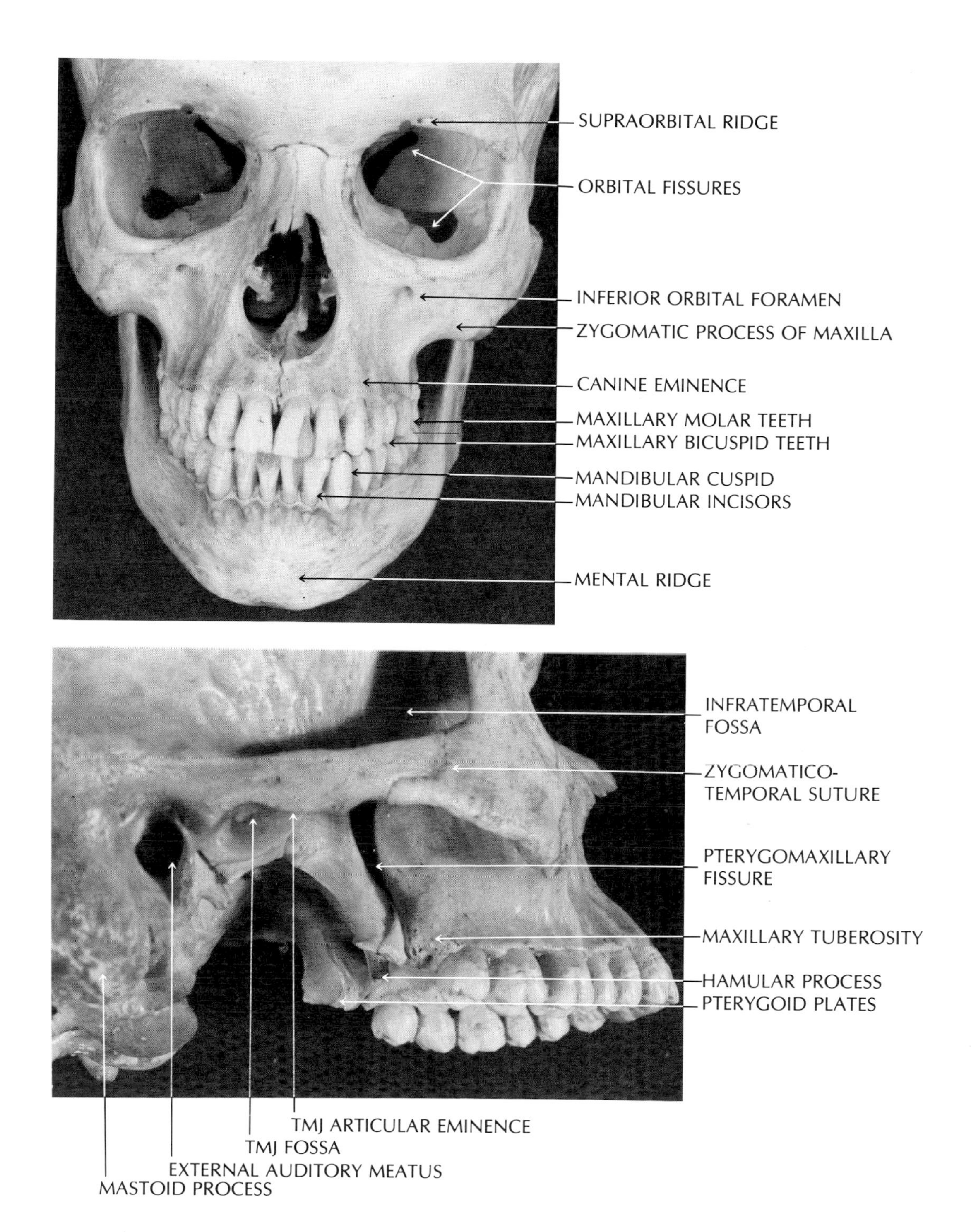

Figure 10–3. Frontal view of facial region and lateral view of maxillary area.

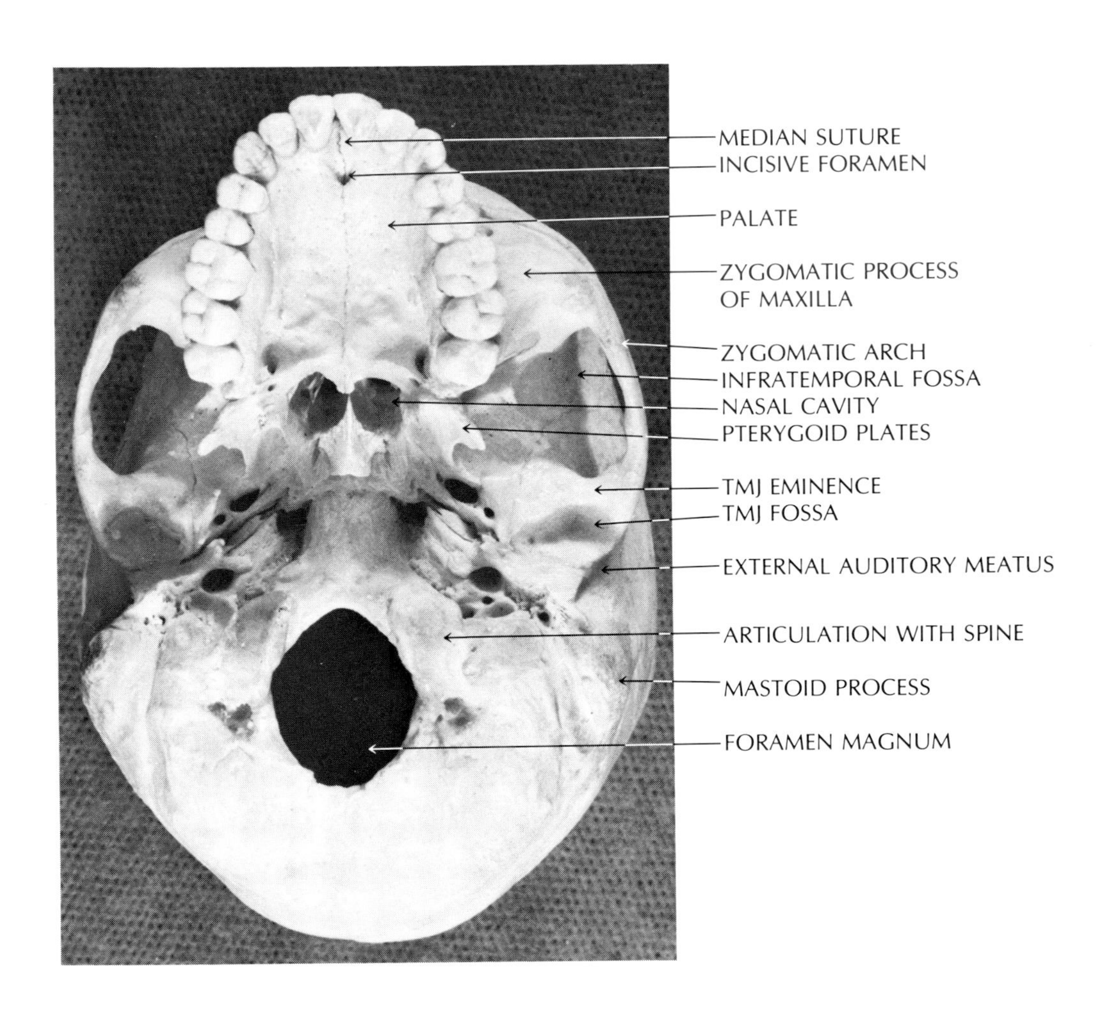

Figure 10–4. Inferior view of skull.

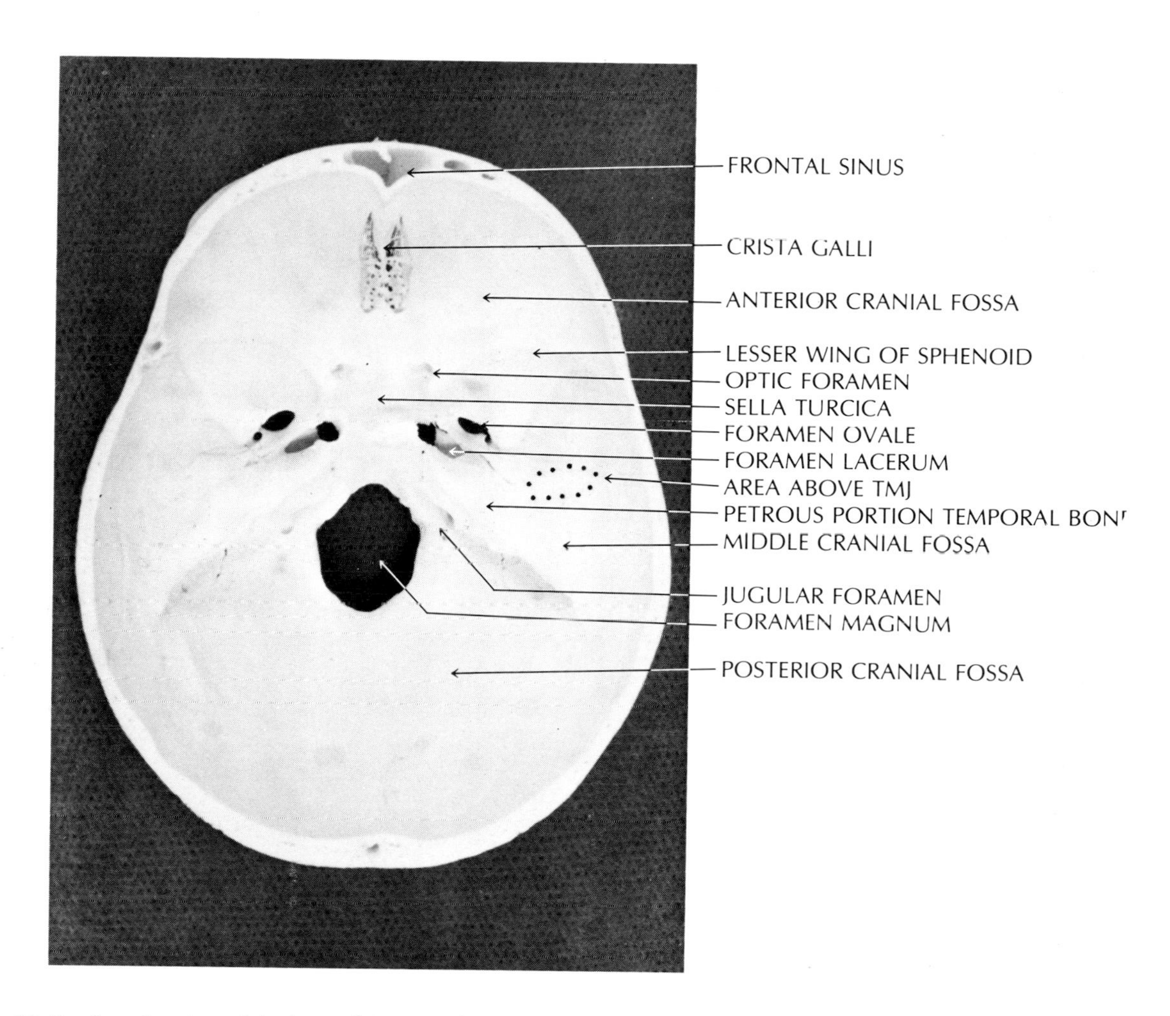

Figure 10–5. Superior view of the base of the cranial cavity. The base of the cavity is divided into three fossae separated by the lesser wing of the sphenoid bone and the crest of the petrous portion of the temporal bone. The orbits lie directly beneath the floor of the anterior cranial fossa.

Chapter 11

Intraoral Radiographic Anatomy and Film Mounting

Radiographic anatomy and film mounting are presented together because film mounting is basically the identification of the anatomic region seen in a radiograph. The subsequent inserting of the identified radiograph in its proper place in a film mount is a simple procedure. In this chapter the radiographic appearance of normal anatomic structures will be presented. In addition, the radiographic appearance of dental restorations and some dental materials will be shown because they are present in most patients and are often helpful in identifying individual radiographs of a complete mouth series for film mounting.

RADIOLUCENT AND RADIOPAQUE IMAGES

Recognition of radiographic images is based upon knowledge of the anatomy of the object, the projection of images by radiation, and the x-ray absorbing ability of the object. Figure 11–1 shows the radiography of two aluminum blocks, one steel ball, and one wax ball. A spherical or ball-shaped object always shows a relatively circular radiographic image; angular or box-shaped objects cast differently shaped shadows relative to their orientation in the x-ray beam.

Steel absorbs x rays more than aluminum, and aluminum more than plastic. Steel is thus a *radiopaque* material and plastic a *radiolucent* material. Radiopaque objects show low density images in a radiograph, whereas radiolucent objects are represented by blacker areas on the radiograph. The density or blackness of any spot on a radiograph results from the amount of x rays absorbed out of the x-ray beam. The amount of absorption is due both to the atomic density (basically weight) of the object material and the amount of the material. Figure 11–2 shows the varying radiographic densities in the images of aluminum tubes oriented differently in an x-ray beam. Note that darker spots on the

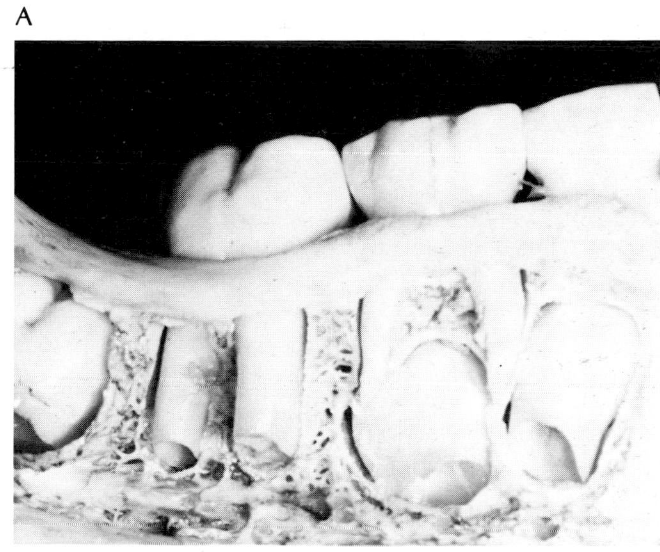

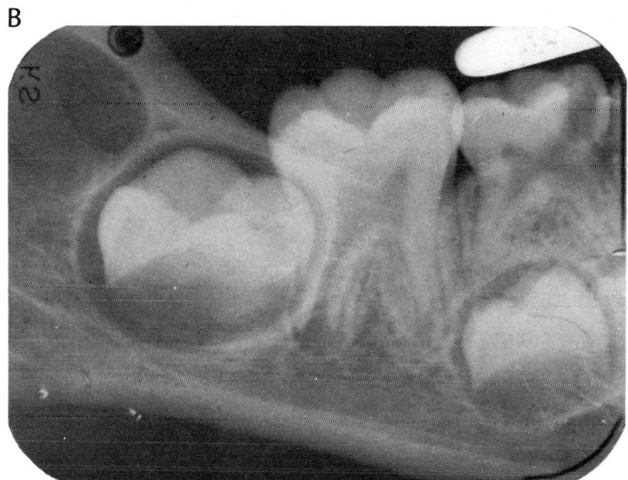

Figure 11–5. A, Photograph of mandibular buccal bone removed to show early stages of tooth development. B, Radiograph of developing second bicuspid and second permanent molar showing calcification of cusps, and of first permanent molar showing formation of root and pulp chamber. Radiolucent tooth follicle of third molar is also seen.

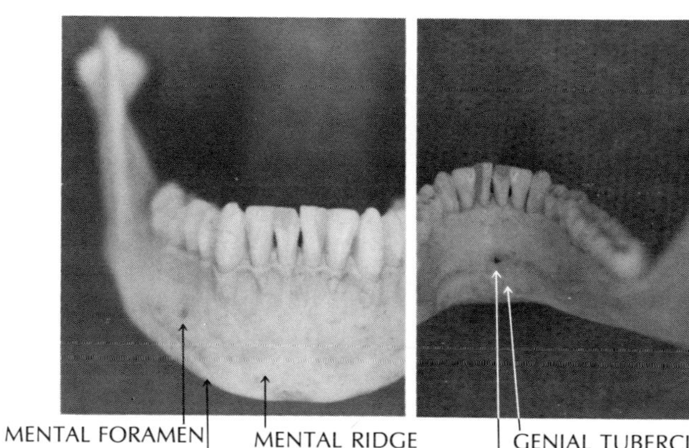

Figure 11–6. Photographs of labial (left) and lingual (right) surfaces of anterior region of mandible.

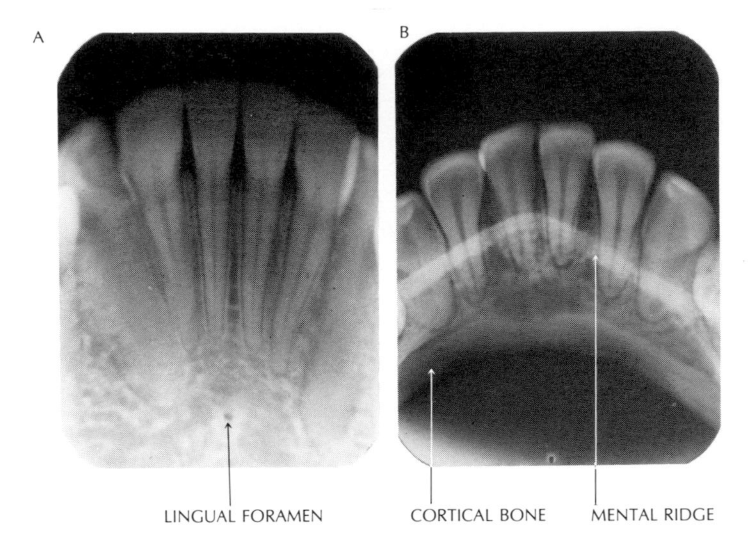

Figure 11–7. Mandibular incisor radiographs made with (A) normal and (B) excessive vertical angulation.

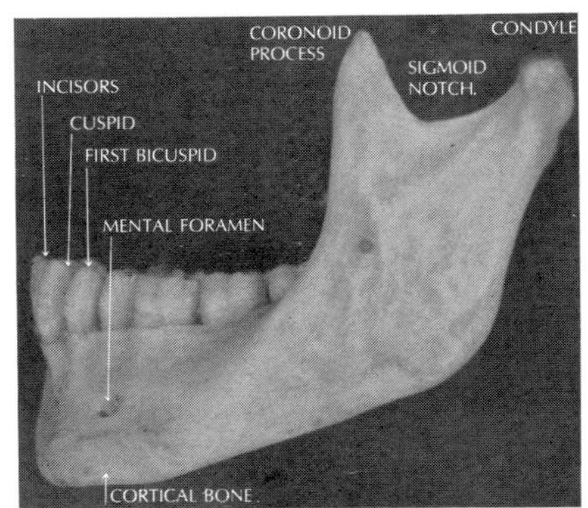

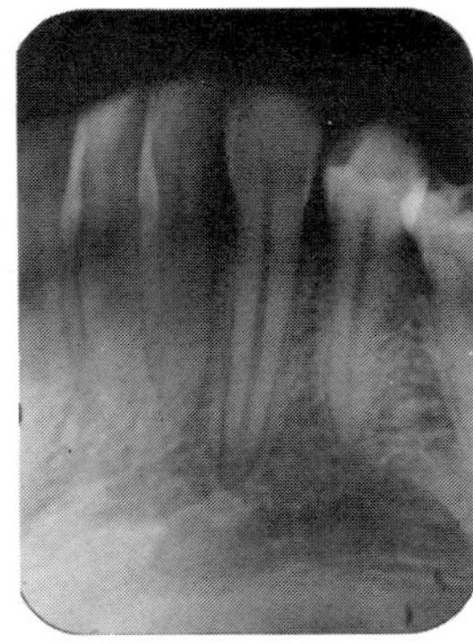

Figure 11–8. Buccal surface of mandible in cuspid region and cuspid radiograph.

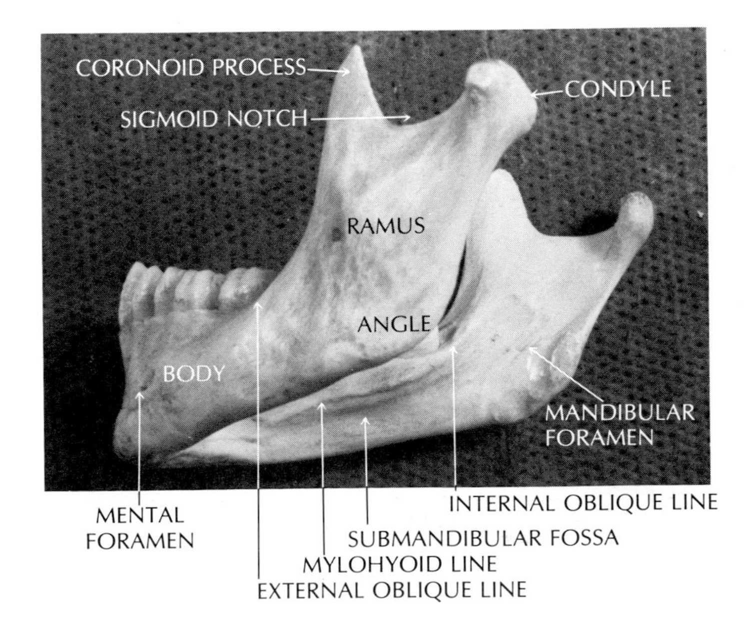

Figure 11–9. Buccal and lingual surfaces of posterior region of mandible.

apices of the bicuspids is often included in this radiograph (Figure 11–8). The mental foramen is located in this area and is thus often shown in the cuspid radiograph.

Figure 11–9 shows the buccal and lingual surfaces of the body and ramus of the mandible. The external oblique and mylohyoid lines are heavy bone ridges on the outer and inner surfaces of the body of the mandible. The mandible in the submaxillary fossa area is thinner and will appear more radiolucent. Within the bone the mandibular canal lies below the apices of the molar teeth between its openings at the inner surface of the ramus and the mental foramen. The canal appears radiographically as a radiolucent band of uniform width; when the wall of the canal is calcified, the radiolucent band will be bordered by two thin radiopaque lines. Figures 11–10 and 11–11 show bicuspid and molar radiographs. The mandibular bicuspids have small lingual cusps and tend to have a single root. However, double rooted bicuspids or teeth with two root canals are not uncommon; the presence of two lamina duras is an indication of this possibility.

Mandibular molars have two roots and many small cusps. The external oblique line crosses the roots of the second and third molars. The mylohyoid line is usually seen when great vertical angulation is used in the radiographic technic; in this instance, the cortical bone plate at the lower border of the mandible is also likely to be seen in the radiograph.

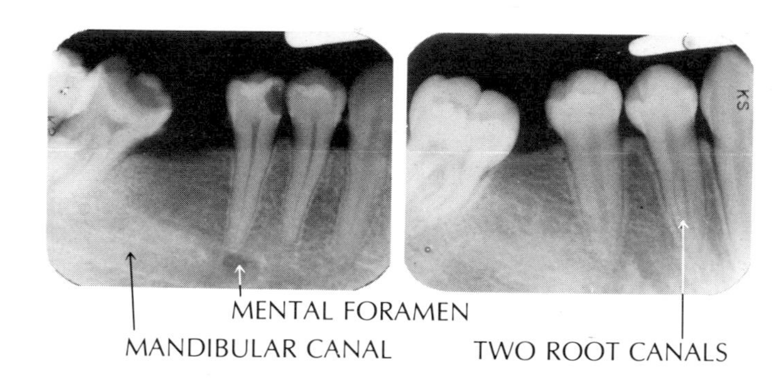

Figure 11–10. Mandibular bicuspid radiographs.

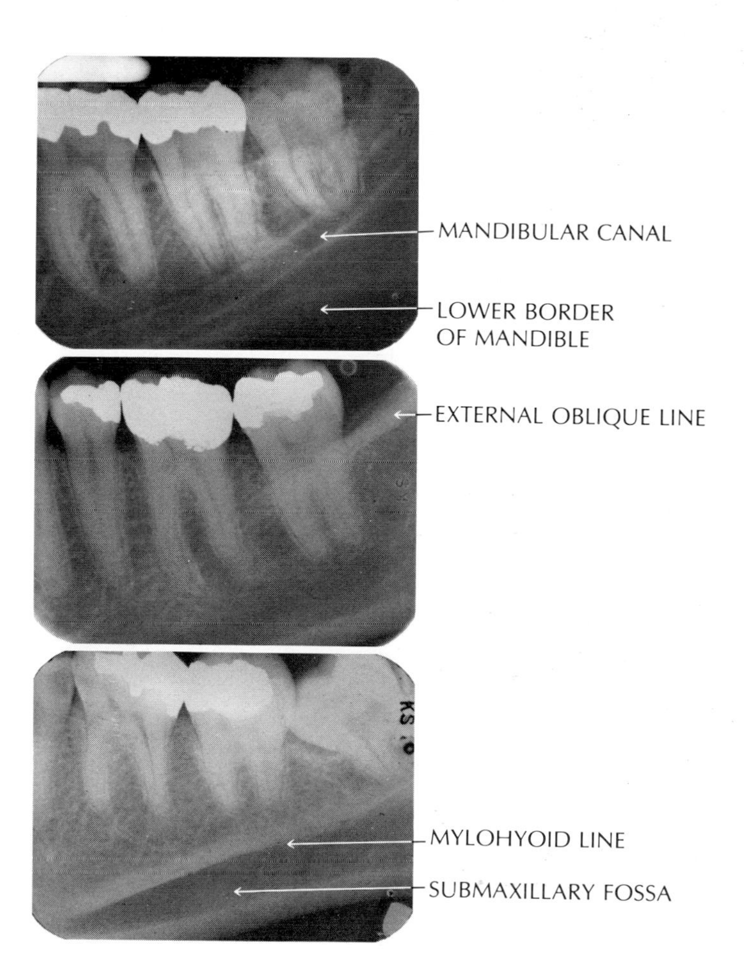

Figure 11–11. Mandibular molar radiographs.

LANDMARKS OF THE MAXILLA

The maxillary incisor region has teeth of different sizes (Figure 11–12). The radiolucent median palatine suture is positioned vertically on the radiograph; the lower part of this suture is sometimes called the median alveolar suture. The incisive foramen is an oval-shaped radiolucency between the apices of the central incisors. The foramen opens on the palatal surface of the maxilla and is connected to the incisive canal which is sometimes seen when the walls of the canal are calcified. The anterior nasal spine is a projection of bone on the labial surface and appears as a V-shaped radiopacity above the incisive foramen. The nasal fossae or cavities, nasal septum and nasal conchae appear

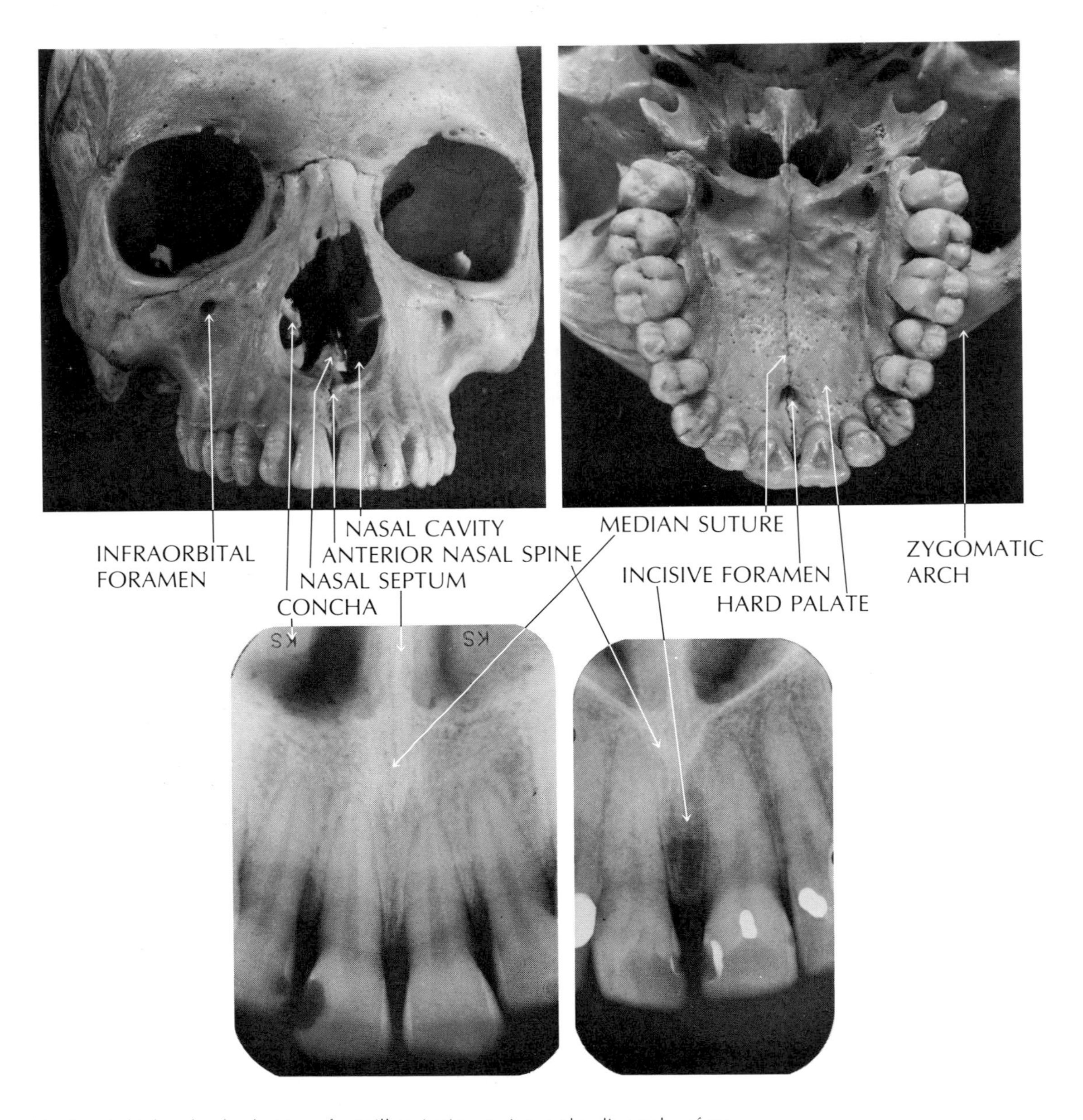

Figure 11–12. Labial and palatal views of maxillary incisor region and radiographs of area.

in the radiograph of the maxillary incisor region when great vertical angulation is used in making the radiograph.

The maxillary cuspid has a root that is much longer than the adjacent lateral incisor and first bicuspid. The apex of this tooth lies at the lateral border of the floor of the nasal fossa (Figure 11–13). The tooth is usually mesial to the maxillary sinus, but in some patients the sinus may extend mesial to the cuspid. The anterior border of the sinus curves upward mesially, whereas the lateral border of the nasal fossa curves upward distally; in the radiograph these radiopaque lines tend to cross each other above the cuspid's apex. The buccopalatal thickness of the alveolar bone at the cuspid is greater than that of the bone immediately mesial and distal to this tooth; this bone elevation on the buccal side is sometimes called the canine eminence and the bone mesial and distal to the cuspid tends to appear more radiolucent.

The maxillary bicuspid and molar regions contain the maxillary sinus, zygomatic arch, pterygoid plates with hamular process, maxillary tuberosity, and sometimes the coronoid process of the mandible. These structures are shown in Figure 11–14. The zygomatic arch forms a U-shaped structure at its anterior attachment to the maxilla above the first and second molar teeth. The arch curves distally to the temporomandibular joint. The maxillary sinus varies greatly in size. The sinus floor may lie above the apices of the teeth or may dip down between the roots of the teeth. The sinus may also have bony partitions or septa dividing it into more than one compartment. The alveolar ridge ends at the maxillary tuberosity and thus the border of bone is directed upward or apically to the maxillary teeth. Immediately distal to the tuberosity are the two thin pterygoid bone plates. These plates are not commonly seen on intraoral radiographs; however, the hamular process of the medial plate may sometimes be seen as a small hook-shaped radiopacity. Note that the coronoid process of the mandible is in the immediate area and may appear in the maxillary molar radiograph.

Figure 11–15 shows maxillary bicuspid and molar radiographs. The maxillary bicuspids tend to have two cusps of approximately equal size and tend to have two roots. Max-

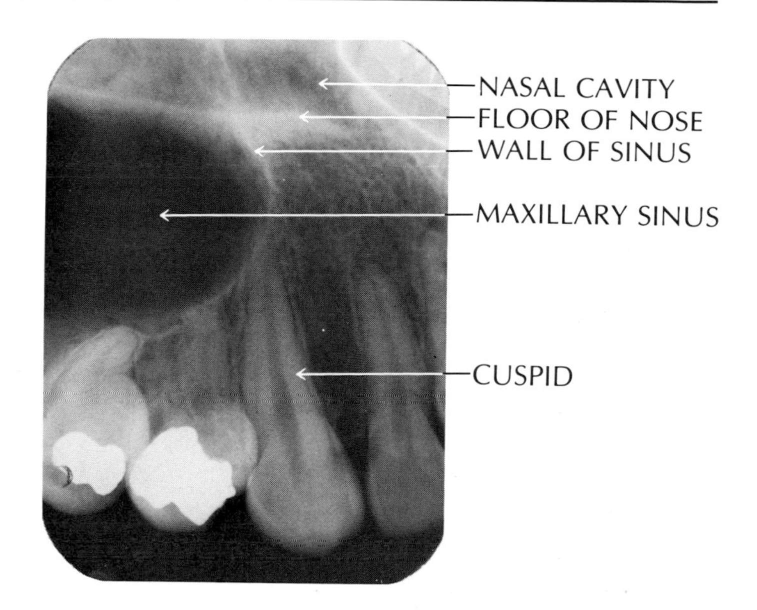

Figure 11–13. Radiograph of maxillary cuspid.

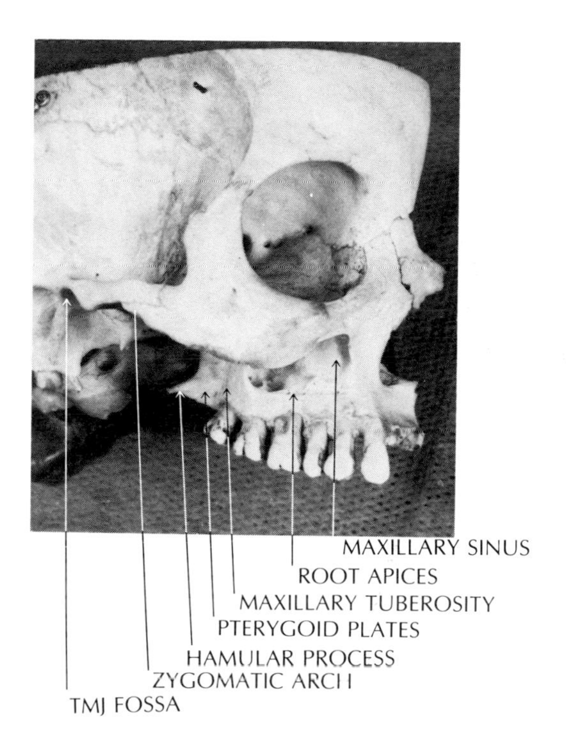

Figure 11–14. Posterior area of maxilla shown with removal of bone overlying sinus.

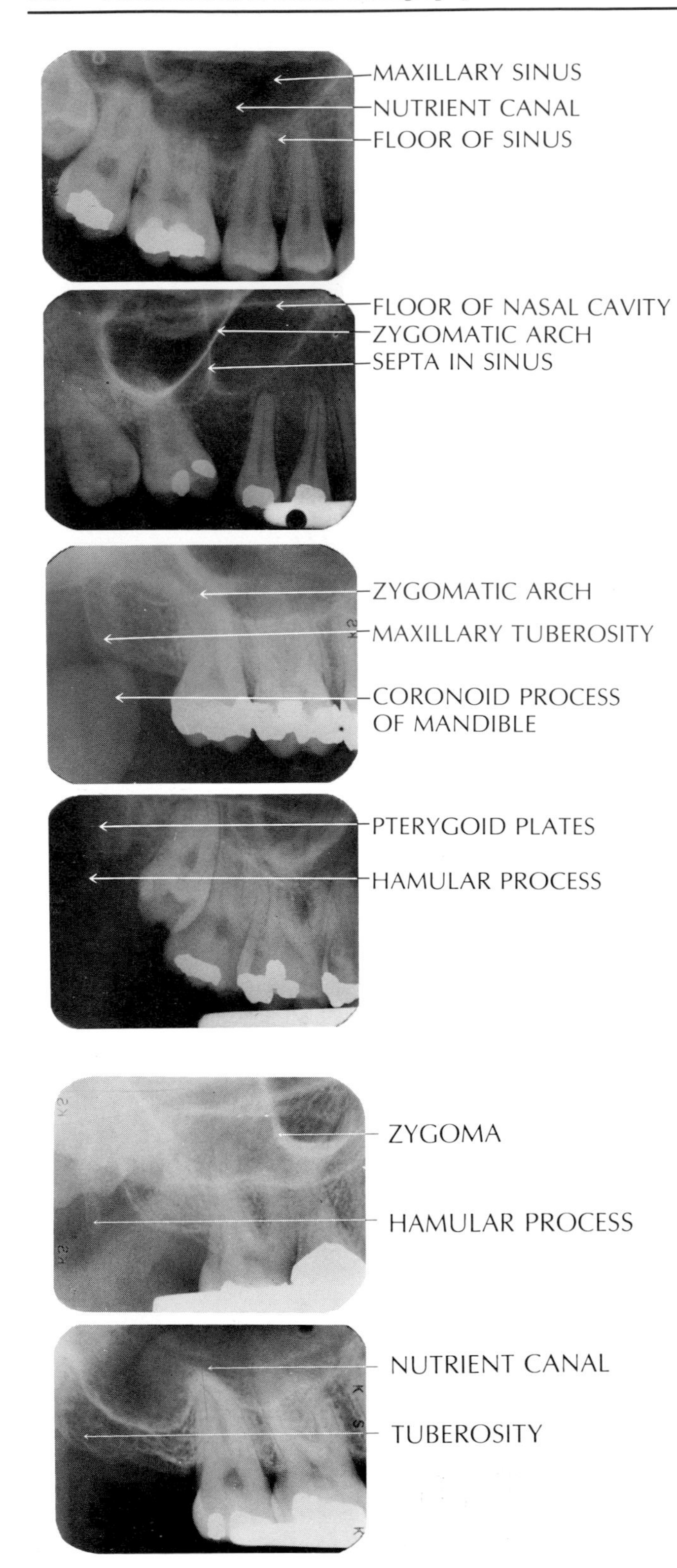

Figure 11–15. Maxillary bicuspid and molar radiographs.

illary molars usually have three roots, two buccal and one palatal.

Sinus septa may or may not be seen in the radiograph, depending on the direction of the x-ray beam during radiography. When the x-ray beam is directed in the same direction as the septa, the septa may absorb enough x rays to appear as a thin radiopaque line. Nutrient canals may be present in the bone or the wall of the sinus and appear as thin radiolucent bands; the radiolucent band may have fine radiopaque borders if the walls of the canals are calcified.

DENTAL MATERIALS

Dental materials, restorations, and instruments are made of radiolucent and radiopaque materials. The film density of restorations seen in radiographs also depends on the thickness of the material in the path of the x-ray beam.

Radiopaque restorative materials are gold, silver amalgam, zinc phosphate cement, zinc oxide and eugenol, silver points, gutta-percha, metal wires, copper bands, and aluminum crowns.

Radiolucent materials are acrylic, silicates, calcium hydroxide, porcelain, and some composite restorative materials.

Some calcium hydroxide pastes and composite restorations contain added radiopaque material that gives the filling material enough x-ray absorbing ability to make it appear radiopaque clinically. The radiographic appearances of dental materials are shown in Figures 11–16 to 11–21.

FILM MOUNTING

Placing films in a film mount is a simple procedure. The problem in film mounting is the identification of the tooth area that is shown in the radiograph.

Individual dentists may wish the radiographs of the left and right side of the patient positioned in the film mount to be on their left and right, respectively, or to be positioned on their right and left, respectively (Figure 11–22). The position of the viewer in the first case is as if he is sitting on the

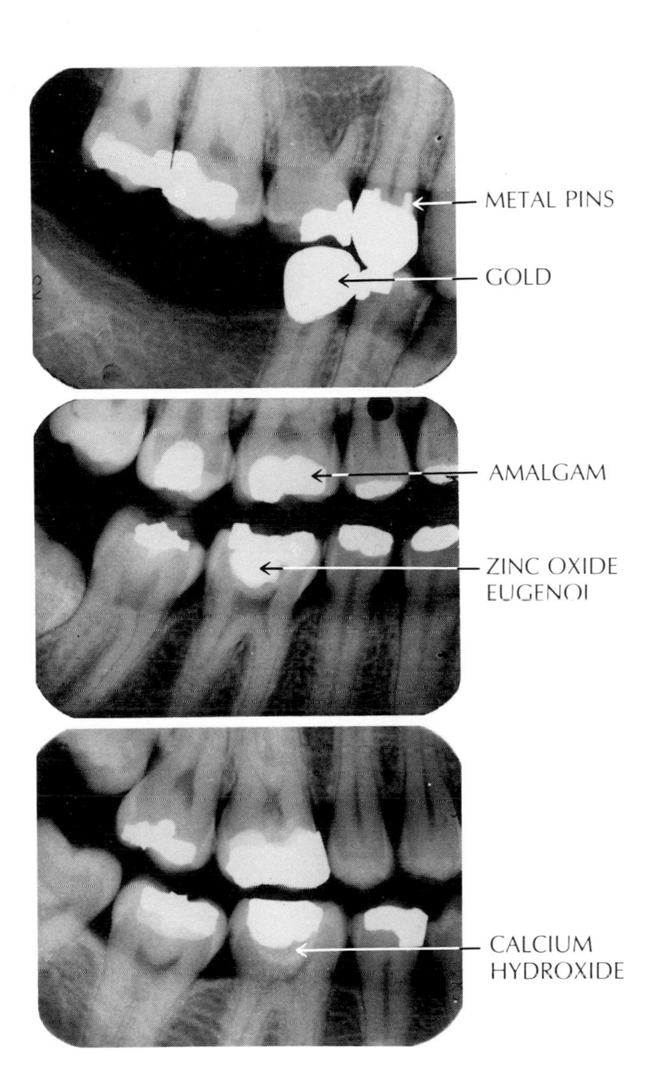

Figure 11–16. Radiographs showing radiographic appearance of metal pins, gold crown, amalgam restorations, zinc oxide-eugenol base, and radiolucent calcium hydroxide subbase.

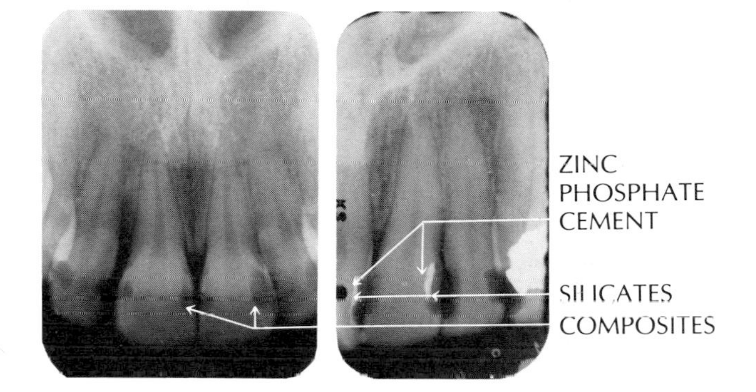

Figure 11–17. Radiographs of anterior teeth showing cement bases and silicate and composite restorations.

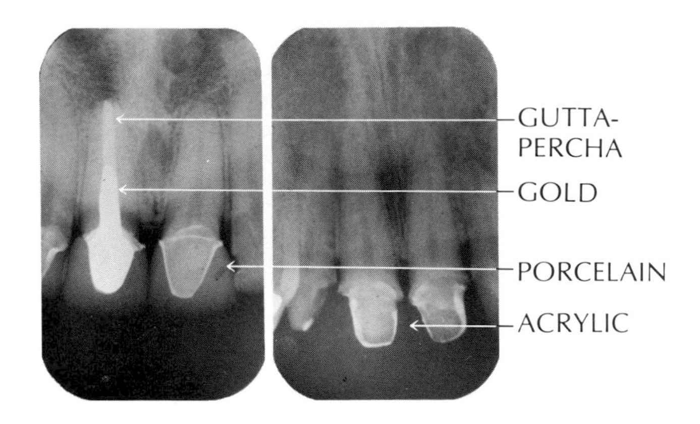

Figure 11–18. Radiographs illustrating different radiopacities of gold and gutta-percha, and different radiolucencies of porcelain and acrylic.

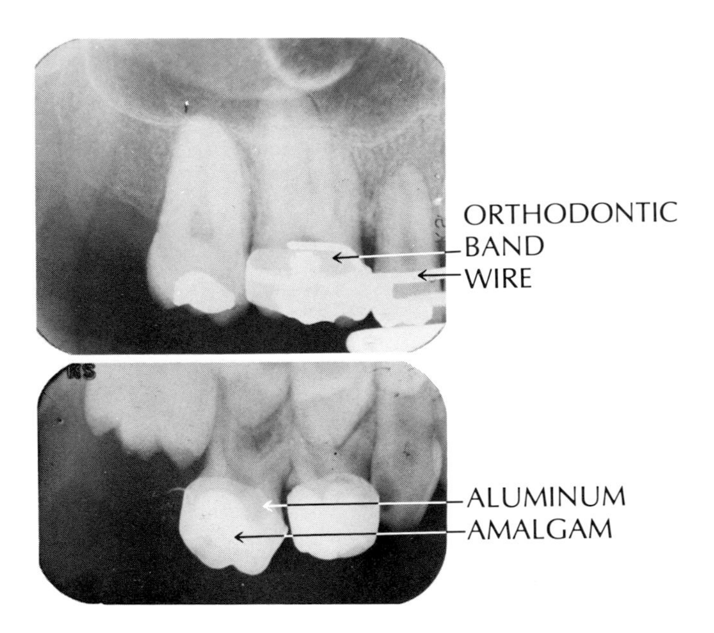

Figure 11–19. Radiographs showing thin steel orthodontic band and orthodontic wires; and aluminum crown over tooth containing amalgam restoration.

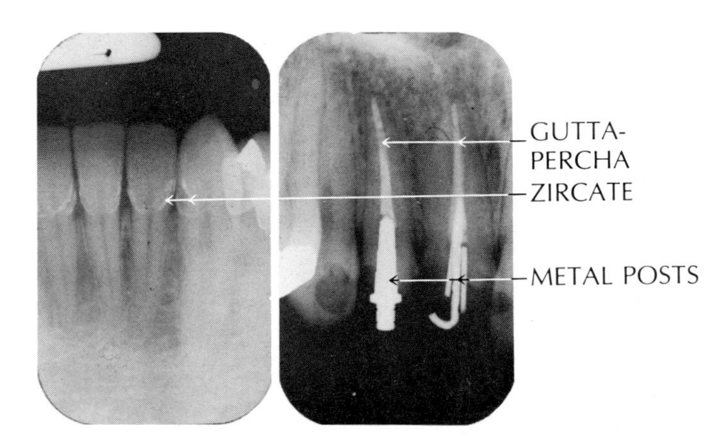

Figure 11–20. Radiographs showing zircate polishing material in gingival sulcus, gutta-percha root canal restoration, and metal posts supporting acrylic restorations.

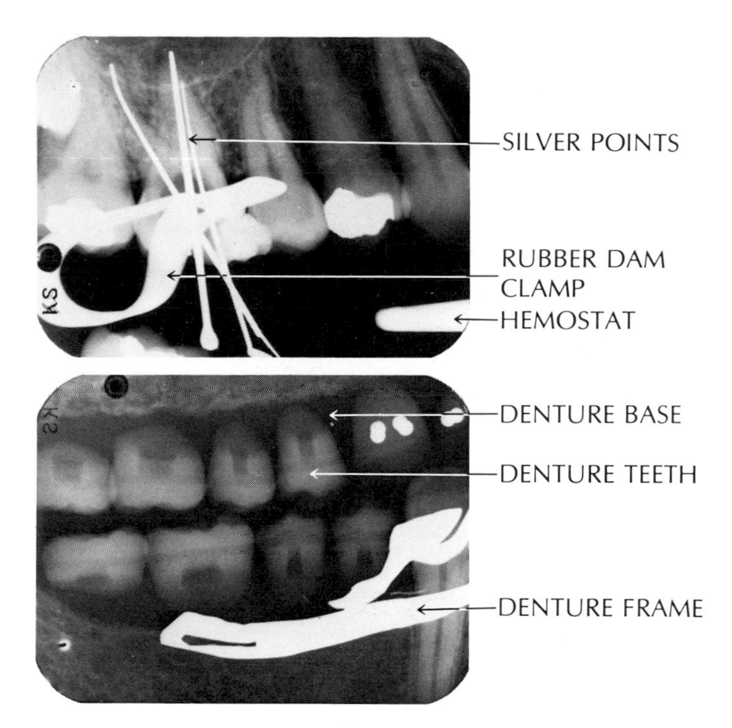

Figure 11–21. Radiographs showing endodontic silver points, steel rubber dam clamp, steel hemostat film holder beak, porcelain denture teeth, acrylic denture base, and gold partial denture frame.

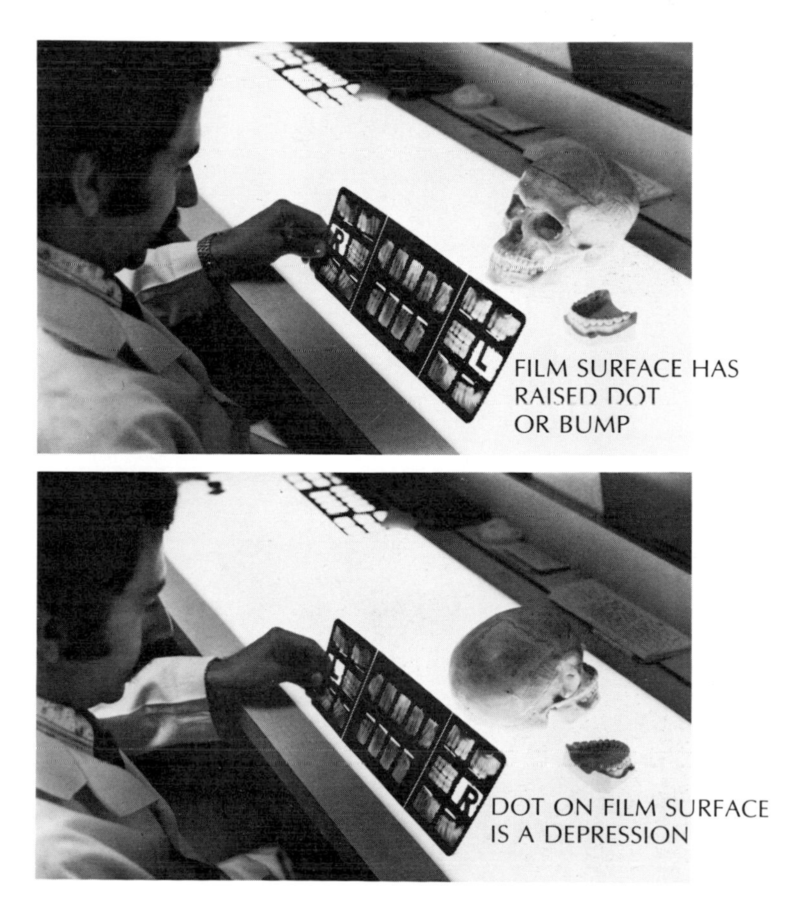

Figure 11–22. Complete mouth radiographs mounted to be viewed (above) with observer facing patient, and (below) with observer positioned behind patient. Note that left (L) and right (R) sides of film mount are different.

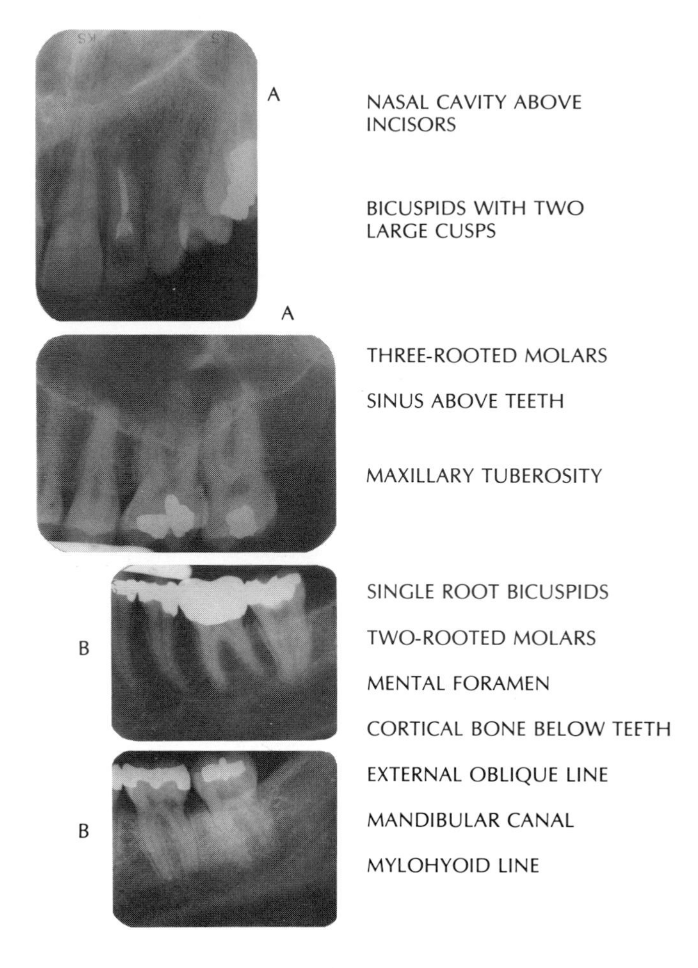

Figure 11–23. Some anatomic landmarks that separate (A) maxillary and (B) mandibular radiographs.

patient's tongue looking out at the patient's teeth; in the latter case the viewer is positioned like the x-ray tubehead facing the patient. In both cases the right and left radiographs are positioned correctly in the film mount; however, in the first method the identifying dot on the film is seen as a depression and in the second method the film's surface shows a bump or raised dot.

The first step in film mounting is to determine where the right and left sides of the patient are to be in the film mount being used and to place the correct film surface towards the operator, whether it be depression or raised dot.

The second step is to determine whether the radiograph is of a maxillary or a mandibular area (Figure 11–23). An image of the cortical plate beyond the apices of the teeth identifies a mandibular radiograph, whereas a similarly positioned radiolucency of the sinus or nasal cavity identifies a maxillary radiograph. A zygomatic arch shadow is seen only in the maxilla. A large canal and cortical bone on the alveolar ridge area distal to the third molar is seen only in the mandible. A tuberosity and hamular process distal to the third molar is seen only in the maxilla. Maxillary teeth have unequally sized incisors, two-rooted bicuspids with two large cusps, and three-rooted molars. Mandibular teeth have small similarly sized incisors, single-rooted bicuspids with unevenly sized cusps, and two-rooted molars.

When the radiograph is identified as a maxillary or mandibular radiograph, it is positioned with the apices of the teeth pointed upward for the maxilla and downward for the mandible. The operator is cautioned not to "turn over" the radiograph as this would reverse the first step of film mounting and identify the patient's side incorrectly in the next step.

The third step in film mounting is to identify the side of the patient seen in the radiograph. This is done by identifying which lateral border of the radiograph is the mesial border and which is the distal (Figure 11–24). In cases of midline incisor radiographs, the midline of the patient is shown in the radiograph and both lateral sides of the radiograph are distal borders. Obviously incisors are mesial to bicuspids and bicuspids are mesial to molars. The roots of teeth tend to curve distally. The zygomatic arch curves distally from its U-shaped image above the maxillary first and second molars. The mandibular canal travels distally from the mental foramen. The maxillary tuberosity and external oblique line are at the distal ends of the alveolar ridges. The incisive and lingual foramen, the anterior nasal spine, and the genial tubercles are all in the mesial midline. When the third step is completed, the radiograph is identified as being in a particular quadrant of the dentition; that is, in the maxillary left or right region or the mandibular left or right area.

The final step is to identify whether the radiograph shows the incisor, cuspid, bicuspid, or molar area. The radiograph is now identified as to area, right or left, and mandible or maxilla. It is now placed in its respective position in the film mount.

When all the films are mounted, the operator should look at the set as a whole and be sure that all the root apices are directed outward and that the area of each radiograph overlaps properly with adjacent radiographs. This procedure will identify one or more radiographs that are mounted upside down or with the dot facing the wrong direction; however, it will not identify radiographs that are mounted incorrectly when all the radiographs have the dot facing the wrong direction.

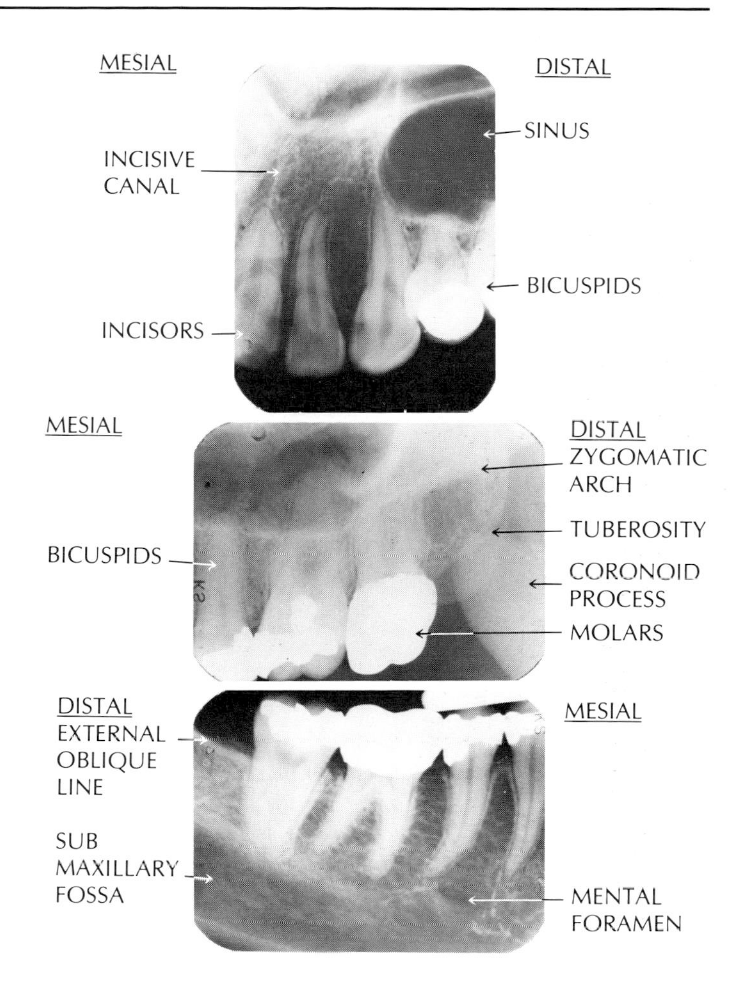

Figure 11–24. Some landmarks assisting identification of lateral borders of radiograph as being mesial or distal.

Chapter 12

Biologic Effects, X-Ray Protection, and Radiologic Health

Soon after the x ray was discovered in 1895, there were reports of erythemas, dermatitis, ulcerations, and neoplastic changes in tissues brought about by exposure to x rays. Many dentists who were ignorant of the early warnings or chose to ignore them suffered the loss of one or more fingers because they used their fingers to hold the film in the patient's mouth and thus exposed the fingers to repeated doses of x-radiation. Since those days information about the biologic effects of radiation upon man has continually increased along with technics for good oral radiography and the safe handling of x-radiation in dentistry. Standards and guidelines have been developed to protect the public, radiation workers and unborn generations from unnecessary exposure to radiation.

BIOLOGIC EFFECTS OF X RAYS

Evidence of the effects of x rays upon humans has been gathered from the damage seen in radiology pioneers, workers in industries using radioactive materials, patients undergoing radiation therapy, and atom bomb victims. Most of this knowledge has been accumulated since 1950. X rays can bring about changes in body chemicals, cells, tissues, and organs; however, the effects of the radiation may not become evident for a great number of years after the time the x rays were absorbed. This time lag is called the *latent period.* An everyday example of a latent period is the few days it takes the skin to tan or darken after it is exposed to the sun at the beach.

Chemical Effects

Chemical effects result from the ability of x rays to ionize atoms and break chemical bonds. Since the structures of many body chemicals are unknown, knowledge of the results of x-ray absorption by body chemicals is limited. However, most of the human body is made of water (H_2O) and the effect of x rays upon water is the production of free oxygen, hydrogen, and hydroxyl radicals; recombination may produce hydrogen peroxide (H_2O_2), or the water parts may combine with other chemicals in the area to form new chemicals (Figure 12–1). The new chemicals may be foreign to the body and may be poisonous. Hydrogen peroxide is an example. When complex body chemicals are irradiated, many unknown radicals and new chemicals may be formed.

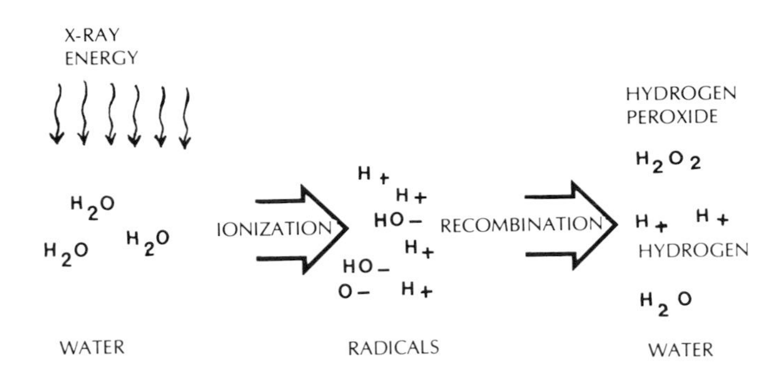

Figure 12–1. Formation of radicals when water (H_2O) is irradiated and possible recombination to form hydrogen peroxide (H_2O_2).

Effects on Cells and Tissues

Not all cells exposed to radiation are damaged; however, some may have broken chromosomes and vacuoles in the nucleus or cytoplasm (Figure 12–2). The damage can be from a *direct* or *indirect* effect. A direct effect is one created by the x-ray photon acting on a cell structure, such as breaking part of the chemical chain forming a chromosome. The same break may be produced by free chemical radicals produced by the x-ray photon being absorbed by nearby water or other chemicals; this is an indirect effect produced by the free radicals acting on the damaged part. Cells may undergo abnormal mitosis and giant cells may be formed. Cells undergoing mitosis at the time of exposure to x rays show greater damage. Tissues that are rapidly growing and have many cells undergoing mitotic division show greater radiation effects; that is, they are more susceptible or sensitive to x-rays. Figure 12–3 lists some tissues in order of radiosensitivity.

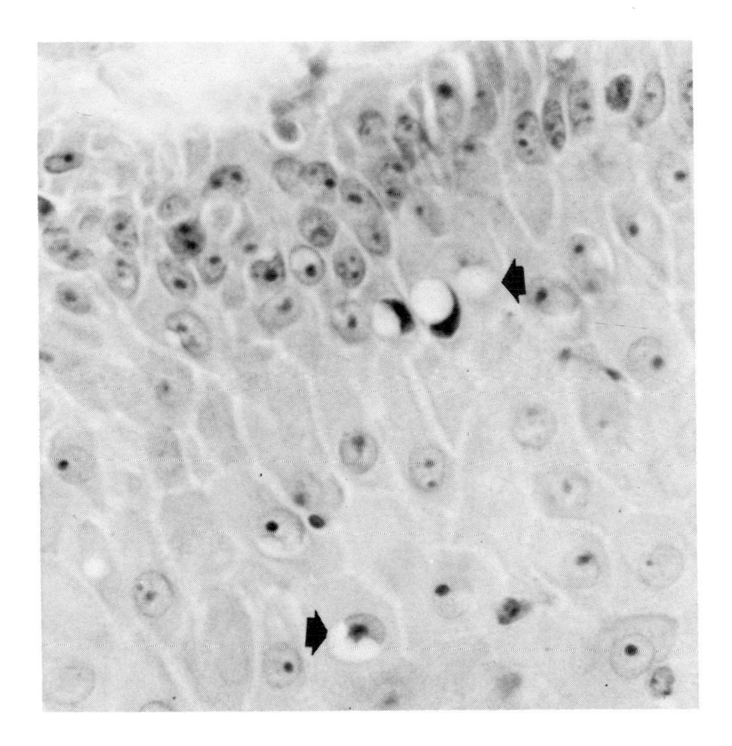

Figure 12–2. Irradiated skin cells showing formation of vacuoles in some cells (arrows).

Malignant tumors or cancers that have many dividing cells are often treated with radiation because they tend to be more sensitive than normal cells to radiation; relatively large doses of radiation are used. Very large x-ray doses may alter the genetic code controlling a normal cell's behavior and can result in a tumor. Thus radiation can treat cancers but can also cause cancers, depending on the amount of radiation and the sensitivity of the tissue. The dose used in cancer therapy is limited by the tolerance of the surrounding normal tissue. Oral cancers are often treated with high x-ray doses of 5,000 to 7,000 rads (50 to 70 grays). Such doses can kill cancer cells; the normal cells are also affected but to a lesser degree.

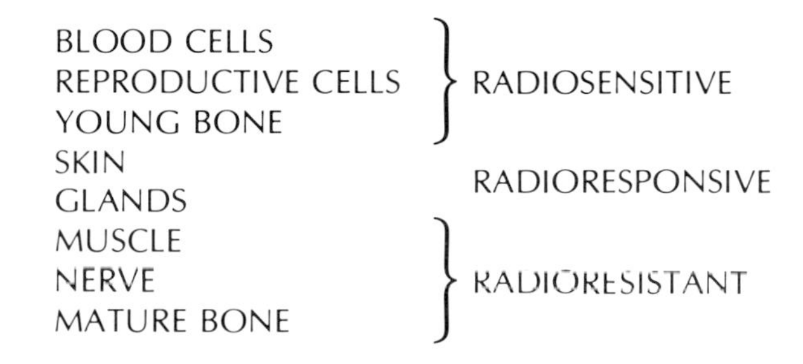

Figure 12–3. List of types of cells in order of sensitivity to x rays.

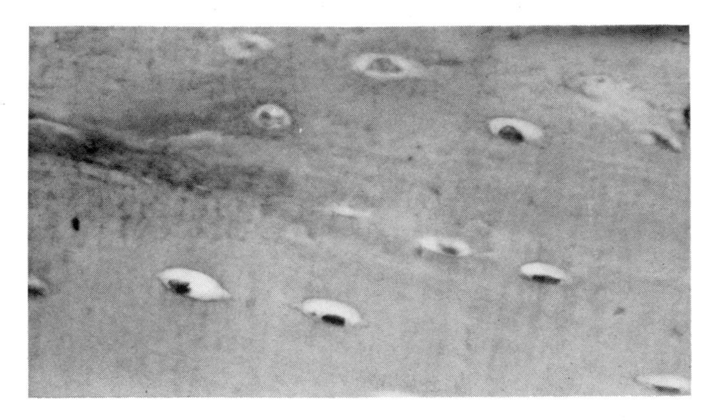

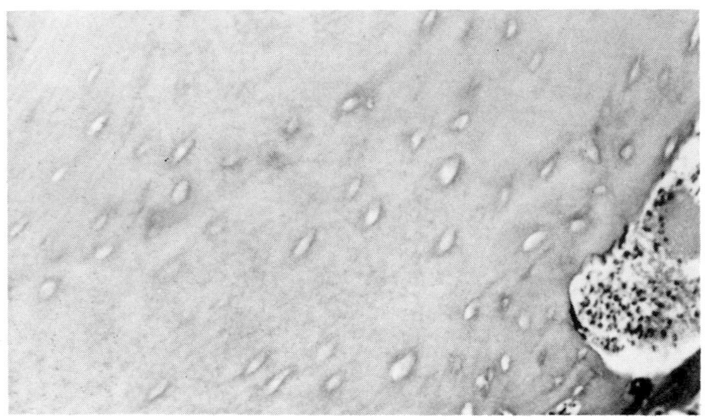

Figure 12–4. Microscopic pictures of normal bone (above) and osteoradionecrotic bone (below) showing missing osteocytes.

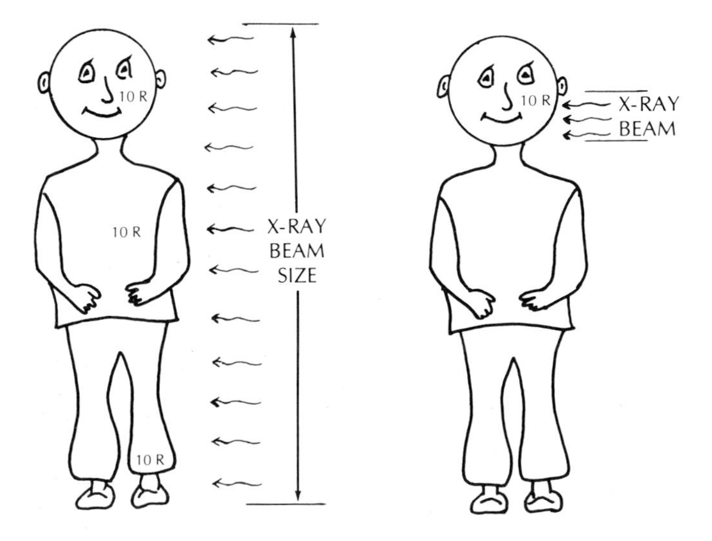

Figure 12–5. Example of same dose (10 rads) being delivered to whole body and to specific area by two x-ray beams of similar x-ray intensity and exposure time but of different size. A dose stated in roentgens or rads does not indicate volume of tissue exposed.

Healed x-ray-treated tissue has fewer, smaller blood vessels, impaired cell function, and poor ability to repair itself. Bone absorbs much more x-ray energy because it is more dense than soft tissue; irradiated bone cells may quietly die and result in a condition called osteoradionecrosis (Figure 12–4). Such x-ray damaged bone and soft tissues are very susceptible to infection.

Acute and Chronic X-Ray Exposure

X-ray exposure produces different effects on humans. Acute exposure occurs when a large dose of radiation is absorbed in a short period of time; such is the case in nuclear accidents and atom bomb victims. These patients exhibit varying degrees of erythema, nausea, bleeding, diarrhea, epilation, fever, and shock; death results in many cases. This acute radiation syndrome is associated with doses of more than 100 rads (1 gray) delivered to the entire body. It does not occur in dentistry because dental diagnostic radiography generally uses less than 5 rads (0.02 gray or 2 cGy) and only to a small specific region of the body (Figure 12–5). If only a small volume of tissue is irradiated, the tissue can withstand much larger doses than if all the body is exposed. (Note that a dose given in rads does not indicate the volume or amount of tissue exposed.) If a dose of 100 rads is received by the whole body, the person may have nausea, vomiting and early signs of radiation sickness; if the same dose is given to an area the size of a dental x-ray beam, none of these effects are produced. A high dose to a small volume of tissue, as is the case in radiation therapy, may produce some effects similar to the acute radiation syndrome but to a much lesser degree.

Chronic x-ray exposure occurs when small amounts of radiation are absorbed repeatedly over a long period of time. With good technic and equipment only a small area of the patient's face is exposed to approximately 250 mR (0.00645 exposure units or 64.5×10^{-4} EU) when an intraoral radiograph is made. Much smaller amounts of x rays reach other parts of the patient and the operator during intraoral radiography from scattered x rays.

Radiation damage caused by a particular dose of acute radiation delivered at one time is usually greater than damage resulting from the same dose delivered in small amounts over a long period. Acute or chronic x-ray exposure and volume of tissue irradiated are only two of many factors (e.g., dose rate or intensity of the x-ray beam and the presence of oxygen and chemical protectors in the irradiated tissue) that vary the amount of tissue damage resulting from a particular dose of radiation.

Cumulative Effect

The cumulative effect of repeated doses of x-radiation is of interest. When tissues are irradiated, the amount of reaction will depend greatly upon the dose delivered. Whatever this reaction is, there will be repair to the damaged tissues as long as complete degeneration has not occurred. The tissues do not return to their original state, however, as there is some irreparable damage and this irreparable damage is what is cumulative (Figure 12–6).

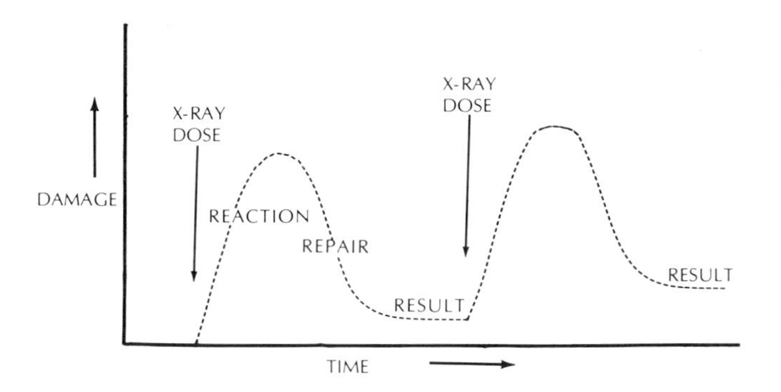

Figure 12–6. Diagrammatic representation of cumulative effect of x-radiation.

Somatic Effects

Radiation affects both genetic and somatic cells. Genetic cells are the germ cells of the reproductive organs, i.e., the eggs of the female and sperms of the male. All other cells belong to the soma or body of the individual.

Clinical effects may be seen on patients who have undergone radiation therapy. The skin in the treated area is tanned and scarred and appears as if a very hot object had been placed upon it. This is often referred to as a *radiation burn* (Figure 12–7). Hair loss also occurs in the irradiated area. When the salivary glands are in the therapy region, the amount and quality of the saliva are affected. A dry mouth and a rampant form of caries often result from these radiation effects. Dental treatment often involves the use of a topical decay preventive agent and liquid preparations to replace the lubricating effect of the lost saliva and alleviate the discomfort of a dry mouth.

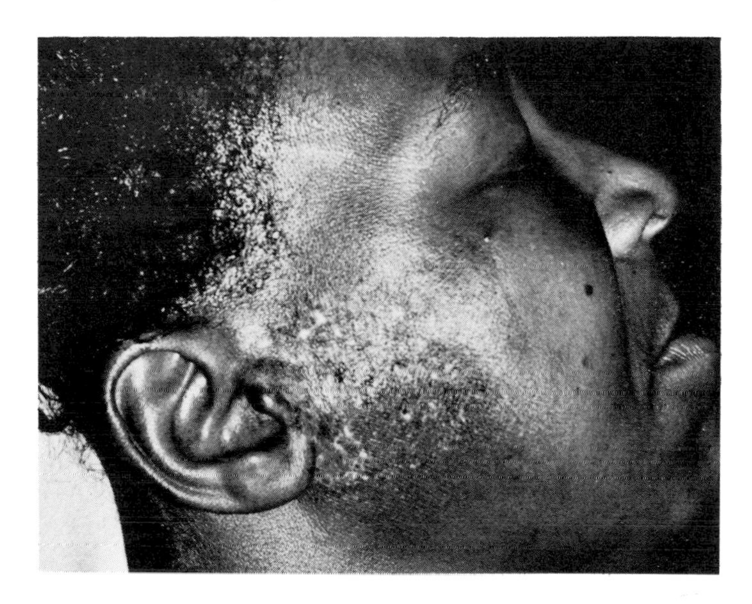

Figure 12–7. Radiation burn showing square shape of collimated x-ray beam on cheek of patient who had x-ray therapy.

In the early days of dental radiography some dentists held the film in the patient's mouth. This dangerous practice resulted in the dentist's hand being exposed to the primary x-ray beam and repeated doses of x rays. Over a period of years the exposed tissues became so damaged that healing of

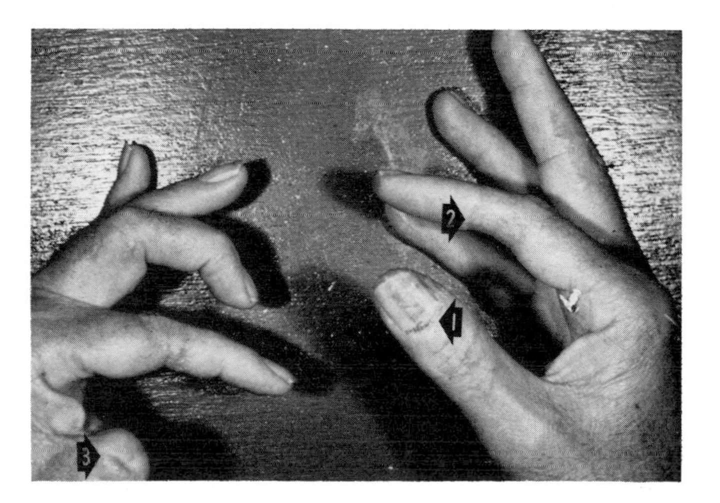

Figure 12–8. Hands of dentist who held films in patients' mouths for many years. Note area of poor healing (1), skin graft (2), and loss of thumb due to radiation damage (3). (Courtesy of Dr. H.H. Hicks.)

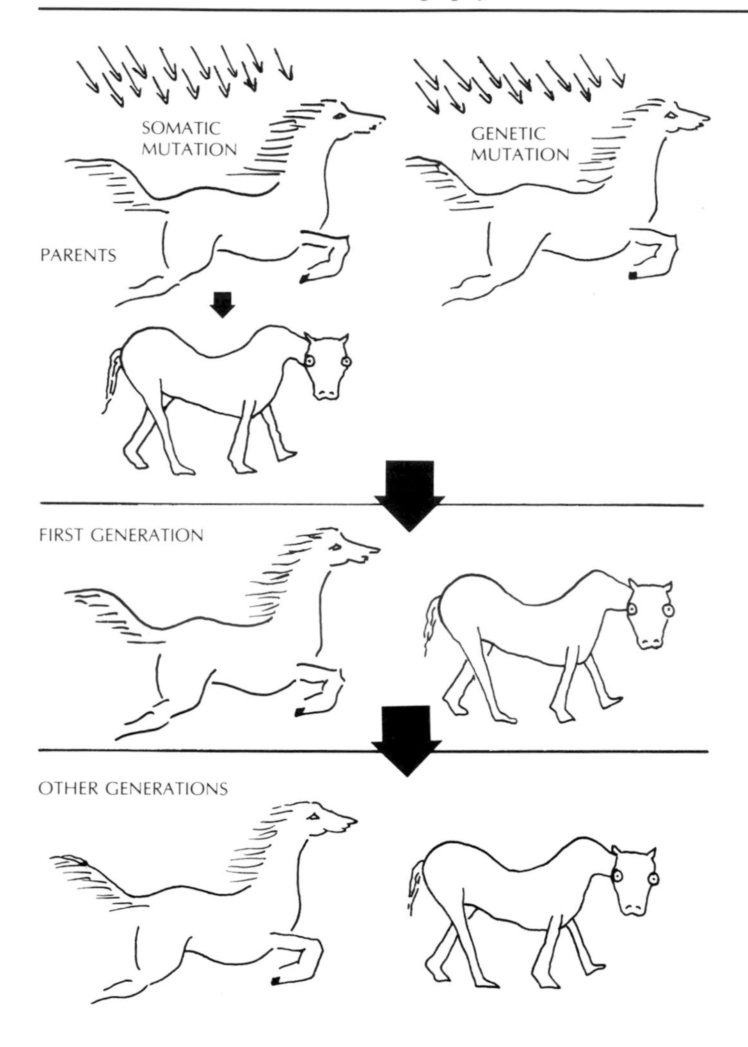

Figure 12–9. Different effects of somatic and genetic mutations. Somatic mutations produce poor health in exposed animal but are not transmitted to subsequent offspring. Genetic mutation does not usually affect exposed individual but affects health of all subsequent generations.

small breaks in the skin was difficult and eventually, in some cases, parts of the hand had to be amputated (Figure 12–8).

Delayed effects appearing many years after the original exposure to x rays may result from a previous acute high-dose exposure or from chronic repeated low-dose exposures. Possible effects include an increased incidence of cancer (especially leukemia), birth defects, cataracts, and lifespan shortening.

There is no real evidence of clinically manifest effects resulting from dental diagnostic radiography. Much more information is needed to accurately establish the effects of small doses of x rays upon humans. Some available information pertinent to dentistry is presented in the discussion on radiation health later in this chapter.

The Genetic Effects

X rays can cause mutations to occur in many types of cells, including the germ cells of the reproductive organs. Mutations in the germ cells that carry the genetic code or hereditary information for making new humans are of special significance. Damage occurring in the somatic cells of living things is removed from the population when the affected organism dies, but damage occurring in the germ cells of males or females can be passed on to succeeding generations (Figure 12–9). Radiation induced genetic changes have been studied in fruit flies and small laboratory animals. Genetic damage can be expressed in congenital defects, depressed growth rates, altered biochemistry, etc. Radiation produces new mutations and an increased frequency of known mutations. The number of produced mutations increases with the dose rate or x-ray beam intensity used in delivering the radiation to the animals. Studies have also shown that many cells appear to have the ability to repair some types of genetic damage to their chromosomes.

A large population of humans was exposed to large amounts of radiation during the atom bomb explosions at Hiroshima and Nagasaki. No measurable evidence of more mutations or increased mortality has been found in the descendants of these people. However, it is possible that effects may take many generations before they become evident. Many professionals believe that low level radiation will produce subtle deleterious changes in health, such as a reduction in life span.

The Dose-Response Curve

A dose-response curve results when one plots on a graph the response of any x-ray effect to the x-ray dose. The resulting curve may be of the threshold or linear type (Figure 12–10A). Many somatic x-ray effects are thought to produce a threshold dose-response curve; this indicates that the earliest evidence does not occur until a minimum or threshold dose is reached; for example, a reddening erythema of the skin and cataract induction. These responses are non-stochastic (effects that require a certain amount of damage before they are observed in whole animals). There is some evidence that genetic effects follow a linear dose-response curve and that regardless of the amount of radiation given to the germ cells a response is produced. These responses are stochastic (an effect that has a probability of occurrence no matter how small the dose). Since there is little available information about the genetic effects of x rays in humans, it is prudent to assume a linear dose-response for genetic tissues and institute radiation protection measures for such tissues for even small x-ray exposures when large numbers of people are involved.

While it is desirable to have a single dose-response curve, the shape of a single curve has not been accepted by all scientists. The difficulty arises because there is not enough research information to establish the shape of the dose-response curve at low radiation levels (in vicinity of diagnostic x rays and permissible occupational doses). However, a majority of radiation scientists agree on a linear quadratic curve (Figure 12–10B) for all human cells or tissues. The unified curve uses a low response to radiation but no threshold in the low dose region. Thus for low radiation doses the response is assumed to be quite small but is never zero. The unified curve promotes the concept that *there is no safe dose of radiation.*

Most geneticists agree that almost all mutations are harmful. Harmful mutations are gradually eliminated from the population when individuals carrying them die without having children. Spontaneous mutations oc-

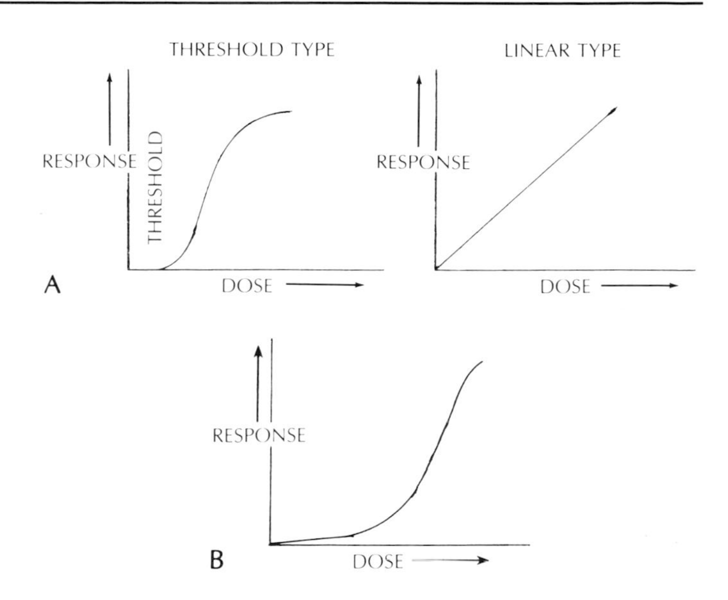

Figure 12–10. A, Threshold and linear radiation dose-response curves. B, Unified concept of the dose-response curve as a linear quadratic relationship.

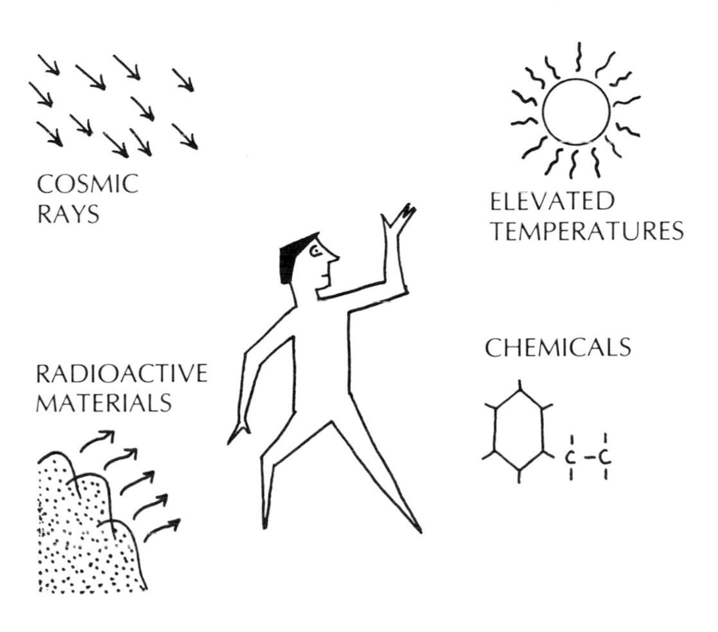

Figure 12–11. Possible sources of spontaneous mutations.

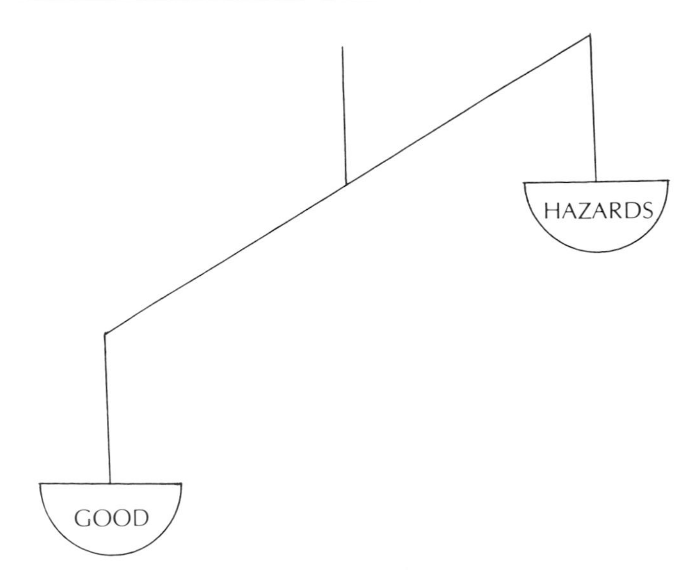

Figure 12–12. Concept for use of x rays in diagnostic radiography.

cur in the population and thus a continuous stream of new mutations is being introduced as old ones are being removed. Natural background radiation in our normal environment probably accounts for a small proportion of the spontaneous mutations, since many other possible factors such as chemicals, drugs, and temperature changes are also involved (Figure 12–11). Gonadal dose from accepted dental radiographic procedures is a small fraction of daily natural background radiation. However, unnecessary irradiation of the gonads should be avoided.

X-RAY PROTECTION

Little concern was shown for exposure of patients and operators to x-radiation in dentistry until 1956, even though there were occasional reports of dentists losing fingers because of overexposure to x rays. The establishment, beyond a reasonable doubt through animal experimentation, of a genetic x-ray hazard that would be passed on to succeeding generations gave rapid momentum to the implementation of protective measures for patient and operator in dental radiology after 1956.

Protective measures that are both useful and practical will be described for (1) the patient, (2) the operator, and (3) the immediate environs (Figure 12–13). Procedures for the patient are described first because any x-ray dose reduction achieved for the patient automatically reduces the dose to all others concerned.

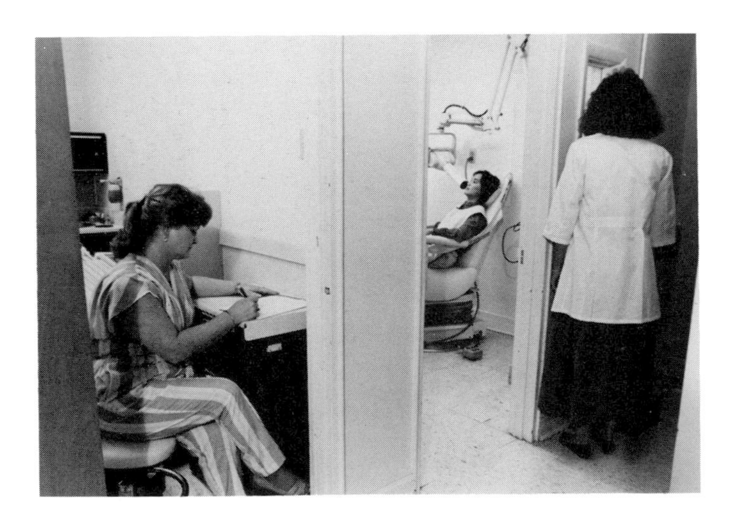

Figure 12–13. Persons to be protected from dental x rays.

Protection of the Patient

The dose of x-radiation to the patient can be reduced to a very small amount. This minimal amount can be lessened by a factor of 20 in some dental offices where good radiation hygiene has not been practiced previously. The procedures are summarized as follows: (1) use of fast film, (2) proper filtration, (3) proper collimation, (4) use of gonadal shields, (5) good film exposure technic, (6) use of open-end cones, (7) increased tube-patient distance, and (8) use of recessed filters and lead-lined cones. The first three procedures are by far the most effective means of reducing the patient's exposure to x rays.

Fast Films: Thirty years ago dental films required an exposure time of 3 or 4 seconds. Today, using the same type of radiation, rate of production, and distance from patient to x-ray machine, it is possible to make similar radiographs in ¼ second (Figure 12–14). This remarkable achievement resulted from the manufacture of faster films that require much less radiation to produce a latent image that can be developed. Many writers consider the use of fast film to be the single most effective method of reducing the patient's exposure to x rays. It must be remembered that when fast film is used, a very light tight and properly safelighted darkroom is necessary, since these films also have increased sensitivity to light; an accurate x-ray machine timer is also needed for the short exposure times used.

Filtration. The beam of x rays emitted by the dental machine consists of x-ray photons of many different wavelengths or energies. The photons thus have different abilities to penetrate human tissues. Those x rays that cannot penetrate the soft tissues, teeth, and bone of the oral region are unable to reach the film. These x rays are therefore useless in making a radiographic image of the teeth; however, they contribute to the dose of x rays received by the patient. In order to remove these useless x rays and prevent unnecessary exposure of the patient, the x-ray beam is filtered. Filtration is accomplished by passing the x-ray beam through aluminum filters placed over the beam's exit port in the head of the x-ray machine (Figure 12–15). The recommended amount of filtration varies with the operating electric potential being used. At or below 70 kVp, the total filtration should be 1.5 mm of aluminum. When the kilovoltage is above 70 kVp, the recommended amount is 2.5 mm of aluminum. The effect of using proper filtration in an older x-ray machine with no filtration can be to reduce the patient's exposure by as much as 50% without any observable loss in the film's exposure to the x rays.

Collimation. The x-ray beam emerges from the machine in the shape of a cone, the apex of which is the source or target of the x-ray tube. The beam's shape is determined by the shape of the exit port in the tubehead which is usually circular. The diameter of the beam or the size of the circular area covered by the

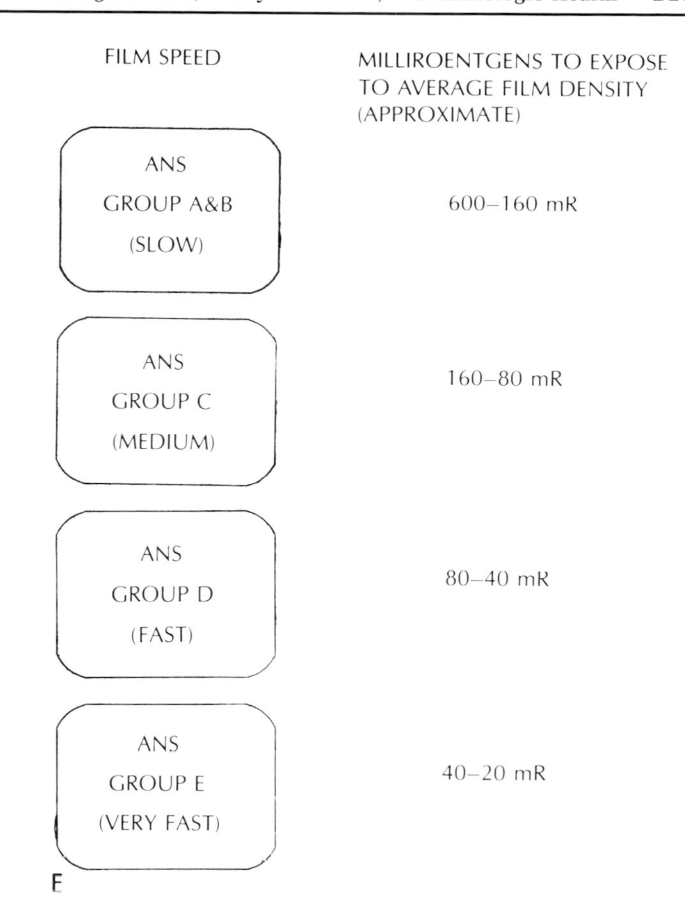

Figure 12–14. Effect of film speed upon reduction in radiation needed to expose film. ANS = American National Standard.

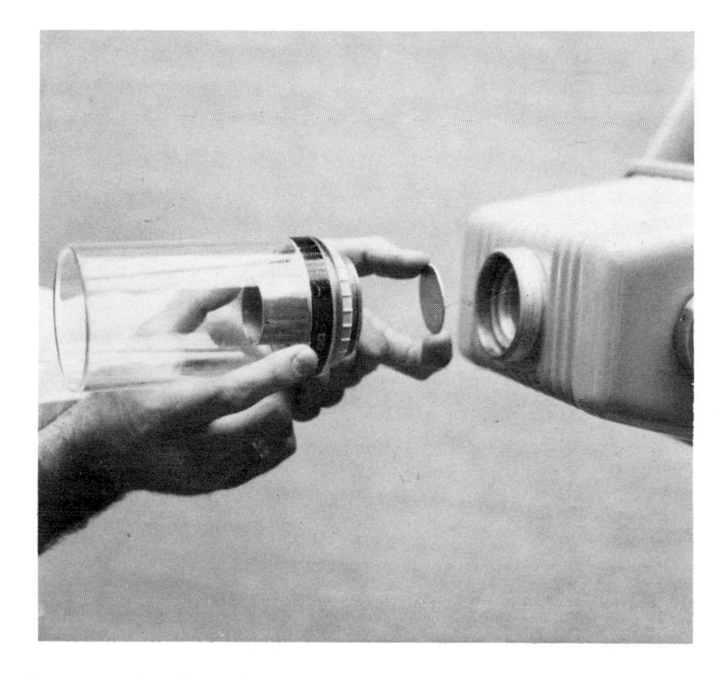

Figure 12–15. Disk of aluminum being placed over exit port of dental x-ray machine to obtain desired amount of filtration.

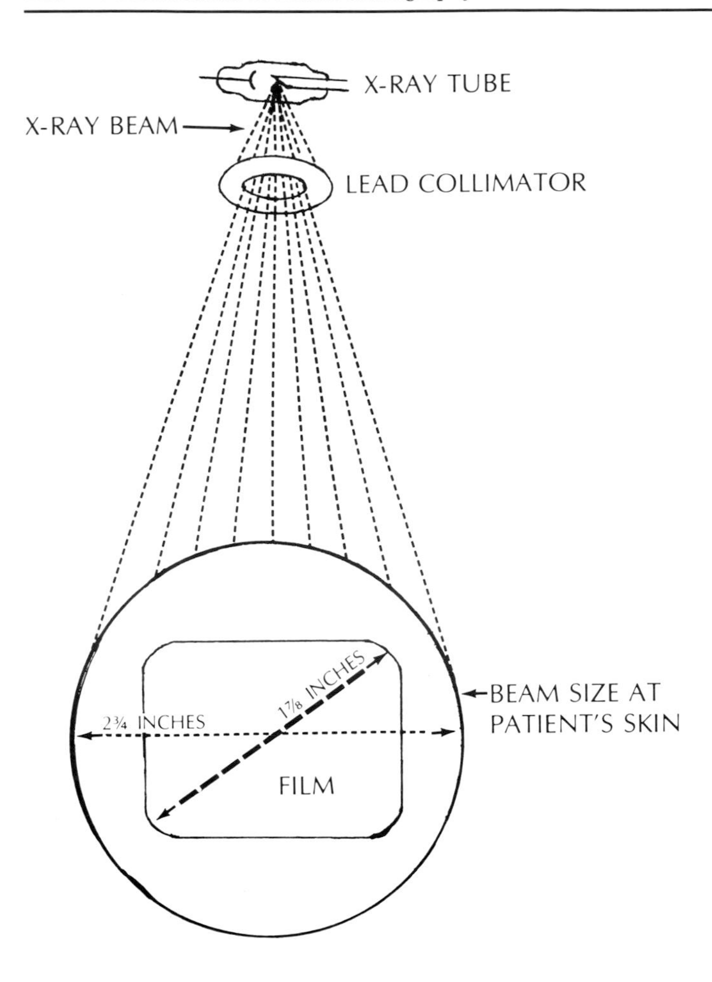

Figure 12–16. Diagram showing collimation of x-ray beam for intraoral radiography. Hole in center of lead disk shapes x-ray beam.

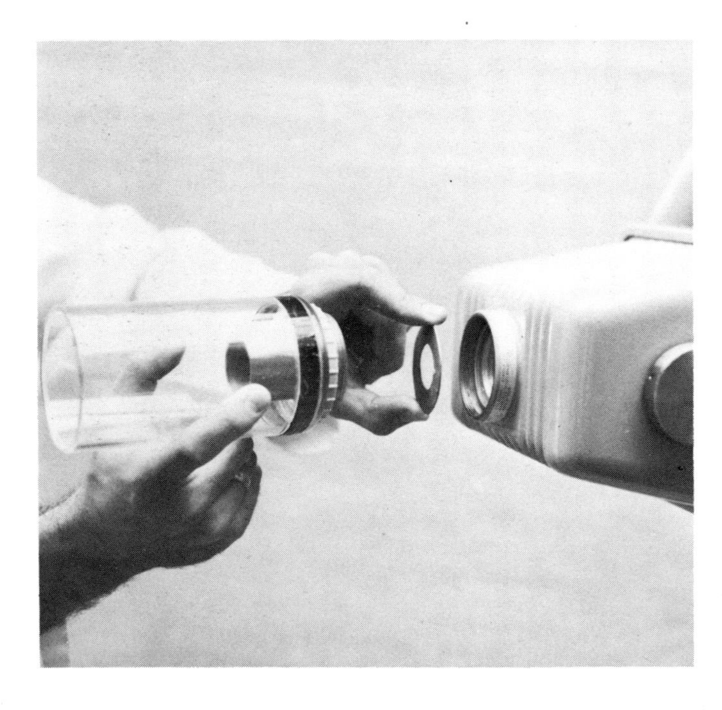

Figure 12–17. Lead collimating diaphragm being placed between exit port and base of cone of dental x-ray machine.

beam is larger the farther it is from the exit port. Different types of intraoral dental radiographic technics employ varying distances between the x-ray tube and the patient's skin. Regardless of the distance, the beam size at the patient's skin should be no more than 2¾ inches in diameter. A beam of this size is quite adequate to cover the regular periapical size of dental film which has a diagonal measurement of less than 2 inches (Figure 12–16). The correct beam size is achieved by placing a lead washer or diaphragm over the exit port (Figure 12–17). The size of the aperture in the diaphragm through which the x-ray beam emerges determines the size of the x-ray beam.

The benefit of reducing the size of the x-ray beam is to reduce the amount of tissue being irradiated. Technical excellence is necessary to avoid cone cutting with a small x-ray beam; however, proper alignment of a 2¾ inch wide x-ray beam to cover the film is easily achieved with little training and unnecessary irradiation of the patient is avoided.

Further collimation of the x-ray beam to the size of the periapical film is achieved with rectangular collimators (Figure 12–18). Rectangular collimators must be capable of pivoting to position the long dimension of the rectangle horizontally and vertically as the long dimension of the film changes position when used in the anterior and posterior regions of the patient's dentition. When rectangular collimation is used, the device holding the film in the patient's mouth must also indicate where the beam is to be positioned relative to the film.

Gonadal Shields. Many types of apron shields are commercially available (Figure 12–19). Some shields cover only the patient's gonadal area; others cover most of the torso. The shields are flexible and are manufactured with different x-ray absorbing abilities. Most dental shields are the equivalent of 0.25 mm thickness of lead. The effect of these shields is to absorb the scattered x rays.

The ratio of x-ray exposure to the patient's face and gonads differs between male and female. In the average male the gonadal exposure without shields is 1/40,000 the facial exposure. In the female, exposure of the reproductive cells is less because these cells lie deep within the body and are protected from scattered x rays originating in the x-ray

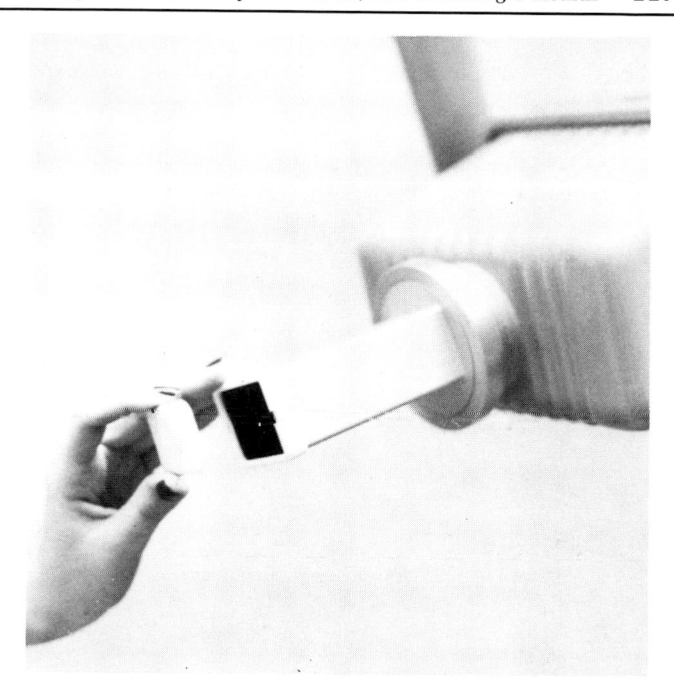

Figure 12–18. Rectangular metal collimator to restrict x-ray beam to size of periapical film.

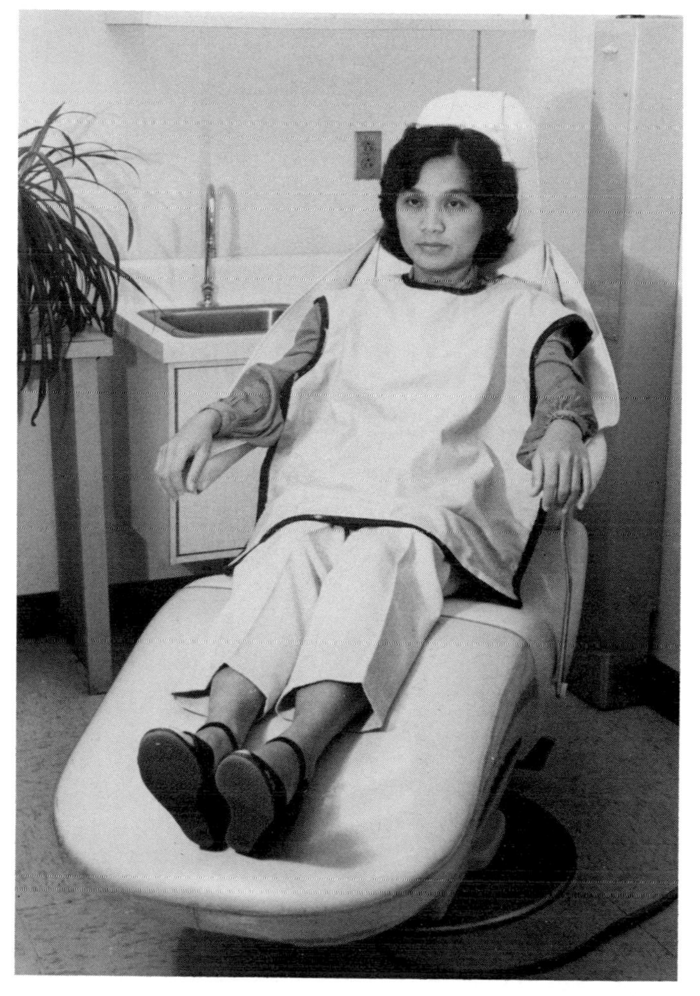

Figure 12–19. Patient prepared for dental radiography using gonadal shield that covers torso.

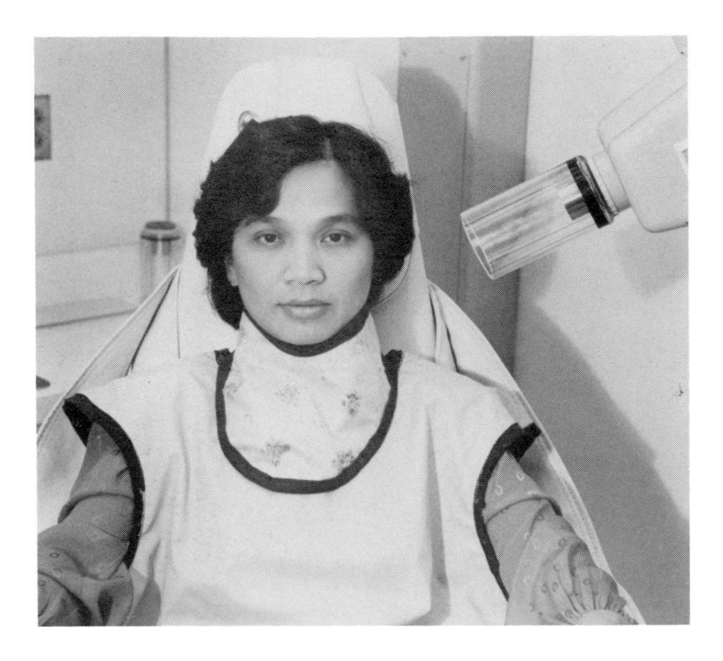

Figure 12–20. A separate thyroid shield used with a torso gonadal shield.

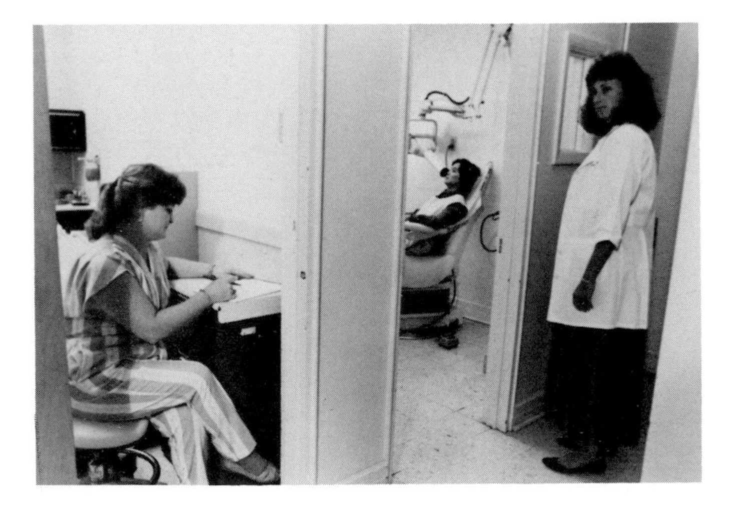

Figure 12–21. Careless technic during film exposure. Operator is not watching patient for movement that produces radiographic errors.

machine or the patient's head. Although the patient's gonadal dose during dental radiography is very small, the use of a gonadal shield will for all practical purposes eliminate this dose.

Thyroid Collars. Thyroid collars are shields similar to gonadal shields. They can be separate shields or be part of a gonadal shield (Figure 12–20). The collar covers the thyroid gland during radiography of the jaws and reduces radiation exposure of the gland. While thyroid disease has not been shown to be caused by the small exposure from dental x rays, collars further minimize patient exposure to x radiation.

Film Exposure Technic. Technical competence of the radiographer is essential. When films are exposed improperly, it is necessary to retake them (Figure 12–21); films that are ruined by improper processing procedures must also be taken again. Retaking radiographs exposes a patient to additional x rays and should be avoided, as the patient receives no benefit from the additional exposure. A good x-ray machine and proper darkroom equipment, in addition to technical competence of the operator, are necessary to achieve the goal of minimizing the patient's exposure to x rays.

Open-End Cones. With a pointed plastic cone on a dental x-ray machine it is necessary for the x rays to penetrate through the plastic of the cone, thus producing a small amount of scattered radiation. The use of an open-end cone achieves the same purpose as a pointed cone of locating the x-ray beam, without requiring the x rays to pass through any plastic material (Figure 12–22). The exposure of patient and operator to cone-scattered radiation is eliminated.

Tube-Patient Distance. Intraoral radiography is usually accomplished through the use of two basic technics, the bisecting-the-angle and the paralleling technics. The paralleling technic requires a distance of 16 to 20 inches between the x-ray tube and the patient's skin. The use of an extended distance reduces the amount of tissue in the primary x-ray beam without reducing the size of the beam at the patient's skin. The reduction is due to the fact that when the tube-patient distance is short the x-ray beam diverges more in the patient (Figure 12–23). It must be remembered that when one changes from the short

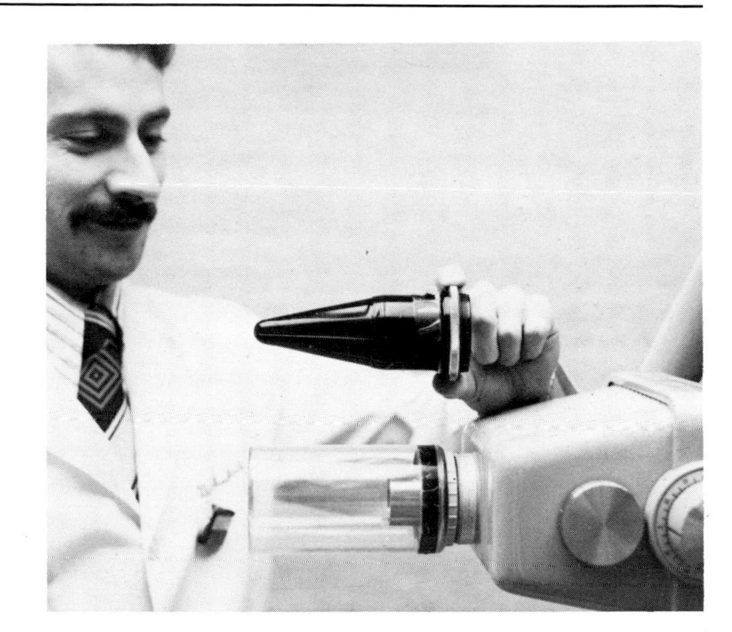

Figure 12–22. Pointed and open-end plastic beam locating cones. X-ray beam does not strike plastic of open-end cone (bottom) as it does in pointed type (top).

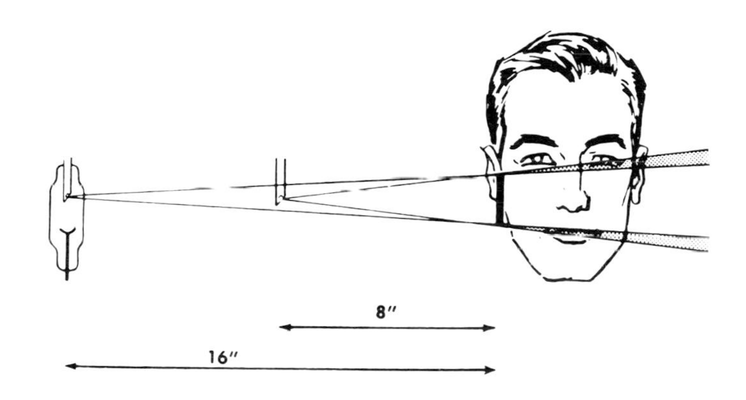

Figure 12–23. Diagram showing effect of using short and long tube-patient distances. Shaded area represents tissue irradiated by short-distance technic that is removed from the primary x-ray beam when long distance technic is used. (From Wuehrmann and Manson-Hing: Dental Radiology, 4th Ed., St. Louis, C.V. Mosby Company, 1977.)

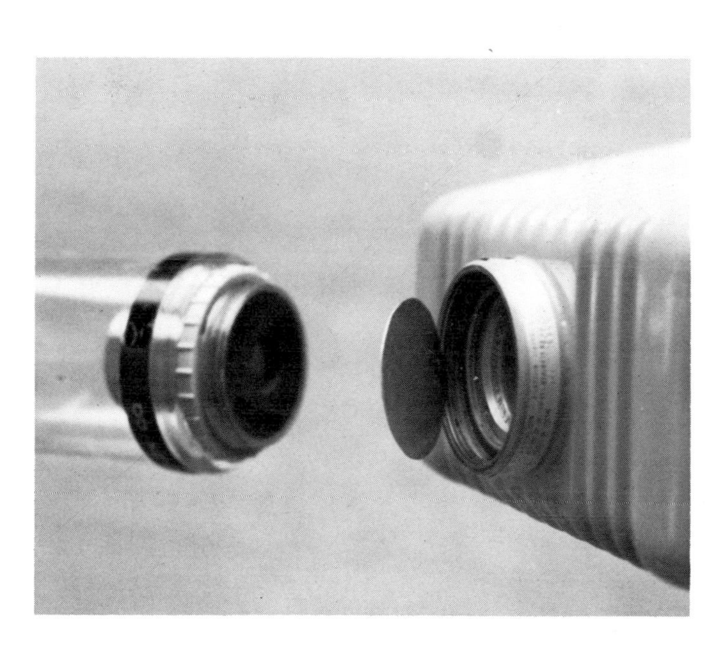

Figure 12–24. Recessing filter behind diaphragm in base of cone to absorb filter and x-ray tube scatter.

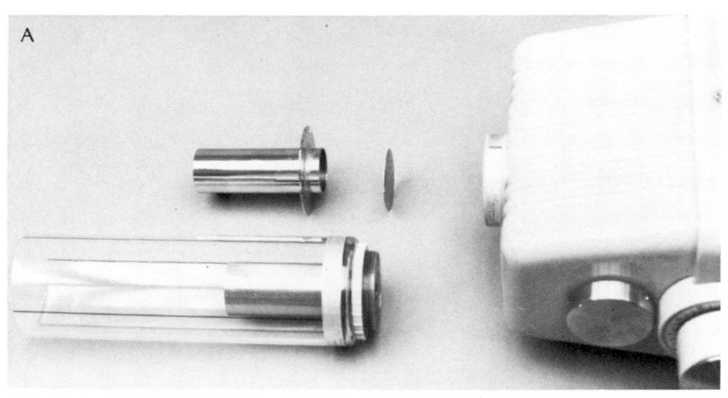

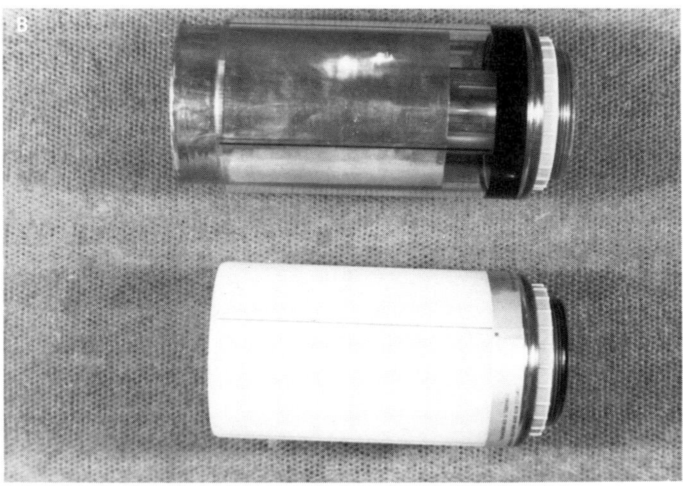

Figure 12–25. Other methods to reduce filter and x-ray tube scatter: A, Recessing filter behind metal cylinder collimator. B, Using either thin lead sleeve in open-end cone or cone made of lead-impregnated plastic.

to the long distance the collimator must be adjusted to maintain the 2¾ inch beam diameter at the patient's skin. In addition, the intensity of radiation is reduced in a ratio relative to the squares of the distances used (the inverse square law) and an increase in film exposure time will be necessary to maintain proper film density. The increased exposure time does not increase the radiation exposure to the patient's skin in this instance, because less intense radiation is being used.

Recessed Filters and Lead-Lined Cones. A certain amount of scattered x rays originates in the head of the machine, mainly through the irradiation of the x-ray tube and filter by the primary beam. Much of this radiation can be absorbed before it reaches the patient by positioning the filter between the collimating diaphragm and the head of the x-ray tube (Figure 12–24). A more efficient method of absorbing these x rays is to place a tube-shaped collimator made of a heavy metal in the plastic beam locating cone. A slight modification of the standard open-end cone can also reduce this scattered radiation; by lining the inside of the open-end cone with a thin sheet of lead or other heavy metal, most of this scatter is absorbed. Figure 12–25 shows such a metal lining.

Protection of the Operator

Before discussing procedures the operator can take to protect himself from dental x rays, it is best to identify the source of x rays to which the operator is exposed. The two most important sources are the primary x-ray beam and scatter radiation originating from the irradiated tissues of the patient. Other sources of lesser importance include leakage of radiation through the tubehead housing, scattered x rays from filters and cones, and scatter radiation coming from objects other than the patient, such as walls and furniture, that the primary beam may strike.

Procedures for protecting the operator include avoidance of the primary beam and contact with the tubehead, distance, shields, and position.

Avoiding the Primary Beam. The first and most important rule is to stay out of the primary x-ray beam. This means not only standing out of the beam but also never holding films for the patient.

Distance. The second important procedure is to move away from the other major source of radiation, namely, the patient's head. A minimum distance of 6 feet is recommended. The x-ray machine must be equipped with a coiled timer cord that can permit this distance. The effect of increasing the distance of the operator from the patient is to reduce the intensity of the scatter radiation reaching the operator (Figure 12–26).

Shields. In the event that the office design does not permit moving 6 feet away from the patient, the operator should stand behind an adequate shield. Such a shield should be at least as effective in absorbing dental x rays as 1-mm thick lead. The operator can still observe the patient during film exposure by having a leaded-glass window inserted in the shield. Such glass will absorb the x rays and still allow visible light to pass through (Figure 12–27).

Operator's Position. In addition to standing 6 feet from the patient, the operator may further reduce exposure by standing in certain areas relative to the patient during film exposure. As a general rule, the areas of least scatter are those that are at right angles to the patient from the x-ray beam and toward the back of the patient (Figure 12–28). Less scatter radiation reaches these areas because the scatter originates in the patient's oral tissues and must pass through the skull of the patient before it can get to these areas of the room.

Avoiding Holding the Tubehead. The x-ray tube housing does not absorb 100% of the x rays around the x-ray tube. A small amount of leakage radiation passes through every dental x-ray machine tubehead. The operator should not hold the x-ray tubehead during film exposure (Figure 12–29). If a machine's tubehead is not mechanically steady, it should be adjusted—a simple procedure.

Protection of the Environs

The primary beam of radiation should never be directed at anyone other than the patient. The patient should be so positioned that the x-ray beam is aimed at a wall of the room and not through a door or other opening to where people may be located.

Radiation Surveys. Dental x rays may pen-

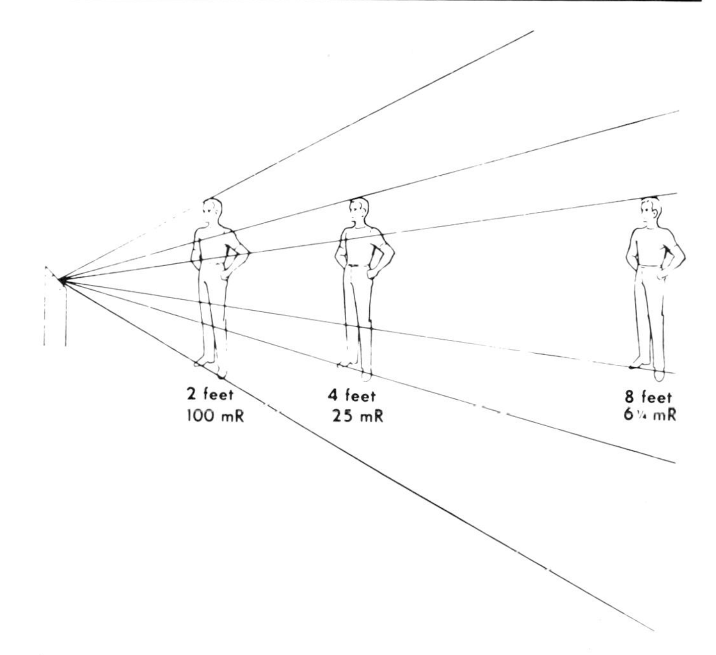

Figure 12–26. Diagram showing reduction in amount of radiation reaching operator when operator moves away from source of radiation. (From Wuehrmann and Manson-Hing: Dental Radiology, 4th Ed., St. Louis, C.V. Mosby Company, 1977.)

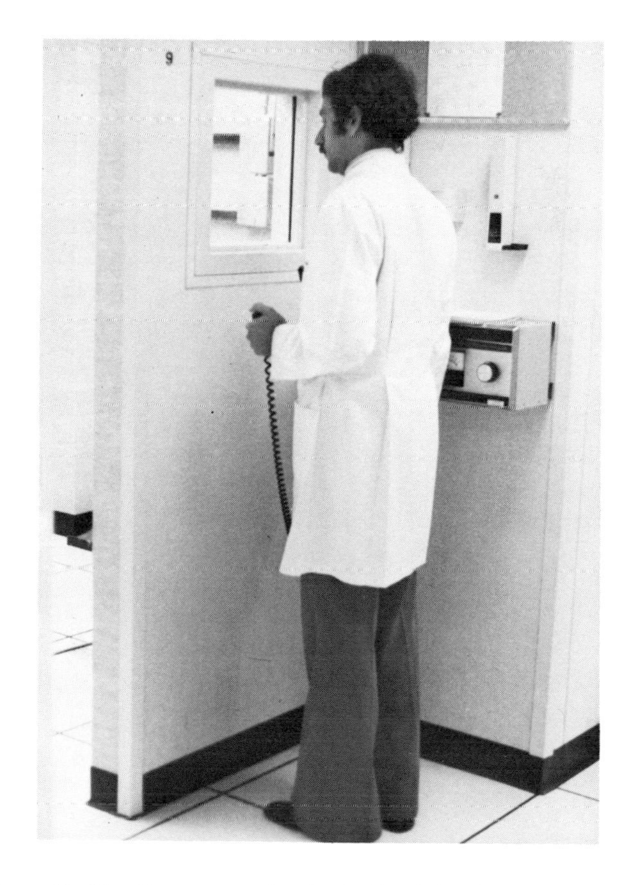

Figure 12–27. Operator standing behind lead shield and observing the patient through leaded glass window.

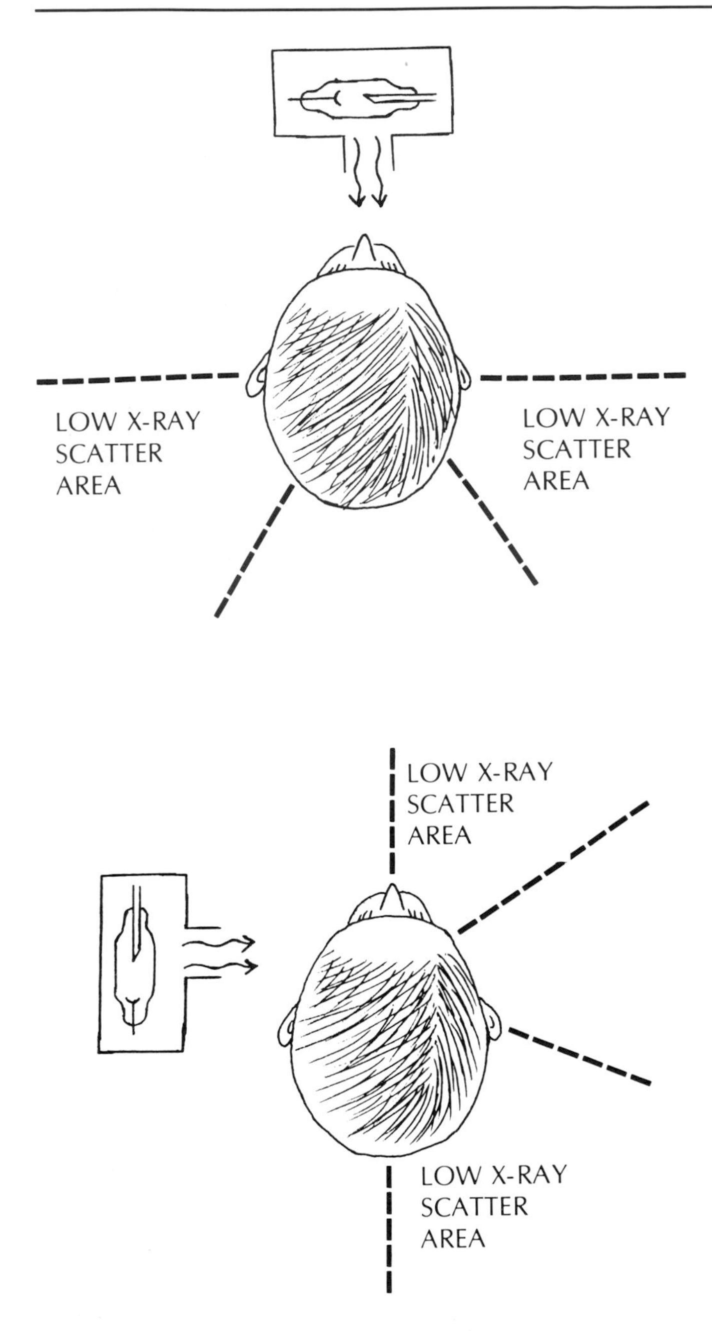

Figure 12–28. Diagram showing areas of less scatter radiation during radiography of anterior (top) and posterior (bottom) teeth.

etrate the walls of the operatory. If this occurs, people in adjacent rooms or corridors may be unnecessarily exposed (Figure 12–13). The amount of exposure is dependent upon many factors, such as the machine kilovoltage used, the work load of the x-ray machine, the x-ray absorbing ability of the walls, and the amount of time the adjacent areas are occupied by people. Due to the existence of so many variables, the exposure of the environs to x rays is best established through a radiation survey of these areas. The x-ray absorbing ability of the walls of any x-ray room can be easily measured with radiation measuring devices. Walls that are made of 3 inches of solid concrete, $\frac{3}{16}$-inch steel, or 1-millimeter lead will provide adequate protection for adjacent areas in even a very busy installation. Radiation surveys of x-ray rooms and x-ray machines are conducted by some state agencies.

Radiation Monitoring. Measuring the x-ray exposure of operators or associated personnel is a good protective measure. Monitoring can be done with small ion collection devices or film badges (Figure 12–30). A film badge uses a film similar to the intraoral dental film. The blackness or density of the processed film indicates the amount of radiation it has received. Many commercial firms supply film badges; the radiation protection committees of state dental societies can usually recommend one or more firms. A radiation measuring system controlled from outside of the dental office is recommended to avoid any bias in the x-ray measurements. It must be remembered that these devices measure x-ray exposure only to that area of the person where the device is worn. These instruments must be removed and placed in a radiation-safe place when the operator has radiographs made of himself. The instruments are designed to measure occupational x-ray exposure and not x rays used when the wearer is a patient.

RADIOLOGIC HEALTH

The use of diagnostic x rays in dentistry is of great value and the information gained through their use benefits the patient, but exposure of the patient to even these small amounts of x rays may involve some element of risk. Thus radiographs are made when it is anticipated that the information they can provide for the good of the patient will outweigh the possible hazard (Figure 12–12). When a dentist prescribes a radiograph for a patient the diagnostic yield can be evaluated in terms of the information gained by the dentist, information altering the patient's treatment or demonstrated patient benefit. While there is a great amount of information showing the value of radiographs in patient care, there is little scientific data measuring diagnostic yield. It is therefore difficult to predict the probability of a particular radiograph, made on a particular patient, to show information that will benefit the patient. Professional judgment is essential in this type of situation.

Patient damage from the low x-ray exposures used in dental radiography has not been observed clinically; thus the risk of a deleterious effect is not directly measurable. The hazard is in the possible occurrence of a harmful effect that could be observed at a later date. The risk of an effect is estimated or predicted from measurements of the effect occurring with high doses of radiation. In projecting (extrapolating) the risk from high dose evidence, a linear dose-response relationship is usually used since this expresses a "worst possible" situation in the unknown region of low dose effects. One example is risk calculations derived from the measured frequency of two cancer cases, per rad, per year, when ten million (10^7) people receive external x-rays to the thyroid gland.*

The calculated prediction is that if 10^7 people receive 1 R (2.58×10^{-4} EU) to the thyroid, there will be 50 cancer cases in the next 25 years or 100 cancer cases in the next 50 years (Figure 12–31). The prediction may also be 1 cancer case in the next 50 years if 10^6 people receive 10 mR (2.58×10^{-6} EU), or 1 cancer case in the next 50 years if 10^7 people receive 1 mR (2.58×10^{-7} EU), or 1 cancer case in the next 50 years if 10^9 people receive .01 mR (2.58×10^{-9} EU). A similar calculation for dental radiographs is 3 cases per 21 intraoral radiographs, per 25 years, per 10^6 people.†

*National Academy of Sciences: The effects on populations of exposure to low levels of ionizing radiation. National Research Council, Washington, D.C., 1972.

†Gregg, E.: Radiation risks and diagnostic x-rays. Radiology, *123*:447, 1977.

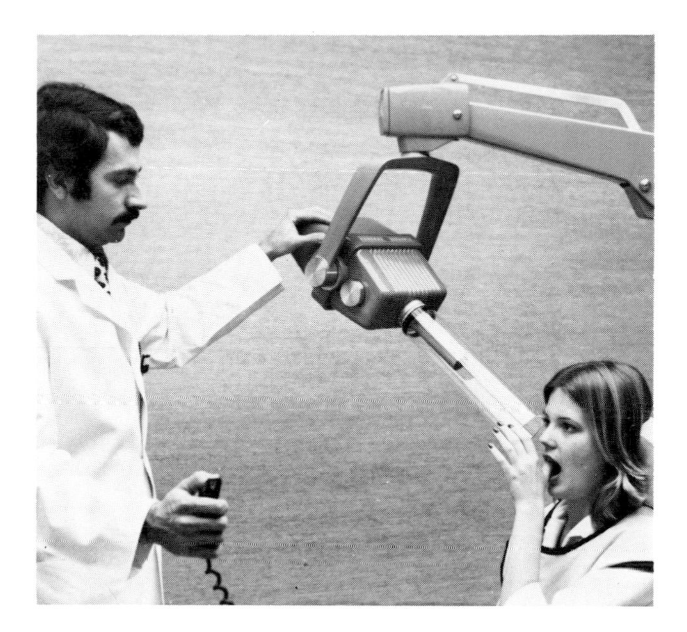

Figure 12–29. Improper technic for stabilizing x-ray tubehead during film exposure. Machine should be leveled and moving joints adjusted.

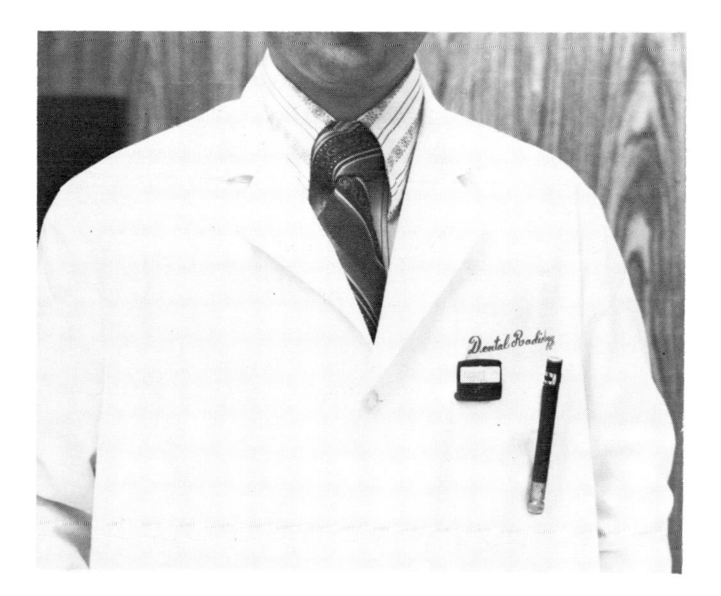

Figure 12–30. Operator wearing radiation film badge and ion collection monitoring device.

Calculated Frequency in 10 Million Exposed People

2 thyroid cancers per rad (1 c Gy) per year
50 thyroid cancers per rad (1 c Gy) in 25 years
100 thyroid cancers per rad (1 c Gy) in 50 years
1 thyroid cancer per 10 mR (0.01 c Gy) in 50 years

Figure 12–31. Examples of the same increase in the frequency of thyroid cancer when ten million people are exposed to x rays.

If the radiation used results in the probability of increasing the number of cancers, by as much as the number of cancers occurring naturally, the use of the radiation would have to be evaluated critically. In general, the calculations for cancers caused by diagnostic x-ray doses increases the possible occurrence of a cancer very little over the number of cancers occurring in patients not receiving the radiation. The small increase over natural occurrence makes it impossible to prove if the type of mathematical projection used is valid.

Regardless of the validity of mathematical projections, investigators continue to apply the calculations to radiation effects; this results in comparisons of the risks of a particular deleterious effect occurring from different causes. For example, a risk estimate of one in a million of dying can be from living 2 days in New York City (from air pollution), living 2 months in Denver (from cosmic radiation), living in a stone building for 2 months (from radioactivity), traveling 300 miles in a car (from an accident), traveling 6,000 miles in a plane (from cosmic radiation), smoking 3 cigarettes (from cancer and heart disease), drinking 30 cans of diet soda (from carcinogens), etc.[z] A similar one in a million risk has been expressed for the chance of a cancer occurring from a dental radiographic examination;* the actual risk may be much less than one in a million. However, since the effects of very low x-ray doses are unknown, it is a prudent public health policy to assume that there is some risk.

Risk assessments vary widely among researchers and cannot be considered very good but is the best that can be done at this time. In everyday living, people are exposed to many dangerous situations involving risks of one in a million. Little attention is paid to situations with such low levels of risk unless someone perceives a risk in a particular situation and ignores the existence of a multitude of similar risks. Dental radiographs are safer than many of the normal risks of daily life. However, dental radiation hazards will

Maximum Permissible Dose (MPD)

1 week	13 wk period	Yearly
100 mR	3 R	5 R
2.58×10^{-5} EU	77.4×10^{-5} EU	129×10^{-5} EU
1 mGy	12.5 mGy	50 mGy

Maximum Accumulated Dose (MAD)
$5 \times (N - 18)R$
N = Operator's age

Maximum Dose During Pregnancy
5 m Sievert (0.5 Rem or 500 mR)

Figure 12–32. Radiation dose limits for operators of x-ray equipment.

[z]Wilson, R.: Risks caused by low levels of pollution. Yale. J. Biol. Med. *51*:37, 1978.

*ADA Council on Dental Materials, Instruments and Equipment: Biological effects of radiation from dental radiography. J.A.D.A. *105*:275, 1982.

remain controversial since it cannot be established when such a biologic risk becomes a human health hazard.

Operator's X-Ray Exposure Guidelines

The United States National Council on Radiation Protection recommends that radiation workers not be exposed to more than 5 R (12.9×10^{-4} EU) per year (or approximately 100 milliroentgens or 0.258×10^{-4} EU per week). This is sometimes called the *maximum permissible dose* (MPD). There is no reason for dental radiographers to be exposed to one-third of this dose, even in a busy office, if proper protective procedures are followed. Should the operator receive more than 3 R (7.74×10^{-4} EU) in any 13-week period, he should avoid further x-ray exposure until his total for the year falls below what he would have received at the rate of 5 R (12.9×10^{-4} EU) per year. Temporarily exceeding these limits does not mean that biologic effects will appear in the exposed person. The limits are designed to keep the mutational effects of x rays on the entire population to a level considered acceptable. In addition to the above guidelines, radiation workers must not exceed an accumulated lifetime exposure of 5 × (operator's age − 18) roentgens. This formula is called the *maximum accumulated dose* (MAD) and indicates that an x-ray worker must be at least 18 years old (Figure 12–32). The unborn baby of a pregnant worker has a special limit of 0.5 rem (5 mSv). Occupational health authorities require radiation workers exposed to more than 25 mR (64.5×10^{-7} EU) per week to wear a monitoring device. Local and state regulatory agencies may establish more stringent and additional guidelines to those presented in this chapter.

Patient Exposure Guidelines

No limit has been established for the amount of radiation the patient is exposed to for diagnostic purposes. However, before prescribing radiographs a dentist must examine the patient to determine if anticipated patient benefit from radiographs will outweigh potential hazards from x-ray exposure.

One guideline for radiology students is that the student should not be used as a patient for x-ray technic training purposes unless the student has a diagnostic need for the radiographs and the radiographs must be interpreted by a dentist.

Organ systems provide vital functions for the human body and information of radiation effects on these organs is of importance in controlling the use of x rays. In dental radiography, the critical organs are the gonads, bone marrow, thyroid gland, and eyes.

Gonadal Exposure. A study in 1958* indicated that the testes of male dental patients receive 1:10,000 of the x-ray dose delivered to the face. A 1970 study† using advanced measuring devices indicated a 1:40,000 relationship of facial to testes dose. Male and female gonadal doses differ due to the external body location of male gonads and the internal body location of female ovaries with protective overlying tissue. The female ovaries receive a dose that is 5 times less than the male testes.‡

Depending on the radiographic technic and equipment used, the patient's face is exposed to 100 to 900 mR (2.58×10^{-5} to 23.26×10^{-5} EU) per intraoral radiograph. Good technic alone (without the use of a gonadal shield) can restrict the male genetic exposure for a complete set of intraoral radiographs to less than 0.3 mR or 7.74×10^{-8} EU (the dose is calculated on a 1:10,000 face to testes relationship and is probably much less). A dose of 0.3 mR (7.74×10^{-8} EU) is the same exposure the average person gets from background radiation every day; background radiation comes from the sun and radioactive materials in the earth and averages 0.3 mR (7.74×10^{-8} EU) per day at sea level. The dose to the female ovaries is equivalent to a few hours of background radiation. Reported estimates of ovaries exposure range from .03 to .1 mR (7.74×10^{-9} to 2.58×10^{-8} EU). A

*Richards, A.G.: Roentgen-ray doses in dental roentgenography. J.A.D.A. *56*:351, 1958.

†Klein, A.B., et al: Dosimetric evaluation of thirty dental facilities in Massachusetts. Oral Surg. *29*:44, 1970.

‡Stanford, R.W., and Vance, J.: Quantity of radiation received by reproductive organs of patients during routine diagnostic x-ray examinations. Brit. J. Radiol. *28*:266, 1955.

medical radiography guide* indicates that in estimating gonadal doses during radiography of the skull with 1 R (2.58×10^{-4} EU), no detectable contribution is made to the testes, ovaries or embryo dose. In complete mouth dental radiography only a small area of the face receives 1 R (2.58×10^{-4} EU). It is possible that the dental radiographic genetic hazard is greatly overestimated when the 1 to 10,000 facial-reproductive organ exposure relationship is used. However, any overestimation would provide an extra margin of safety for dental radiography. The use of a gonadal shield would, for all practical purposes, eliminate this already small possible hazard.

Bone Marrow Exposure. Severe injury to the bone marrow or blood forming organ occurs when the entire body is exposed to more than 200 R (5.16×10^{-2} EU). A small increase in the number of leukemia cases has been reported when the entire blood or a large portion of the bone marrow has been exposed to radiation doses approaching the diagnostic range (e.g., chest radiography). These data give some cause for concern regarding bone marrow exposure. The chest contains 50% of the body's bone marrow while the head contains 13% and the mandible 1.2%. A bone marrow dose of 13 milliRads (13×10^{-5} Gy) for complete mouth radiographs and 147 mRads (147×10^{-5} Gy) for a chest survey have been reported.† It appears that the risk of leukemia from dental x rays is small.

Thyroid Exposure. Patients receiving radiation therapy to the head in childhood appear to have a small increase (about .0006%) in the occurrence of thyroid cancer. Some patients had calculated thyroid doses as low as 10 rads (10 cGy). This has produced some concern regarding radiation exposure of the thyroid during dental radiography. In complete mouth dental radiography the reported thyroid dose is approximately 40 mR (40×10^{-5} Gy). The risk of serious injury to a pa-

*Handbook of selected organ doses for projections common in diagnostic radiology. HEW Publication (FDA), 76–8031, May, 1976.

†US Dept. HEW. The mean active bone marrow dose to the adult population of the United States from diagnostic radiology. FDA Pub. 77–8013, Washington, D.C., 1977.

tient from thyroid exposure during dental radiography is small.

Eye Exposure. Cataracts of the lens of the eye can occur at x-ray doses above 500 rads (5 Gy). In complete mouth radiography using high speed film the total amount of radiation measured at the end of the cone is 3 to 4 roentgens (7.74×10^{-7} to 10.32×10^{-7} EU). Proper radiography would expose the lens of the eye to only scatter radiation of a few mR. If the eye is in the primary beam, the exposure will be a few hundred mR during the exposure of a single film. There has been relatively little concern expressed about eye x-ray exposure.

Parotid Gland Exposure. A recent study has statistically associated parotid gland tumors with dental x-ray exposures of 50 rads (0.5 Gy) or more. There was no association with cumulative doses below 50 rads of radiation. This dose is far in excess of the approximately 0.1 rad (1×10^{-3} Gy) that part of the parotid receives in present day complete mouth and panoramic radiography. No real concern for the parotid glands has been expressed relative to properly made dental radiographs.

The ALARA Concept. Research studies measuring the risks of x-ray exposure for increased occurrence of cancers, birth defects, cataracts, and lifespan shortening have been controversial and are not conclusive. However, the information does indicate that there is a relationship between x-ray exposure and deleterious effects. The information is obtained mainly from animal experiments designed to identify such a relationship and from mass surveys of humans who have been exposed to x rays for other purposes. In 1968 the American Dental Association had no knowledge of any death or serious injury resulting to a patient from a dental radiographic examination.* While clinical cases of radiation damage from dental x rays have not been reported, it cannot be proved that there is no possibility of a hazard to the patient. This situation has produced the concept of keeping radiation exposure *as low as reasonably achievable.* The concept is commonly referred to as the ALARA principle. It obviously involves dentists who prescribe

*ADA criticizes magazine article on radiographs. J.A.D.A., *76*:1310, 1968.

radiographs and auxiliaries who make radiographs. Radiation hygiene must be practiced in the dental office to minimize the use of x rays and maximize the diagnostic information obtained from radiographs. When discussing the subject of low level radiation hazards, it must be noted that one is dealing with estimates and personal perceptions since few established scientific facts are available.

Procedures to minimize x-ray use have already been presented in this chapter. Maximizing diagnostic information include proper viewing and interpretation of the radiographs by a knowledgeable diagnostician. In minimizing the use of x rays attention is now being paid to the prescribing of radiographs. Guidelines have been developed to prevent the radiography of patients when the patient does not receive benefit from the radiographs. The guidelines indicate that dental radiographs are not to be made for administrative purposes and that radiographs should be prescribed with the use of patient selection criteria. Some criteria recommended are as follows:

For new patients, (1) posterior bitewing radiographs for children with primary dentition, (2) an individualized periapical/occlusal examination with posterior bitewing radiographs or a panoramic examination with posterior bitewing radiographs for children with transitional dentition, (3) selected periapical films with posterior bitewings for adolescents with unerupted third molars, (4) selected periapical films with posterior bitewings for dentulous adults, (5) complete mouth intraoral or a panoramic radiographic examination for edentulous patients.

For recall patients, (1) posterior bitewings at 6-month intervals for children with clinical caries or with increased risk of developing caries, (2) posterior bitewings at 6- to 12-month intervals for adolescents with clinical caries or with increased risk of caries development, (3) posterior bitewings at 12- to 18-month intervals for adults with clinical caries or increased risk of developing caries, (4) no radiographic examination for edentulous adults without clinical signs or symptoms, (5) posterior bitewings at 12- to 24-month intervals for children with primary or transitional dentition without clinical caries and high risk for caries development, (6) posterior bitewings at 18- to 36-month intervals for adolescents without clinical caries and high risk for caries development, (7) posterior bitewings at 24- to 36-month intervals for dentulous adults without clinical caries and high risk of caries development.

For patients with periodontal problems an individualized radiographic examination consisting of selected periapical and/or bitewing radiographs of areas with clinical evidence or a history of periodontal disease is recommended. Radiographs made for assessment of growth and development (i.e., in patients without clinical signs or symptoms) are limited to the initial diagnostic survey in children with primary dentition; a periapical, occlusal or panoramic examination after eruption of the first permanent tooth, and a single set of periapical films of the third molar areas or a single panoramic examination between ages 16 and 19.

Chapter 13

Fast Exposure and Localization Technics

Many patients, for a variety of reasons, require the operator to place the film in the mouth, align the x-ray beam, expose the film, and remove the film from the mouth in a very short period of time. The patient may be a gagger, spastic or hyperactive, or may be under general anesthesia. Modification of the standard intraoral technics for quick film exposure will be discussed in this chapter. In addition, the technics often needed to locate the position of objects within bone will be presented.

FAST EXPOSURE TECHNIC

Preset Patient and Machine

To minimize the time that the film is in contact with the patient's oral tissues the operator should correctly position the patient, make all necessary machine kVp, mA, and time adjustments, and position the x-ray beam in the probable beam alignment before placing the film in the patient's mouth (Figure 13–1). The patient must be taught ahead of time what he or she will be required to do to keep the film in position (Figure 13–2). The operator must be knowledgeable and technically proficient to position the film quickly and accurately in the proper position with the minimum shifting of the film around the patient's mouth.

Quick Angulation Technic

When the film has been placed in the patient's mouth and is being held in position by the patient, the operator must very quickly position the x-ray beam. Some technical accuracy is sacrificed in order to obtain quick x-ray beam alignment.

The horizontal angulation is achieved by placing the horizontal edge of the open end of the cone parallel to the buccal surfaces of the teeth being radiographed (Figure 13–3). This method can be applied in all areas of

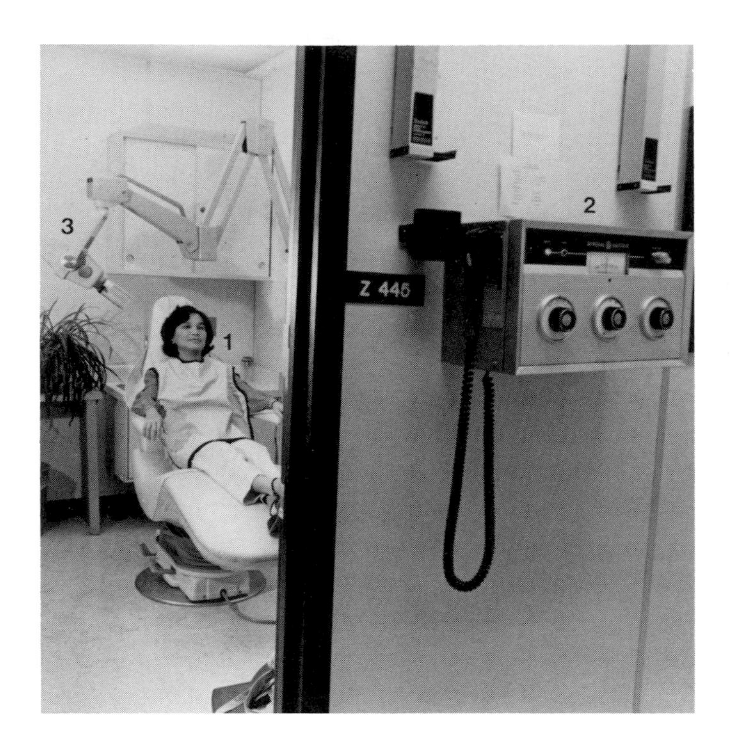

Figure 13–1. Pre-film placement procedures for fast film exposure: (1) position patient, (2) adjust machine factors, (3) align x-ray beam.

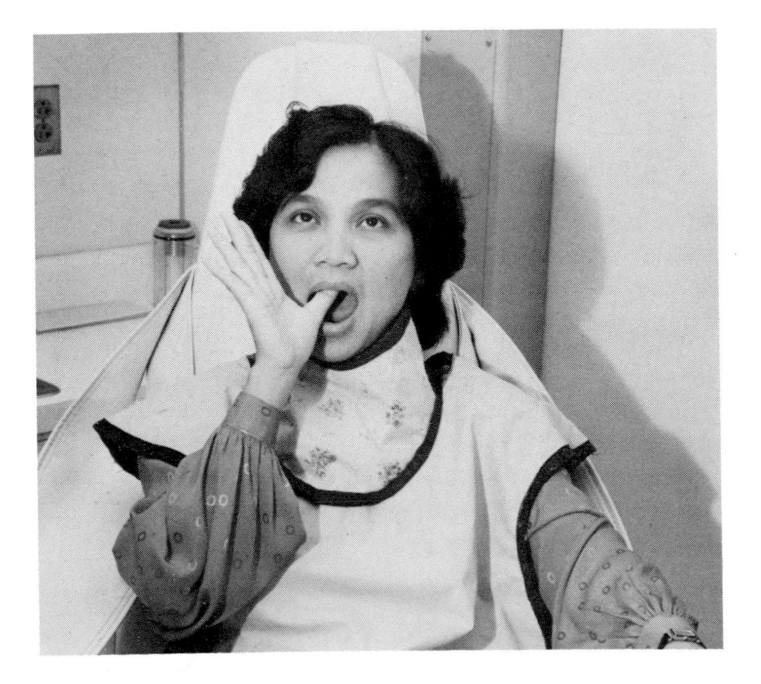

Figure 13–2. Patient ready to hold film in place prior to insertion of film into mouth.

the mouth to produce useful radiographs in most cases.

The vertical angulation is achieved through knowledge of the approximate anatomic position of the long axes of the teeth (review Chapter 4) and an observation of the film's position. For maxillary molars and bicuspids the vertical angulation is obtained by placing the vertical edge of the open-end cone parallel to a line joining the inner or medial corner of the opposite eye to the crowns of the molars (Figure 13–4). This line of the patient's face is quickly identified. It is close to the bisector of the angle formed by the film and long axes of the teeth. The line is approximate to the bisector of the angle because the inner corner of the opposite eye is between the top of the head (where the long axes of the teeth are directed toward the sagittal plane from the crowns) and the top of the palate (where the film is directed toward the sagittal plane from the crowns of the teeth). This technic tends to produce a slightly greater than normal vertical angulation. The greater angulation gives a margin of error to avoid retakes caused by underangulation; however, it is usually not the ideal angulation.

Quick vertical angulation for the maxillary cuspid is similar to that for the bicuspids and molars, but the vertical edge of the cone is placed parallel to a line joining tooth's cusp to the outer edge of the opposite eye of the patient (Figure 13–5).

Quick vertical angulation for maxillary and mandibular incisors cannot use anatomic landmarks unless the long axes of the teeth are in normal positions. Since the direction of the long axes of anterior teeth vary greatly among patients, another method is used to obtain the approximate vertical angulation. This involves two steps. First, the vertical edge of the cone is positioned parallel to the film; this procedure locates the vertical angulation as being greater than the angle needed and is accomplished quickly. Secondly, the vertical angle is reduced by approximately 15 degrees; the reduction is half of the average angle existing between the long axes of the teeth and the film (Figure 13–6). These steps can be accomplished in a few seconds. If the operator can quickly assess the tooth-film angle as being larger or smaller than normal, he can adjust the an-

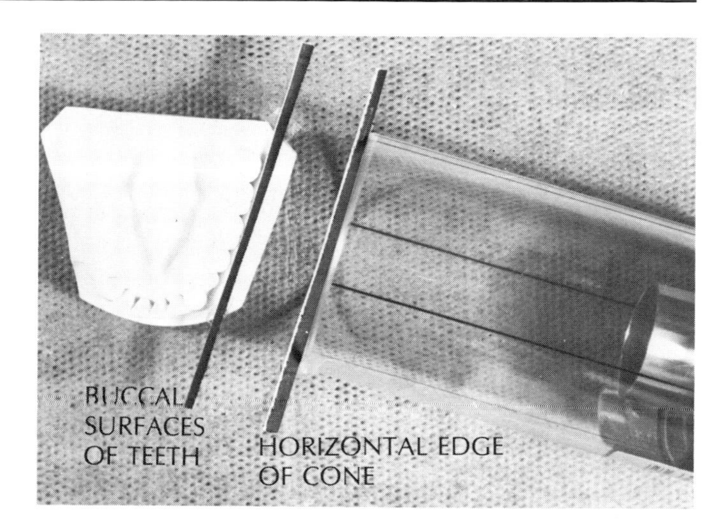

Figure 13–3. Alignment of horizontal angle.

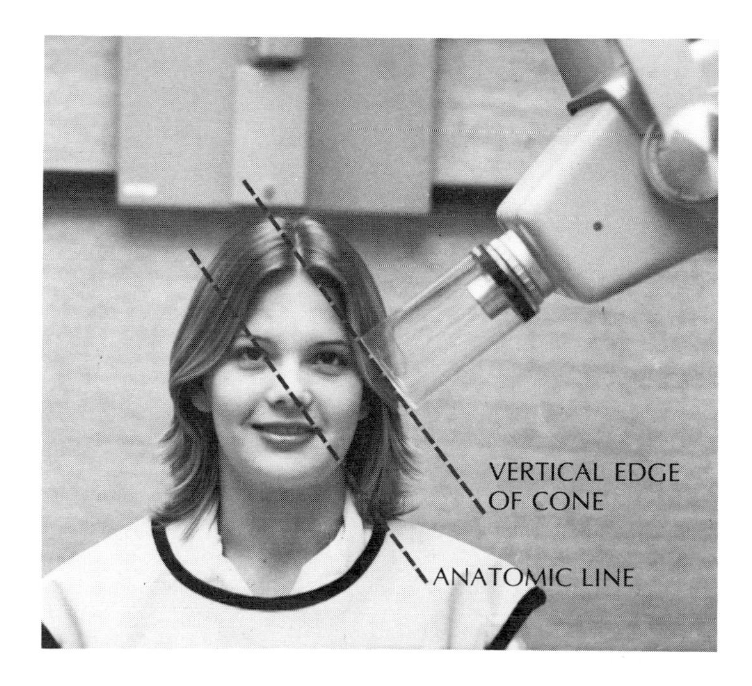

Figure 13–4. Quick alignment of vertical angle for maxillary posterior teeth.

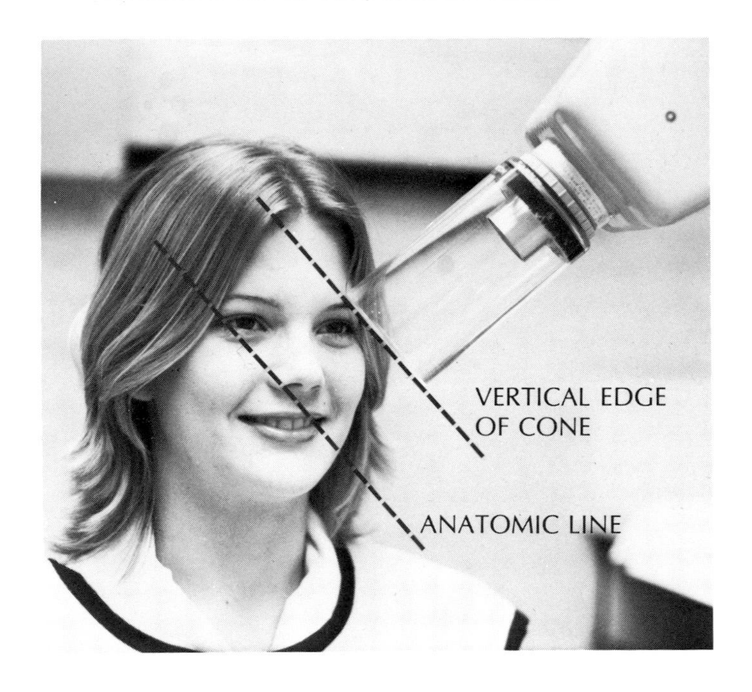

Figure 13–5. Quick alignment of vertical angle for maxillary cuspids.

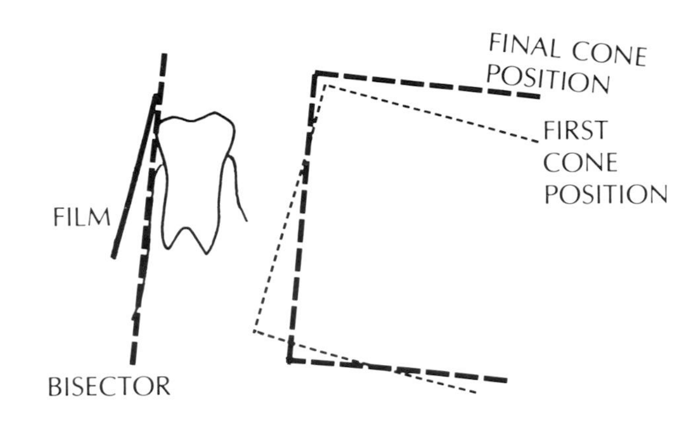

Figure 13–7. Quick vertical angulation for mandibular posterior teeth.

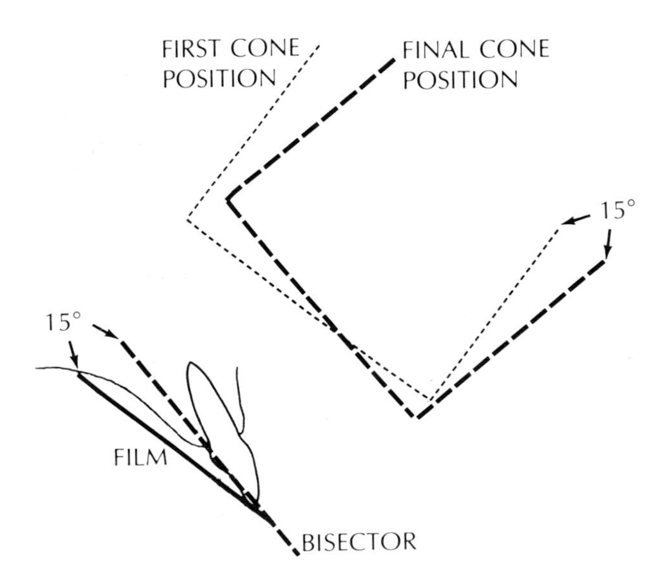

Figure 13–6. Quick vertical angulation for maxillary anterior teeth. A similar procedure is used for mandibular anterior teeth.

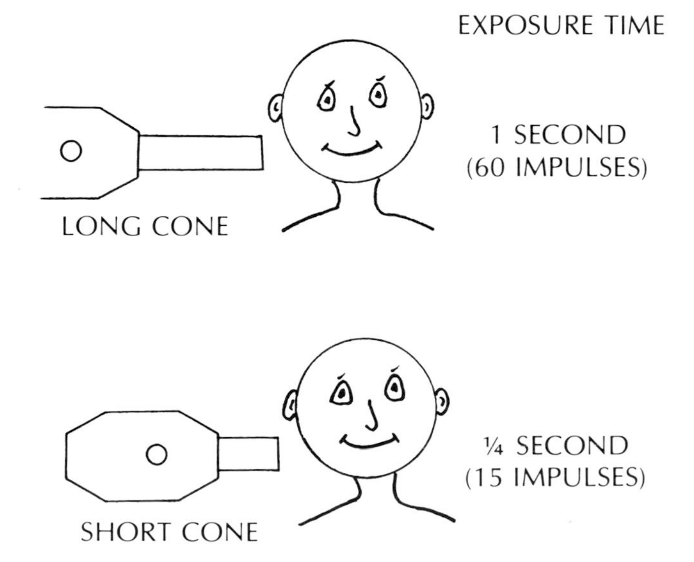

Figure 13–8. Use of short cone distance to reduce film exposure time.

gular change from step 1 to step 2 much more accurately.

Quick vertical angulation of mandibular posterior teeth is accomplished in a manner similar to that for anterior teeth, but the angular reduction between steps 1 and 2 is only a few degrees (Figure 13–7). There is usually only a small tooth-film angle in this region of the mouth. In most instances a useful diagnostic radiograph can be made with the vertical edge of the cone parallel to the film.

Short Film Exposure Time

The patient, film, and x-ray tubehead need to be motionless only during film exposure. At other times, the patient's movement does not produce a blurred radiograph. There are many patients who cannot hold perfectly still or cannot remain motionless for the film exposure time used with the normal radiographic technic. With such patients it is often advantageous to use a short exposure time.

Film speed directly affects exposure time. The fastest film that can produce good quality radiographs should be used. Using a fast, instead of a slower speed dental film can reduce exposure time as much as 75%.

If the operator normally uses a 16-inch tube-film distance, the use of an 8-inch distance with a short cone will place the film in the x-ray beam where the radiation is more intense; thus a shorter film exposure time can be used (Figure 13–8). Since the intensity of radiation is inversely proportional to the square of the distance, the exposure time is reduced to ¼ of the time used at 16 inches when the film is placed 8 inches from the x-ray tube. When distance is changed and all other factors remain constant, the new exposure time can be calculated from a simple formula (new distance^2 divided by old distance^2 multiplied by old time equals new time).

The ability to increase milliamperage and kilovoltage is available on some dental x-ray machines. When mA is increased, more x rays per second are produced and exposure time can be reduced accordingly. For example, if an exposure of 1 second is used at 10 mA, then ⅔ second can be used with 15 mA (Figure 13–9).

Increased kilovoltage results in the production of x rays having greater energy,

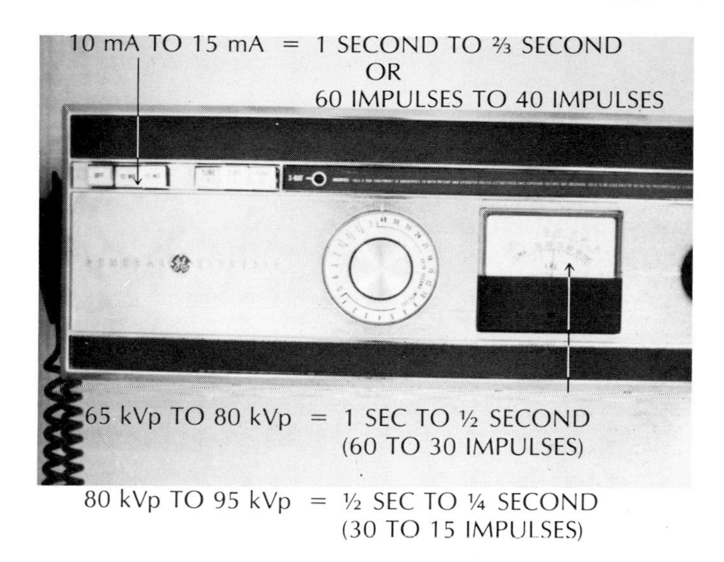

Figure 13–9. Reduction in exposure time by increasing milliamperage and kilovoltage.

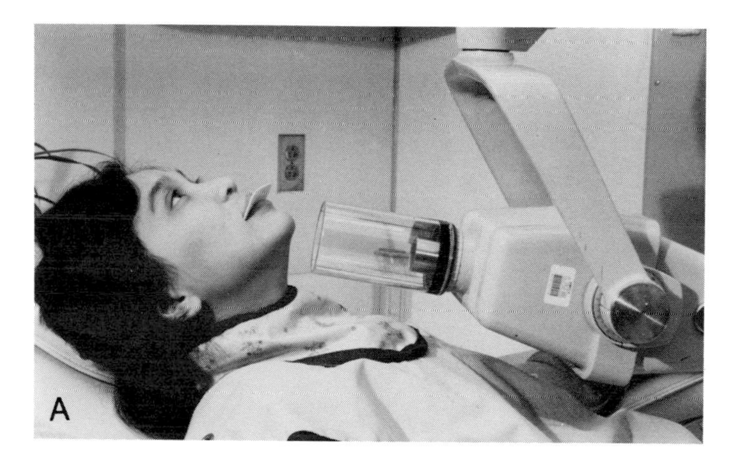

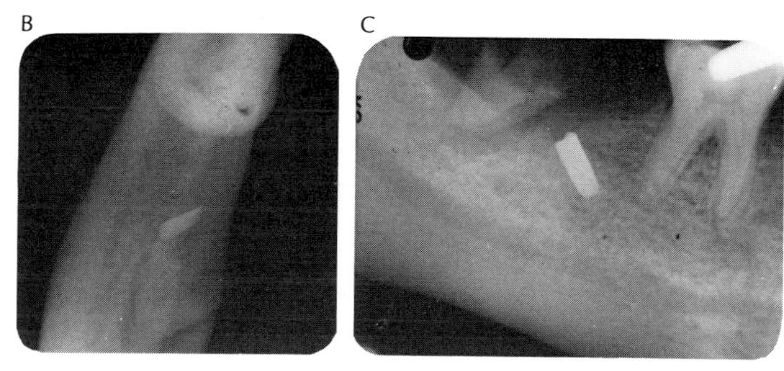

Figure 13–10. A, Technic for making cross-section view of body of mandible. B, Resultant radiograph showing medial-lateral positions of teeth and other structures. C, Standard periapical radiograph of area shown in B. Viewing B and C together helps to identify location of broken instrument within bone.

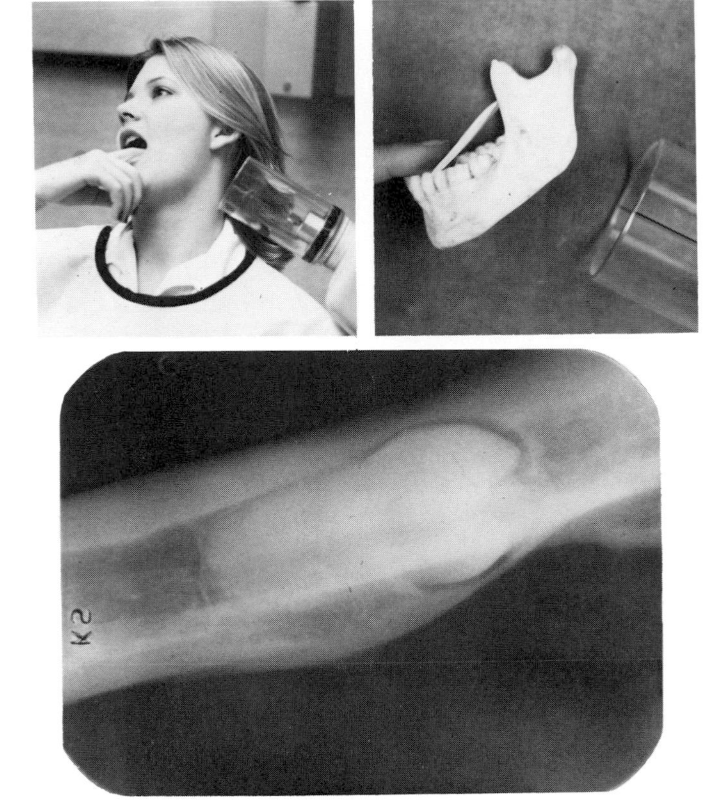

Figure 13–11. Modified cross-section technic for impacted mandibular third molar; cross-section radiograph.

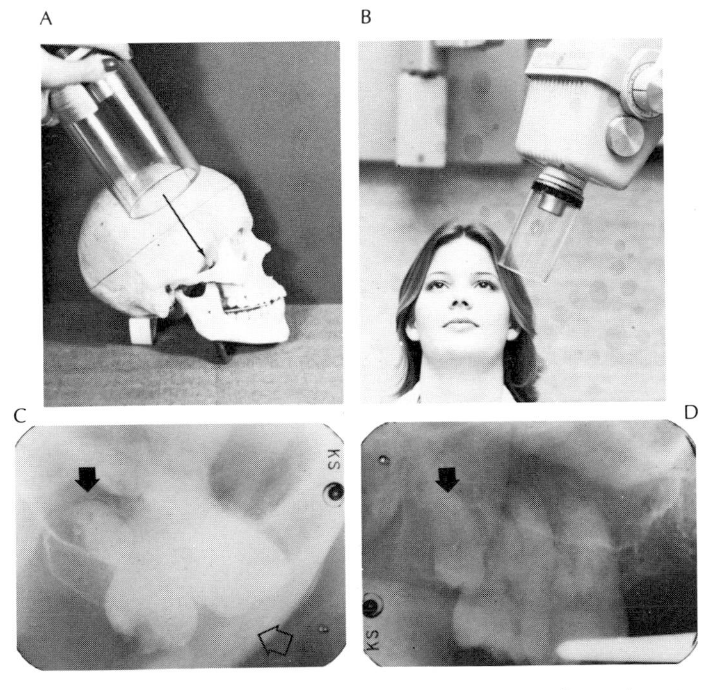

Figure 13–12. Modified cross-section technic of maxillary tuberosity area. A, Direction of central ray. B, Position of x-ray cone and patient. Film is in occlusal plane in molar region. C, Radiograph made with modified cross-section technic showing zygomatic arch (outlined arrow) buccal to erupted molars and palatally positioned impacted third molar (solid arrow). D, Standard periapical radiograph showing impacted third molar without information about palatal or buccal location of impacted tooth.

shorter wavelength, and more penetrating power. An increase of 13 to 15 kVp (depending upon the efficiency of the x-ray machine being used) permits a reduction by 50% in the exposure time (Figure 13–9).

When fast film (ANS speed group D) is used with an 8-inch tube-film distance, 15 mA, and 100 kVp, the exposure time is reduced to between $^{1}/_{30}$ and $^{1}/_{8}$ second (2 to 7 impulses) depending upon the size of the patient. To use these short exposure times the operator must have available an x-ray machine that has an accurate electronic timer. Note that if 1 impulse is needed and the machine produces 2 instead, the error in film exposure is 100%.

LOCALIZATION TECHNICS

It is often important to establish the location of objects seen in intraoral radiographs. The standard periapical radiograph shows teeth, bone, and foreign objects in only two dimensions, namely, superior-inferior and anterior-posterior relationships. The medial-lateral relationships of the objects are not seen. Two basic technics are used to obtain the needed information, the right-angle technic and the tube-shift technic.

Right-Angle Technic

The technic uses two radiographs made separately with the films positioned at right angles to each other. One film is usually the standard intraoral radiograph. The other radiograph is made with the film positioned in the occlusal plane and the x-ray beam directed perpendicular to the film (Figure 13–10). This projection is often called a cross-sectional or cross-fire view and shows the medial-lateral positions of the teeth and adjacent objects.

When the mediolateral position of an impacted mandibular third molar needs to be determined, the technic is slightly modified. The film cannot be placed posteriorly enough to be over the impacted tooth because of interference by the anterior border of the ramus. The posterior border of the film is thus elevated above the occlusal plane on the anterior border of the ramus and the central ray is directed perpendicular to the film from the angle of the mandible (Figure 13–11). The film is held in position by the patient. It is often advantageous to turn the patient's head away from the side being examined to produce adequate space behind the ramus where the cone of the x-ray machine must be positioned.

The right-angle technic can be used in locating objects in the mandible; it cannot be used in the maxilla because to make the cross-sectional radiograph the x-ray beam would have to pass through the anterior part of the skull, plus the nasal and maxillary bones. The resultant radiograph would have too many superimposed images and be of little diagnostic use. In the maxilla the tube-shift technic is a more effective localization procedure. However, a modified cross-sectional projection is sometimes useful for impacted maxillary third molars (Figure 13–12). The film is positioned in the occlusal plane with the exposure surface toward the maxilla. The central ray is directed toward the film through the zygomatic arch. The resultant radiograph shows distorted images due to the oblique angulation; however, the zygomatic arch is easily identified and this locates the lateral border of the area. The buccopalatal position of an impacted tooth relative to the erupted teeth can now be identified.

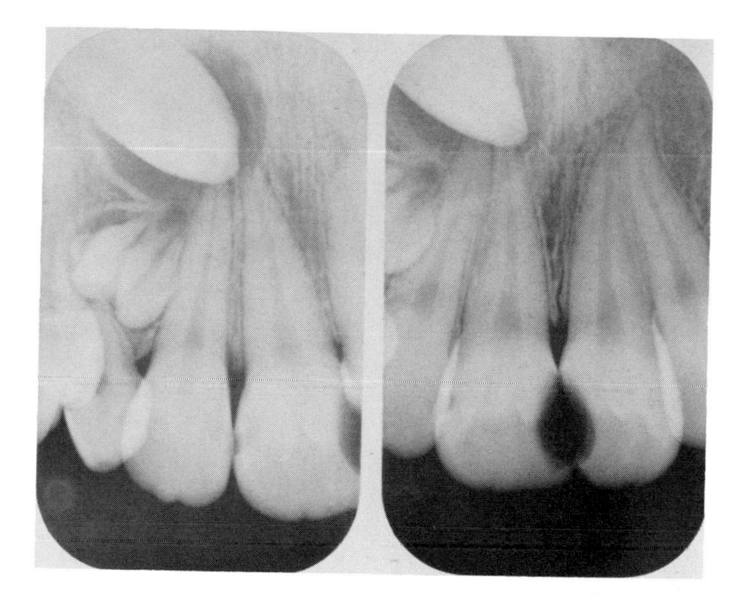

Figure 13–13. Periapical radiographs of a maxillary central and lateral incisor made with different horizontal angulation of the x-ray beam. Note that the odontoma and cusp of the impacted cuspid are located at different positions relative to the lateral incisor in the two radiographs.

Tube-Shift Technic

The tube-shift technic utilizes two periapical radiographs made with different horizontal angulations; a standard radiograph and a second one of the area made with a shift in the horizontal angulation. The medial-lateral position of an unknown object is located relative to the known position of an object such as an erupted tooth (Figure 13–13). (When teeth are not present, known objects, such as different-shaped radiopaque wires, can be placed in a sheet of wax that is molded over the edentulous area like a denture base.) Shifts in horizontal angulation of the x-ray beam move the position of objects on the x-ray film in a mesial or distal direction (Figure 13–14). When the x-ray tubehead is positioned more distally, all shadows of objects move mesially, that is, in the opposite direction to the tubehead. The shadows of objects closer to the film move less than the images of objects farther away; thus

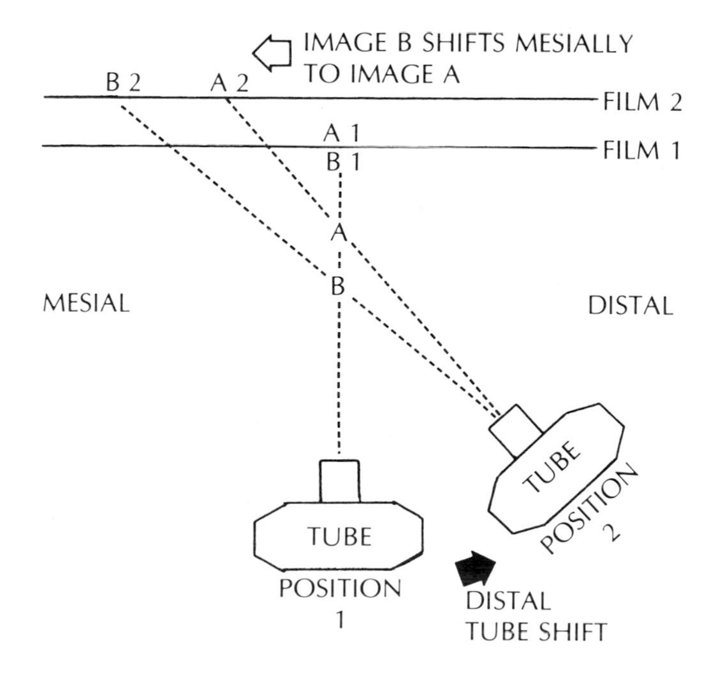

Figure 13–14. Diagram showing mesial shift of images of objects A and B when tubehead is moved distally. Note that image of object A (which is closer to film) shifts less than image of object B. In other words, image B shifts mesially relative to A when tubehead shifts distally.

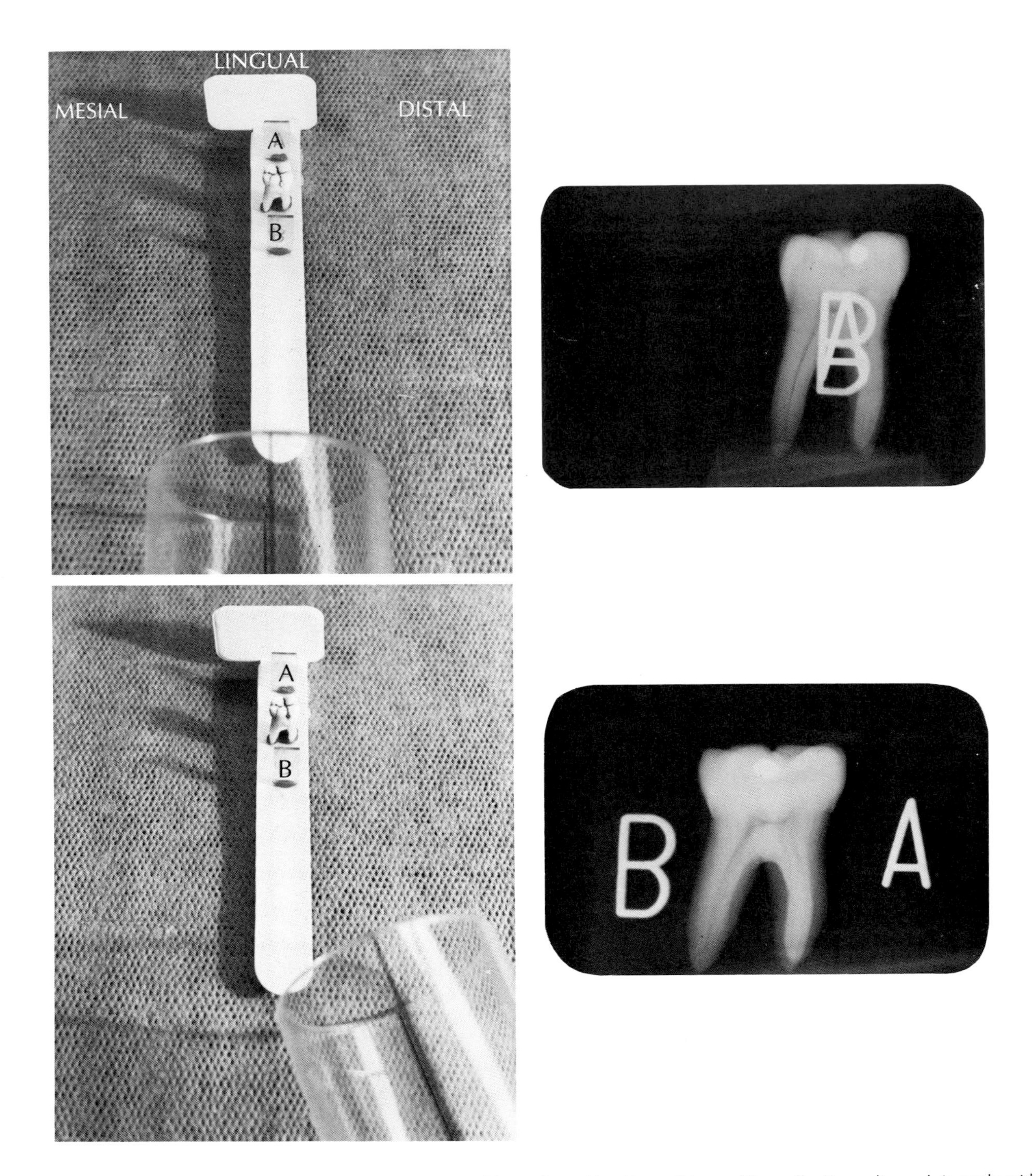

Figure 13–15. Two radiographs of a tooth, lead letter A located lingually and lead letter B located buccally. Top radiograph is made with x-ray beam directed horizontally along line joining three objects. Lower radiograph is made with x-ray tube positioned distal to position used in making top radiograph. Observation of positions of objects A and B relative to tooth in both radiographs enables dentist to locate object A as being lingual to the tooth and object B as buccal to the tooth.

shadows of objects far from the film tend to shift in the opposite direction of the tube-head movement relative to the shadows of objects that are closer to the film. When the position of one object is known and the second object unknown, the mesial or distal direction of shift of the unknown object's image relative to the known object's image identifies whether the unknown is located lingual (closer to the film) or buccal (farther from the film) to the known object. If the tubehead is moved distally and the unknown object's image moves medial to the known object's image, then the unknown is buccal to the known object or farther from the film. If the unknown image moves in the same direction as the tubehead's shift, then it is located closer to the film or lingual to the known object (Figure 13–15).

The tube-shift technic is often referred to as the "buccal rule" and may be described differently by individuals as "the buccal object moves opposite to the tube-shift direction" or "buccal always moves away." Such descriptions of this localization procedure may not apply to radiographs made with the x-ray beam aimed at the patient from a posterior or inferior direction.

The use of the tube-shift technic is most important when a cross-sectional or right-angle view to the periapical radiograph is unobtainable. Such is the case in locating the exact positions of objects in the maxilla (Figure 13–16); in this case the cusp of the impacted tooth is seen to move distal to the mesial border of the lateral incisor as the x-ray tube shifts distally, thus placing the cusp of the impacted tooth in a palatal location relative to the lateral incisor. The apex of the impacted tooth moves from above the second bicuspid to a position above the first bicuspid as the x-ray tube moves distally; this identifies the apex of the impacted tooth as being located buccal to the bicuspids. With the buccal palatal position of the impacted tooth identified and the radiographs showing the superior-inferior and anterior-posterior positions of all teeth, the exact location of the impacted tooth is identified.

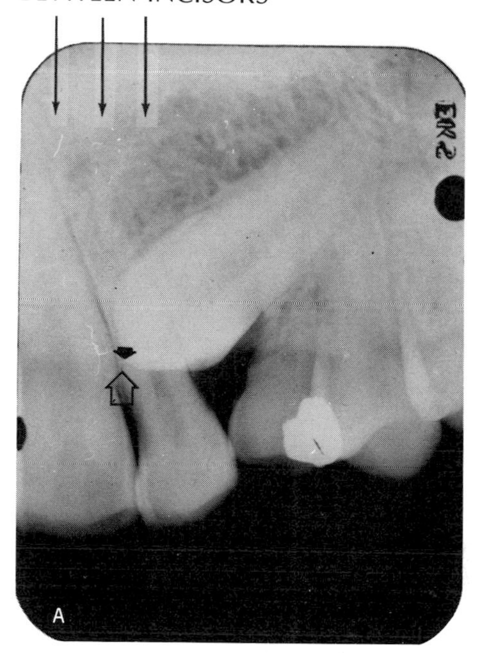

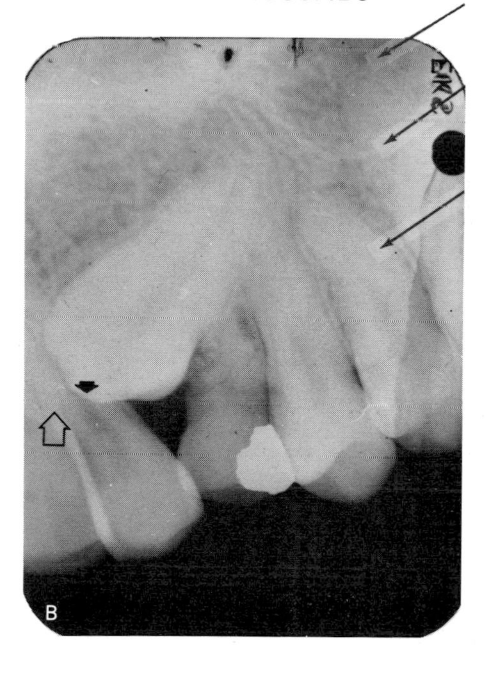

Figure 13–16. Periapical radiographs of maxillary cuspid area made with different horizontal directions of x-ray beam. A, X-ray beam directed between incisor teeth. Image of cusp tip of impacted tooth (solid arrow) is seen in same position as mesial border of erupted lateral incisor (outlined arrow). B, X-ray tube positioned more distally and x-ray beam directed between bicuspid teeth. Image of cusp of impacted tooth (solid arrow) shifts to more distal position on radiograph relative to mesial surface of lateral incisor (outlined arrow). Cusp tip of impacted tooth is thus located palatal to erupted teeth. Location of apex of impacted tooth can be found in similar manner.

Chapter 14

Occlusal Film and Extraoral Radiography

The intraoral periapical radiograph examines a small area of the dentition. In many cases these films do not show the entire lesion that needs to be observed. Proper oral diagnosis requires the use of radiographs that not only depict a lesion in its entirety but also determine if there are similar lesions in and around the jaws. This is accomplished by using larger radiographs. The films used are occlusal films and screen films in cassettes (Figure 14–1).

OCCLUSAL FILM RADIOGRAPHY

The occlusal film is packaged like a periapical dental film and is approximately 3 × 2¼ inches in size. The film's speed is similar to that of fast speed periapical films, that is, ANS speed group D. The film is made to be placed inside the oral cavity in the occlusal plane and thus is sometimes called a "sandwich" film.

The film in introduced into the mouth the same way as a sandwich. It is then gently held between the teeth. If the patient is edentulous, the film can be held in place by the patient's thumbs for the upper jaw and the forefingers for the lower jaw. If the edentulous patient for some reason cannot use his hands, then cotton rolls, a bar of wax, or some other like substance can be placed in the intermaxillary space formerly occupied by the teeth in order to support the film.

The film is placed as far back into the mouth as can be tolerated by the patient, with the stippled surface facing the beam of radiation. The lateral position of the film is determined by the area of interest, i.e., whether the right, middle, or left side of the jaw is being examined. Basically, occlusal radiography is used to get a topographic projection or a cross-sectional projection of an area.

Topographic Projections

Topographic projections are possible in the entire upper jaw and in the anterior area of

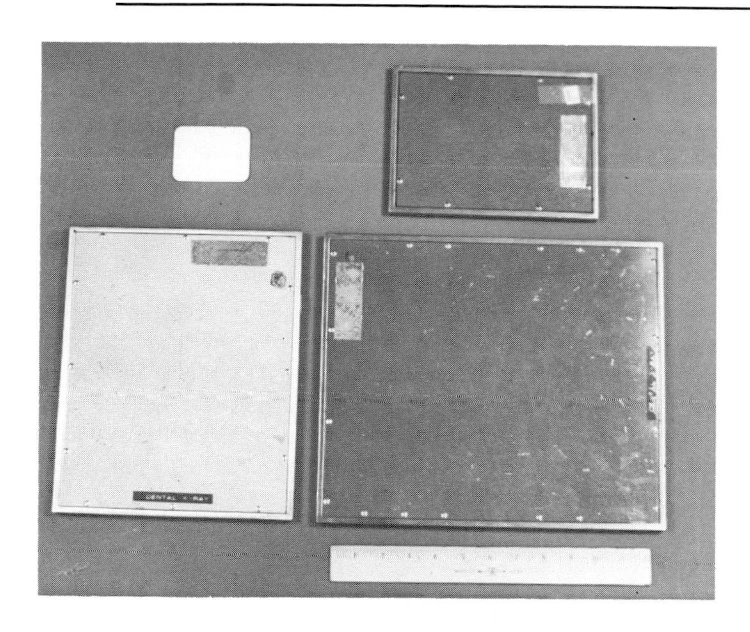

Figure 14–1. Occlusal film and cassettes of various sizes.

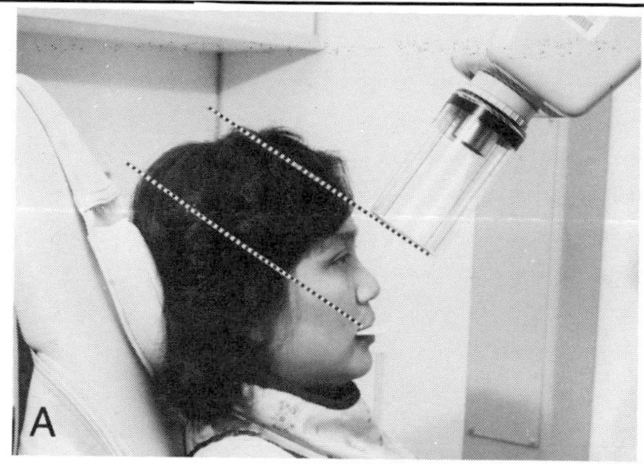

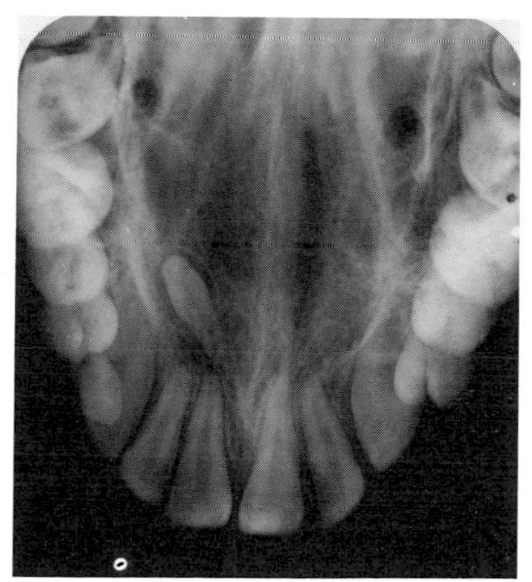

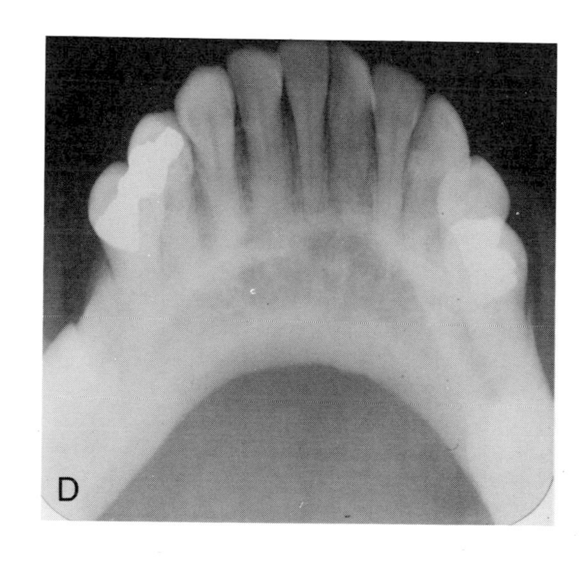

Figure 14–2. A, Technic for topographic occlusal radiograph of the maxillary anterior region. Film is held gently between teeth. The vertical edge of the cone is parallel to a line drawn from the incisal edge of the teeth to the top of the external ear. Cone of radiation covers area measuring 2¾ inches in diameter at patient's skin. With 10 mA and 65 kVp, exposure time is approximately ⅓ second. B, Topographic occlusal radiograph showing supernumerary tooth that was first partially seen in periapical radiograph of area. C, Diagram of film cone positions for a topographic occlusal radiograph of the mandibular incisor area. The vertical edge of the cone is parallel to a line drawn from the incisal edge of the teeth to the antegonial notch (located just anterior to the angle of the mandible). D, Topographic occlusal radiograph of the mandibular incisor region.

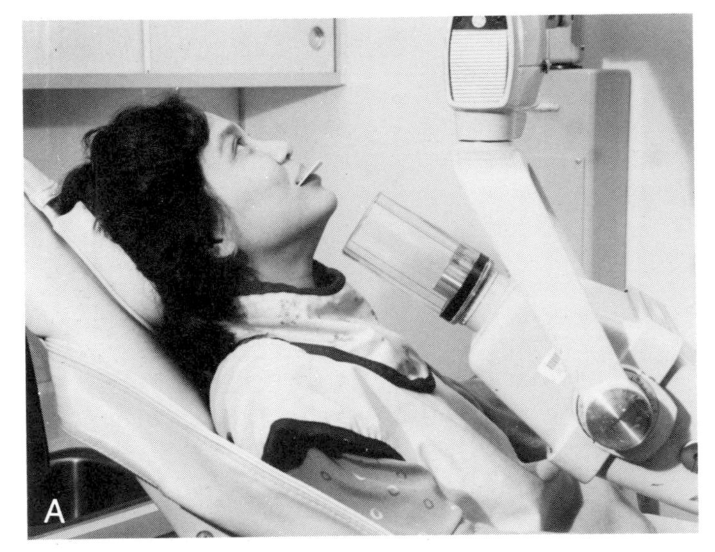

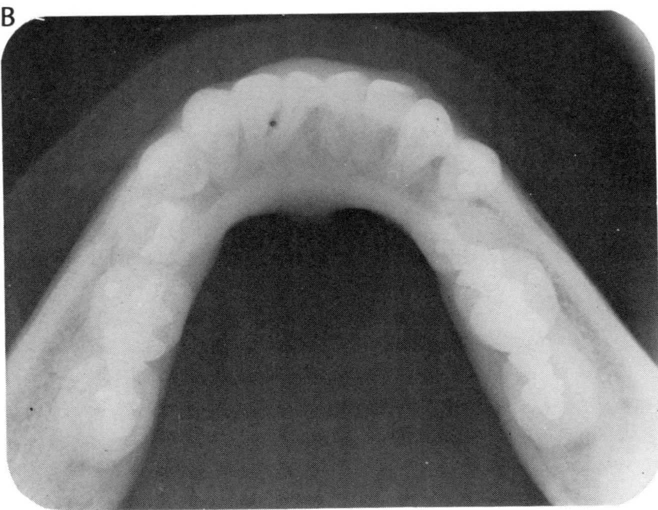

Figure 14–3. A, Patient-tube relationship for making cross-section occlusal radiograph of lower jaw. B, Cross-section occlusal radiograph of lower jaw. When the presence of objects in soft tissues is suspected, it is advisable to use less exposure time than is normally used to examine bony structures.

the lower jaw. These radiographs are made with the patient in the dental chair in the same position generally used for intraoral radiography (Figure 14–2A).

The principle involved in the topographic projection is the same as that used in the bisecting-angle technique of intraoral radiography. The bisector of the angle formed by the film and the long axes of the teeth is first determined; then the central ray of the cone of radiation is directed through, or at the level of, the apex of the tooth or teeth in question so that it is perpendicular to the bisector. When no teeth are present, the operator can use the buccal or labial surface of the alveolar bone as a guide for the other side of the angle. In most cases the vertical edge at the cone is parallel to a line drawn from the incisal edge of the teeth to the top of the external ear. The horizontal angulation of the x-ray beam is similar to that used in intraoral radiography. In other words, the operator directs the central ray between the teeth that he is interested in.

It is obvious that to obtain a good topographic radiograph, an acute angle must be formed between the film and the teeth. In the lower jaw the long axes of the posterior teeth tend to be tilted in such a manner that their crowns are tipped inward. This produces an obtuse angle between the long axes of these teeth and the film in the occlusal plane position; this angle is so great that more often than not a topographic projection of this area on the occlusal film is of little value. An example of the topographic projection and its use in radiographically depicting a supernumerary tooth above the apices of the erupted teeth is shown in Figure 14–2B.

In the mandibular incisor region the vertical angulation of the x-ray beam will position the vertical edge of the cone parallel to a line drawn from the incisal edge of the teeth to the angle of the mandible (Figure 14–2C).

Cross-sectional Projections

Cross-section occlusal radiographs are used mainly in localizing objects or lesions, such as impacted teeth, root tips, fractures, and foreign bodies that are first detected on standard periapical radiographs. These radiographs can be made for the mandible and maxilla; however, for the maxilla a screen film in a special small cassette is needed and thus cross-sectional projections of the maxilla are not commonly made. The regular occlusal film is not used in a cross-sectional projection of the maxilla because the x-ray beam has to penetrate through the cranium and the exposure time would have to be about 8 seconds. The maxillary projection will not be discussed in this chapter.

Cross-sectional projections of the lower jaw are easily accomplished. The film is placed in the mouth in a position similar to that used for the topographic projection (Figure 14–3A). The central ray is directed along the sagittal plane as nearly perpendicular to the film as possible. In this instance the patient's head must be tipped backward. This radiographic projection shows most of the lower jaw (Figure 14–3B).

When the buccolingual position of an object within the jaw is to be determined, the central ray should be directed along the long axes of the teeth present in the particular area (Figure 14–4). This projection shows the relationship of the object to the teeth in the horizontal plane buccolingually and thus provides the information which, when coupled with that obtained from the intraoral periapical survey, accurately localizes the position of the object within the jaw.

The cross-sectional projection of the lower jaw is important in the diagnosis of sialoliths in the submaxillary gland duct and of calcifications within the gland itself. Here, however, the tissue under examination is actually the soft tissue and not the bone, and the exposure time thus has to be reduced if the area under examination is not to be overexposed.

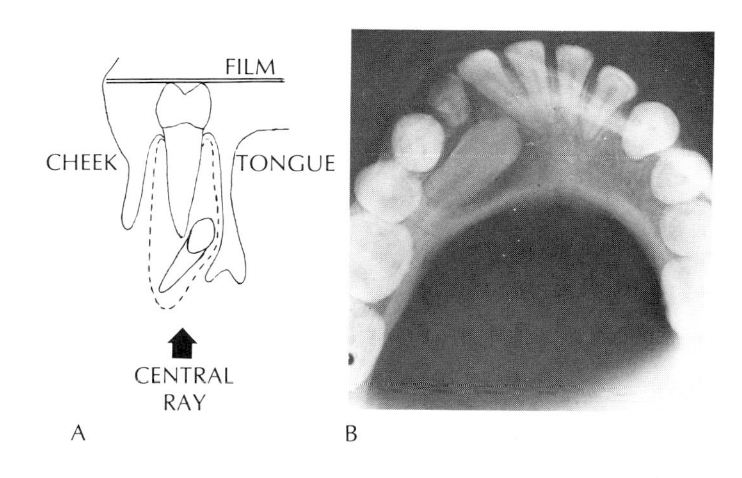

Figure 14–4. A, Diagram showing the film, object, and x-ray beam positions for making cross-section occlusal radiograph of body of mandible. B, Cross-section radiograph showing buccolingual position of permanent cuspid and dentigerous cyst within mandible.

Occlusal Film Used Extraorally

Some dentists use the occlusal film extraorally or outside of the oral cavity. The extraoral use of the film should be avoided if possible because the speed of the film is slower than that of a screen film in a cassette that is designed to be used extraorally. Screen film should be used whenever possible to keep the patient's x-ray exposure at a minimum.

Lateral Jaw Radiography with Occlusal Film. The lateral jaw projection is sometimes made on small children because the film is

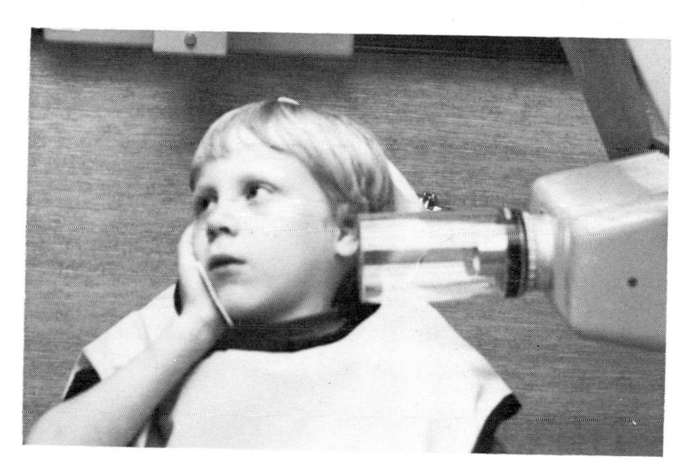

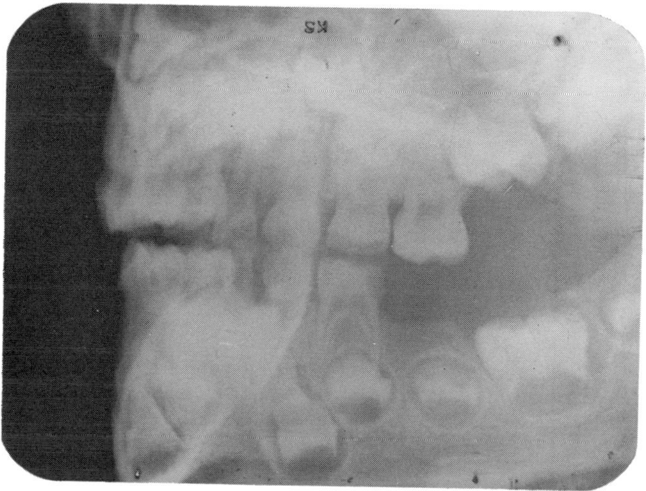

Figure 14–5. Technic for lateral jaw radiograph using occlusal film on young child.

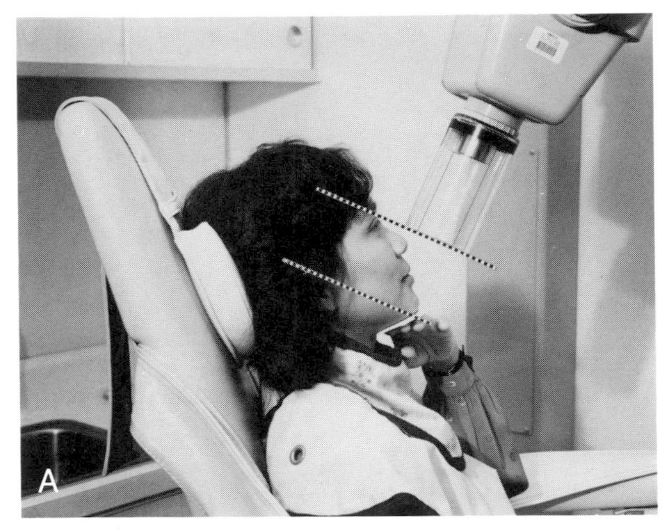

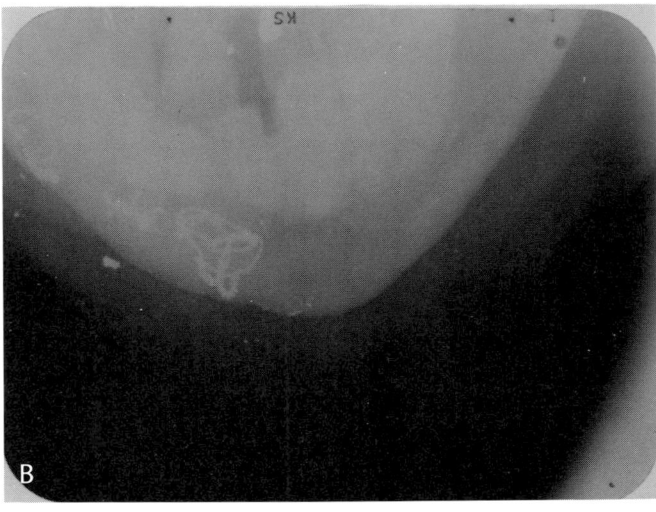

Figure 14–6. A, Reverse topographic projection of mandibular incisor area and B, Radiograph made on patient with jaws wired together because of fracture.

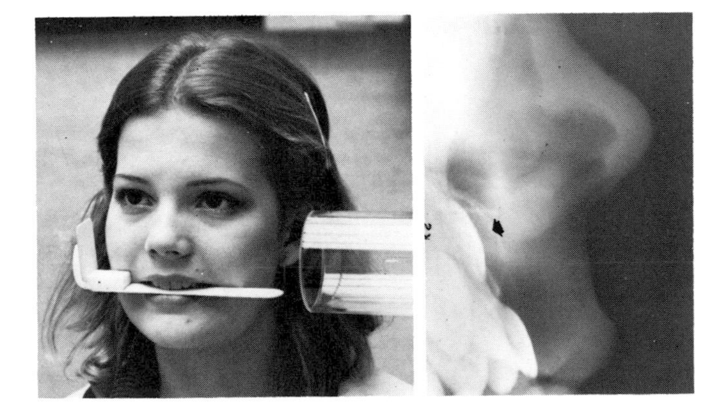

Figure 14–7. Tangential projection of maxillary anterior region and radiograph showing buccopalatal position of impacted tooth.

large enough to cover most of jaw area and the amount of tissue that the x-ray beam has to penetrate is not great (Figure 14–5). The technic is the same as that using 5 × 7 inches screen cassette; the screen-film lateral jaw technic is described later in this chapter.

Reverse Topographic Projection. The occlusal film can be used to make a topographic radiograph of the mandibular anterior region by placing the film under the patient's chin (Figure 14–6A). The central ray is directed perpendicular to the bisector of the angle formed by the teeth and film. The vertical edge of the cone is parallel to a line drawn from the chin to the external auditory meatus. A reverse topographic radiograph is shown in Figure 14–6B. The projection is useful when a topographic radiograph is needed and the patient's mouth cannot be opened because of trismus, wiring together of the jaws, or some other reason.

Tangential Projection. The intraoral periapical film and the occlusal film in the occlusal plane positions two films at right angles to each other. The occlusal film can be positioned extraorally at right angles to both of these two film planes (Figure 14–7). The film is held in the groove of a wood or plastic stick (a bite-block taped to a throat stick is adequate). The stick is held by the patient between the teeth with the film turned upward or downward, depending upon which jaw is being examined. The central ray is directed perpendicular to the film in both the horizontal and vertical planes in such a manner that it basically forms a tangent of the curve of the jaw at the point of interest. The radiograph can thus be called a tangential projection in order to distinguish it from lateral projections of the jaws. Some operators prefer to call the projection by other names, such as profile view or mesial-distal projection. The tangential radiograph is especially useful in localizing objects in the anterior area of the jaws.

EXTRAORAL RADIOGRAPHY

Extraoral radiographs are made to examine large areas such as the face or skull. Whenever periapical and occlusal radiographs do not show the entire picture of a pathologic condition, extraoral x-ray projections are necessary. These radiographs may be not only an adjunct to intraoral radiography but also may be the only radiographic survey possible, for example when the patient cannot open the mouth or a child will not open the mouth.

Many extraoral projections are designed to examine the entire skull or specific parts of the skull. Only those basic projections useful and practical for the dental practitioner will be discussed in this text.

Equipment

Extraoral radiography utilizes screen film in cassettes equipped with screens. Screen films need much less exposure to x-radiation to produce the desired film density for viewing. This fact allows the operator to make these films with exposure times that are short enough to be practical (less than 2 seconds) thus minimizing the blurring effect caused movement of the patient.

Lightweight, thin cassettes are recommended because the patient in many instances has to hold the film in position. To examine large and small parts of a patient's skull various sizes of cassettes are needed. The most commonly used films are 5 × 7 inches and 8 × 10 inches; occasionally a 10 × 12 inches radiograph is needed (Figure 14–8). The cassette must be larger than the x-ray beam wherever the cassette is positioned. The x-ray beam is collimated to be slightly larger than the area of the patient being examined. When variable collimators are unavailable, the desired x-ray beam size can be obtained by using the standard collimator in the short cone and varying the distance between the x-ray tube and the patient.

Cassettes need to have R and L letters made of lead placed on the exposure side. These letters appear in the processed radiograph and indicate whether the lateral view radiograph is made of the right or left side of the patient, or which side of the frontal view radiograph is the patient's left and which side is the right. For some projections a stand or cassette holder mounted on the wall is advantageous (Figure 14–9). Note that skull projections described later in this chapter show the use and non-use of this device.

Most processing tanks designed for dental offices will accommodate film 8 × 10 inches; when larger films will be used, the darkroom

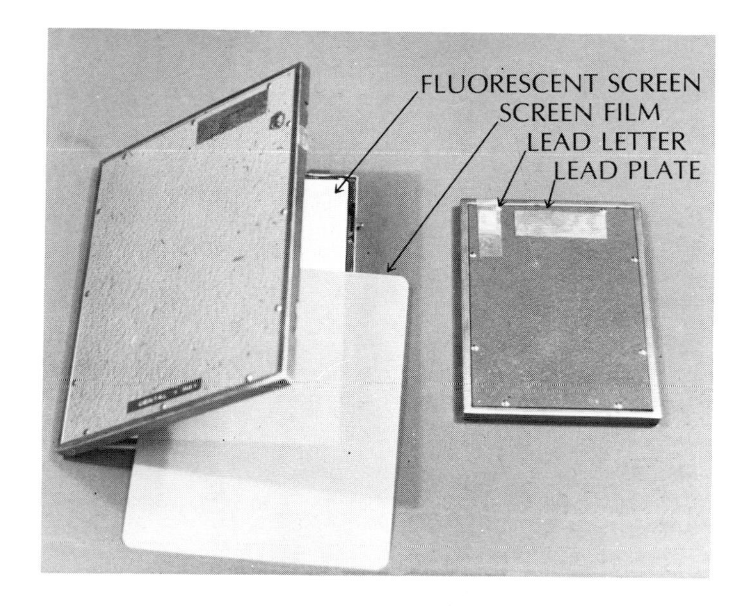

Figure 14–8. Open and closed cassettes showing screens, film, and lead (R and L) markers.

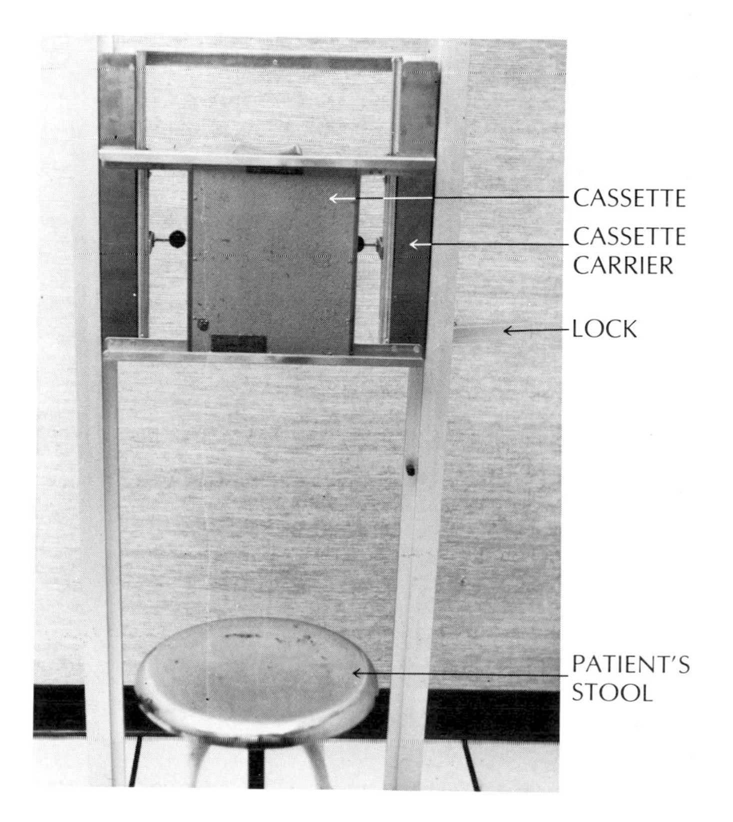

Figure 14–9. Screen film cassette holder mounted on wall. Cassette can be positioned vertically at any level.

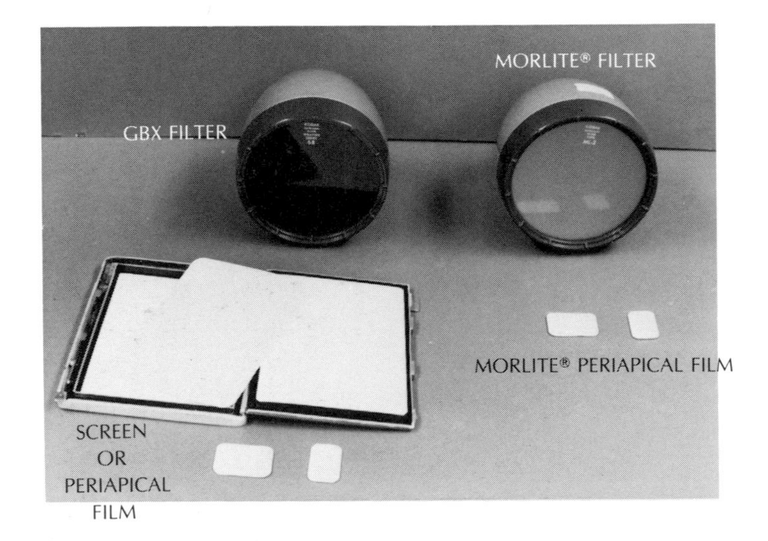

Figure 14–10. Safelights needed for periapical film and screen film.

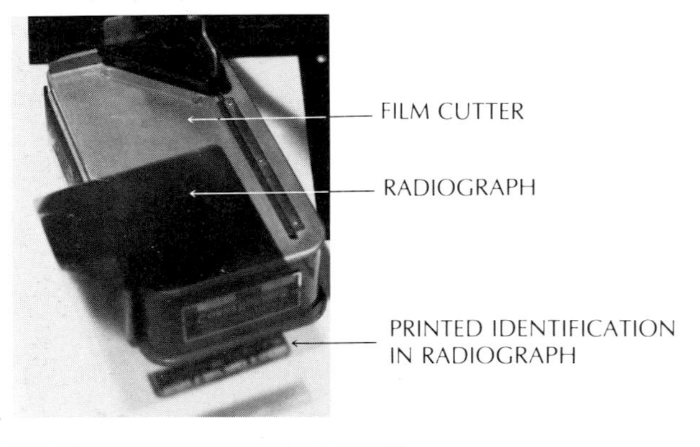

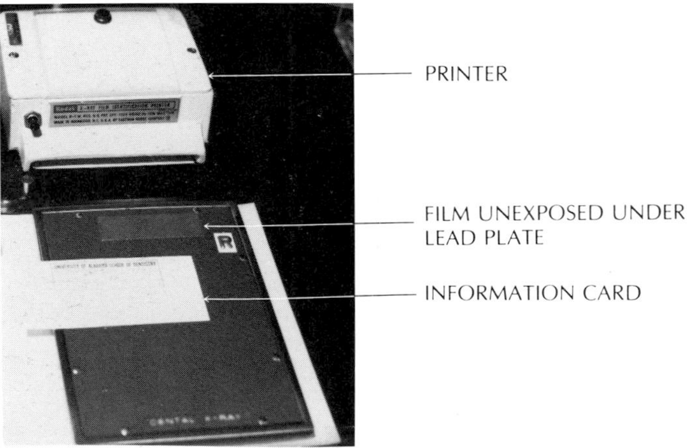

Figure 14–11. Identification printer, semitransparent card, and radiograph with desired information.

facilities must be designed to accommodate them. Film hangers must be available for tank processing of the various sizes of films. Available automatic film processors vary in the maximum width of film they can process. Extraoral film size must be matched to the type of automatic processor being used.

Darkroom safelights must be of a type recommended by the screen film's manufacturer (Figure 14–10). Safelight filters specially made for intraoral film usually allow light in the darkroom that is unsafe for screen film. Safelights designed for screen film are also safe for intraoral film; they allow much less light in the darkroom. When both screen and intraoral films are to be processed in the darkroom, both types of safelights should be provided to obtain the most efficient darkroom working conditions. Some automatic processors have daylight loaders. The filters used with daylight loaders are usually not safe for screen films; information of the capabilities of a daylight loader must be obtained before it is used with any film.

Additional equipment that can be of assistance are a film cutter, a large viewbox, and a machine for printing the patient's name and other information on the film (Figure 14–11). The printer is used in the darkroom with a semitransparent card on which the operator writes the information to be placed in the radiograph, such as the patient's name and date. The information is printed on the undeveloped film on a part of the film left unexposed to x rays by placing a small piece of lead on the exposure surface of the cassette. The developed radiograph has the printed information permanently fixed in the film.

Lateral Jaw Radiography

Lateral jaw radiography is the term usually used to describe lateral projections of the mandible and/or maxilla on films that are usually 5 × 7 inches in size. A true lateral projection of an entire side of a jaw is not possible, since the opposite jaw would be superimposed upon the same area of the film. Thus at best this projection entails a certain degree of oblique angulation. If the beam of radiation is directed underneath the mandible opposite the side under examination, a large area of the mandible and maxilla can be examined; however, the roentgen shad-

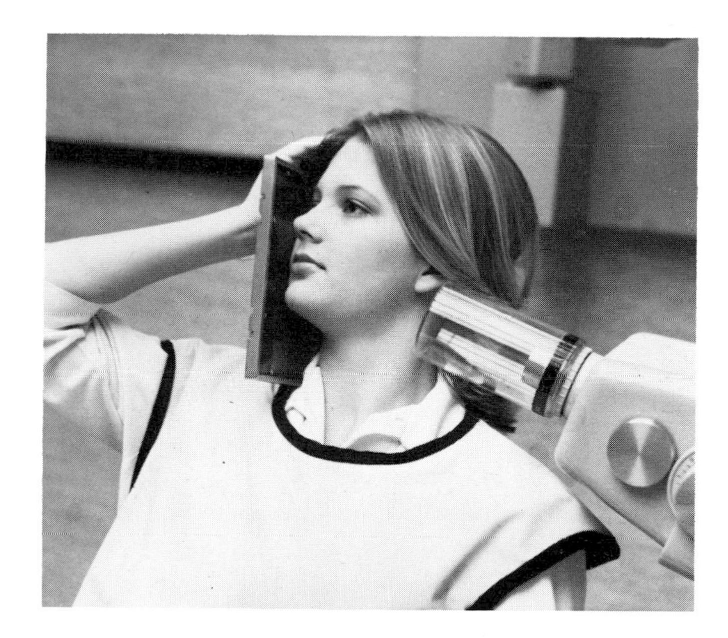

Figure 14–12. Positions of patient, film, and x-ray machine for lateral jaw radiography.

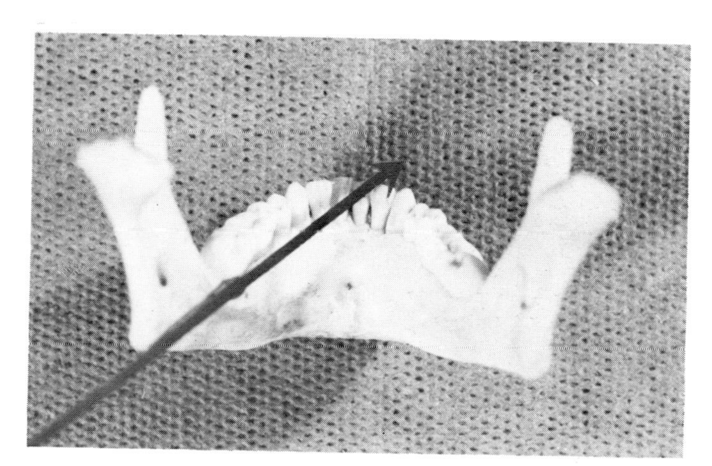

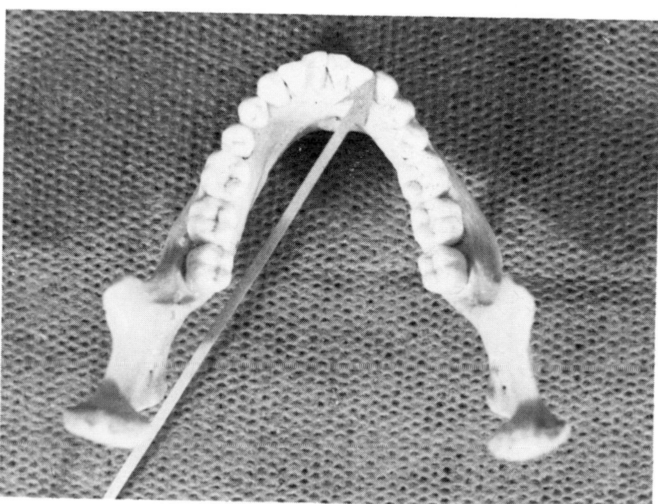

Figure 14–13. Direction of central ray of x-ray beam for bicuspid region lateral jaw radiograph. Top, central ray as seen from behind mandible. Below, central ray as seen from above mandible.

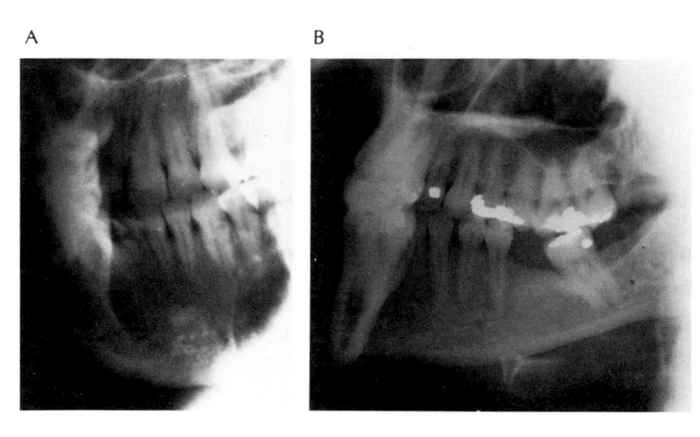
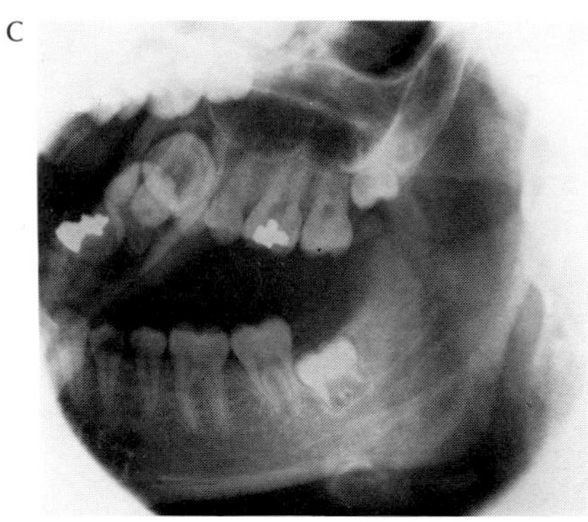

Figure 14–14. Lateral jaw radiographs of anterior (A), bicuspid (B) and ramus (C) regions of jaws.

ows thus obtained suffer much from distortion caused by the great degree of oblique vertical angulation necessary for this projection. If the x rays are directed from behind the angle of the mandible opposite to the side under examination, the distortion is held to a minimum, but the area that can be examined is reduced. The x-ray beam in this second technic has to pass between the ramus on the opposite side and the vertebral column. The latter method is preferred and the first method should be used only when circumstances make the second method impractical.

The technic for lateral jaw projections is not difficult if certain basic rules are followed. The patient is seated in the chair with the occlusal plane as nearly parallel to the floor as possible (Figure 14–12). The patient is then asked to project his chin directly forward as far as is comfortable. This position places the jaws away from the vertebral column. The x-ray machine, using an 8-inch cone, is positioned so that the central ray is directed to a point just medial to the angle of the mandible opposite the side being examined. The vertical and horizontal angulation of the x-ray beam is so adjusted that the central ray is directed to exit from the patient's head at a point just anterior to the area of interest and at the level of the alveolar ridge or necks of the teeth of the maxilla (Figure 14–13). With the beam projected in this manner only a section of the jaws can be examined with any one radiograph. However, any section examined in this manner will have well-proportioned images of both the upper and lower jaws.

Separate lateral jaw radiographs should be made for the ramus, molar area, bicuspid area, and anterior area of any one side. Figure 14–14 shows three radiographs of such a series. Note that a lateral jaw film of the anterior area of one side of the jaw also shows teeth that are on the other side. Two film exposures, one made of each side, will thus show the entire anterior area of the jaws without the vertebral column superimposing its image upon this area. The ability of this projection to show areas past the midline is useful, since most projections of this area using a beam of radiation originating from this general direction will superimpose the vertebral

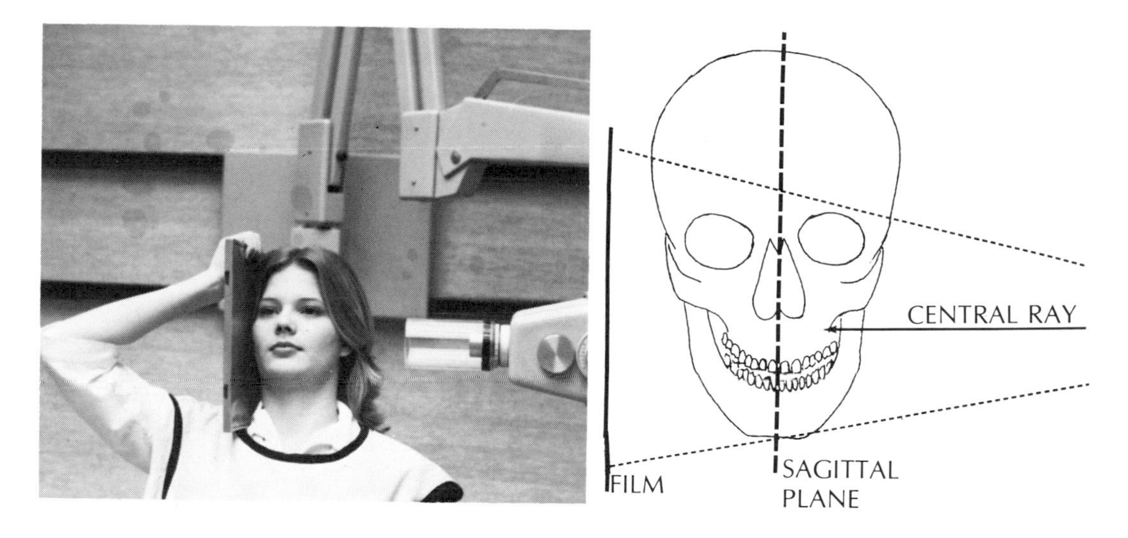

Figure 14–15. Position of patient, film, and x-ray tube for lateral sinus radiograph. Cassette is being supported by patient. A cassette holder can also be used.

column upon the anterior areas of the jaws and make interpretation difficult.

The patient's head can be turned slightly away from the x-ray tube in the bicuspid and incisor area projections; this head position increases the space between the ramus and vertebral column. The patient's head must not be turned for the molar and ramus projections because turning the head will place the ramus being examined behind the vertebral column.

The positioning of the film is important. The operator should strive at all times to have the film perpendicular to the central ray in both the horizontal and vertical planes. Acceptable film positions for examining the various areas of the jaws can be achieved without the use of any accessory equipment by having the patient hold the lightweight cassette between the heel of the hand and the malar or cheek bone. In the posterior areas the zygomatic arch and in the anterior area the nose will assist in stabilizing any horizontal movement of the film. In all instances the patient curves and rests the tips of the fingers on the cranium. This position of the hand assists in preventing any movement of the film holder in the vertical plane.

Exposure times for an average adult patient using medium speed film and screens, 10 mA, and 65 kVp are as follows: ramus and molar areas, 10 impulses; bicuspid area, 15 impulses; anterior areas, 24 impulses.

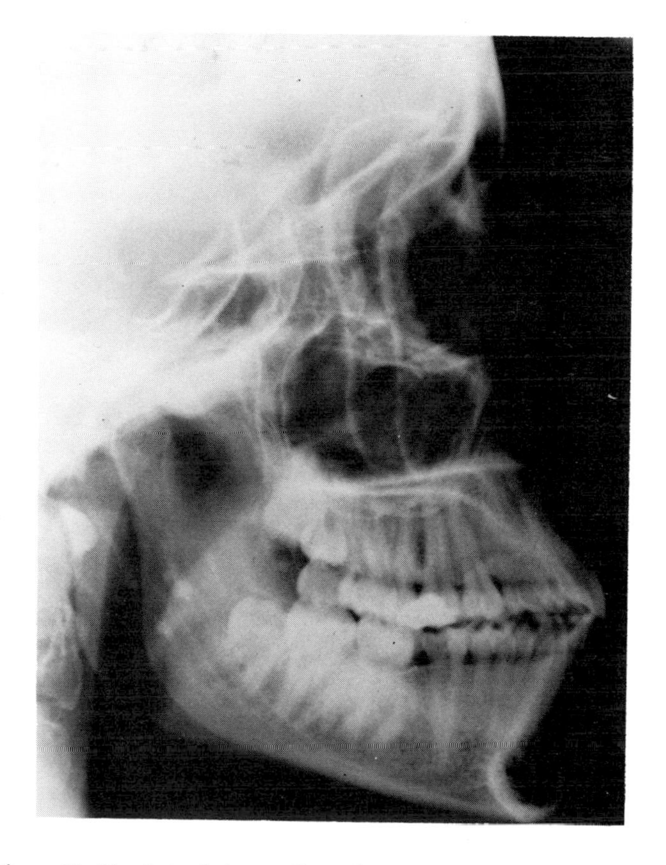

Figure 14–16. Lateral sinus radiograph.

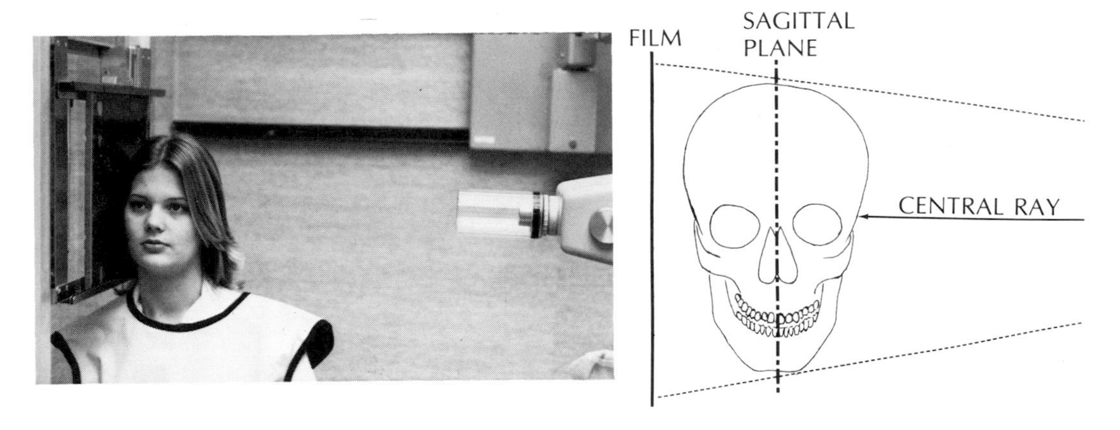

Figure 14–17. Technic for lateral skull projection. Cassette is being supported by wall-mounted cassette holder.

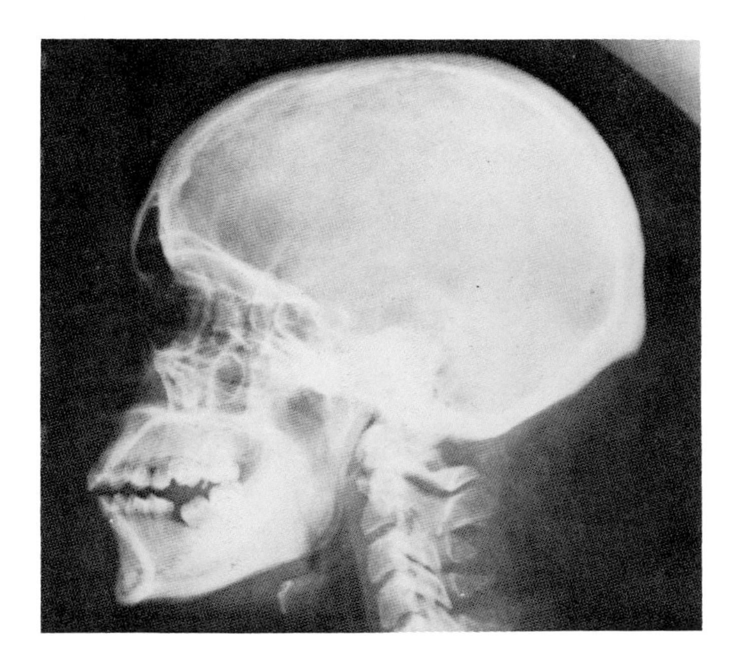

Figure 14–18. Lateral skull radiograph.

The Lateral Sinus Radiograph

The projection is made with the cassette placed plano-parallel to the midline or sagittal plane of the patient's head (Figure 14–15). A film 5 × 7 inches or 8 × 10 inches can be used with the patient supporting the cassette on the shoulder and holding it against the side of the head. The cassette can also be placed in a wall-mounted holder. The central ray is directed perpendicular to the film horizontally and vertically and enters the patient at the apices of the maxillary first molar. Using the short cone, a 20-inch target-film distance, medium speed film and screens, 10 mA, and 65 kVp, the exposure time is approximately ¼ second (15 impulses).

Figure 14–16 shows a lateral sinus radiograph. The radiograph evaluates most of the face from the lateral aspect but is particularly useful for the maxillary sinus region and the nasal bones.

The Lateral Skull Radiograph

The film is positioned plano-parallel to the sagittal plane of the skull (Figure 14–17). The central ray enters at or a few inches above the auditory canal. The central ray is perpendicular to the film in both the horizontal and vertical planes. Using a short cone, 36-inch tube-film distance, medium speed film and screens, 10 mA, and 65 kVp, the approximate exposure time is ½ second (30 impulses).

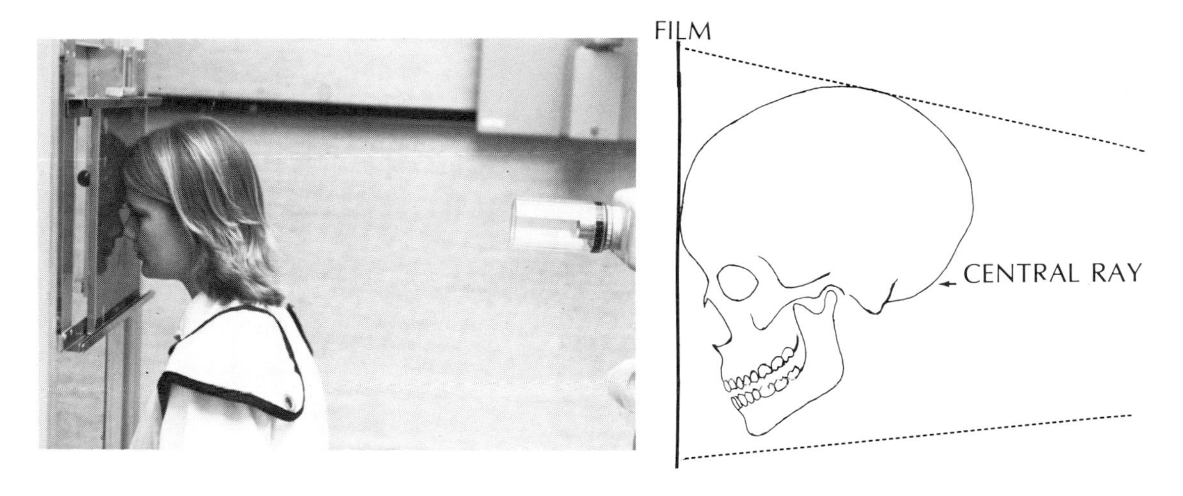

Figure 14–19. Technic for P-A skull radiograph. A cassette holder is being used.

The lateral skull radiograph is shown in Figure 14–18. Structures on the right and left of the skull are superimposed upon each other, with those on the side near the x-ray machine being magnified to a somewhat greater extent. If the exposure time is reduced by 50% or more, the osseous structures will be underexposed, but soft-tissue structures will become visible. This technic is used by some orthodontists and prosthodontists to obtain soft-tissue profiles of their patients. The radiograph is used to survey the entire head and shows the anteroposterior and superior-inferior positions of objects or lesions affecting osseous structures.

Posteroanterior Skull Radiograph

In the posteroanterior (P-A) skull projection, the cassette is perpendicular to the sagittal plane of the skull. The patient's forehead touches the film and the orbitomeatal line is perpendicular to the cassette (Figure 14–19). The x-ray beam travels from the posterior to the anterior of the patient. (When the x-ray beam travels in the opposite direction, the projection is called an A-P radiograph.) The x-ray beam is positioned with the central ray in the sagittal plane, perpendicular to the film and at the level of the orbitomeatal line. Using a short cone, 36-inch tube-film distance, medium speed film and screens, 10 mA, and 65 kVp, the approximate exposure time is $\frac{4}{5}$ second (48 impulses).

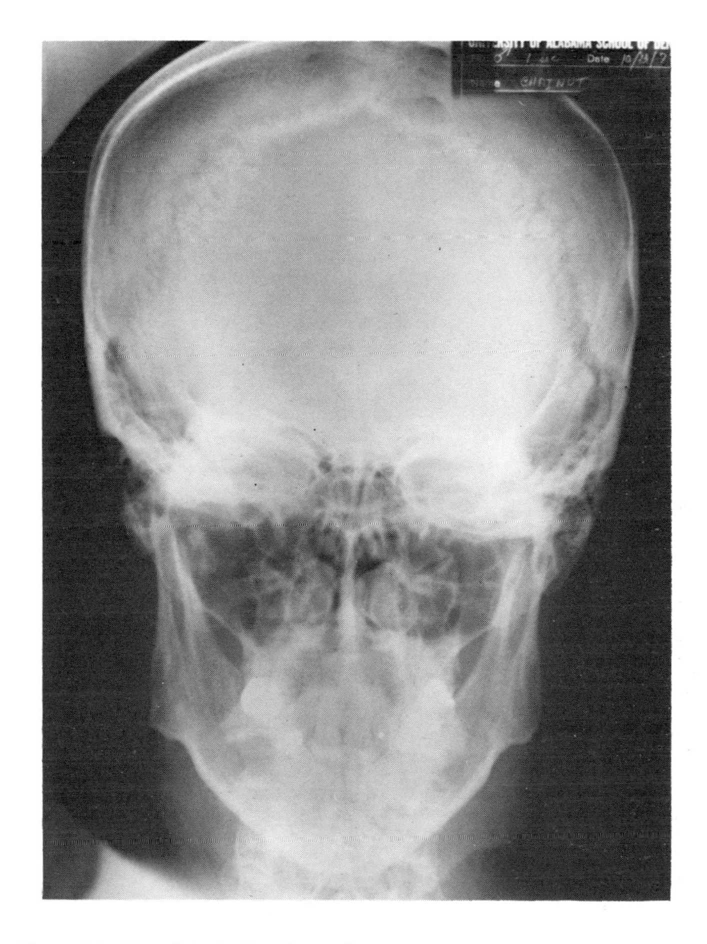

Figure 14–20. P-A skull radiograph.

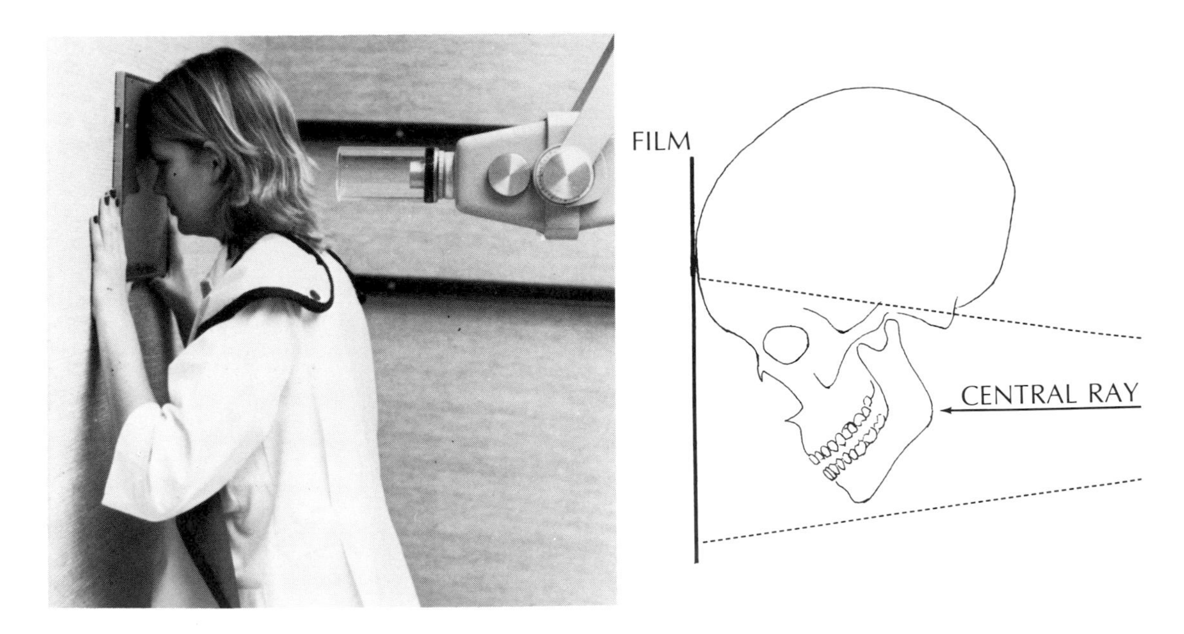

Figure 14–21. Technic for P-A mandible radiograph. Cassette is supported by patient who is standing and facing wall. A cassette holder can be used with the patient seated.

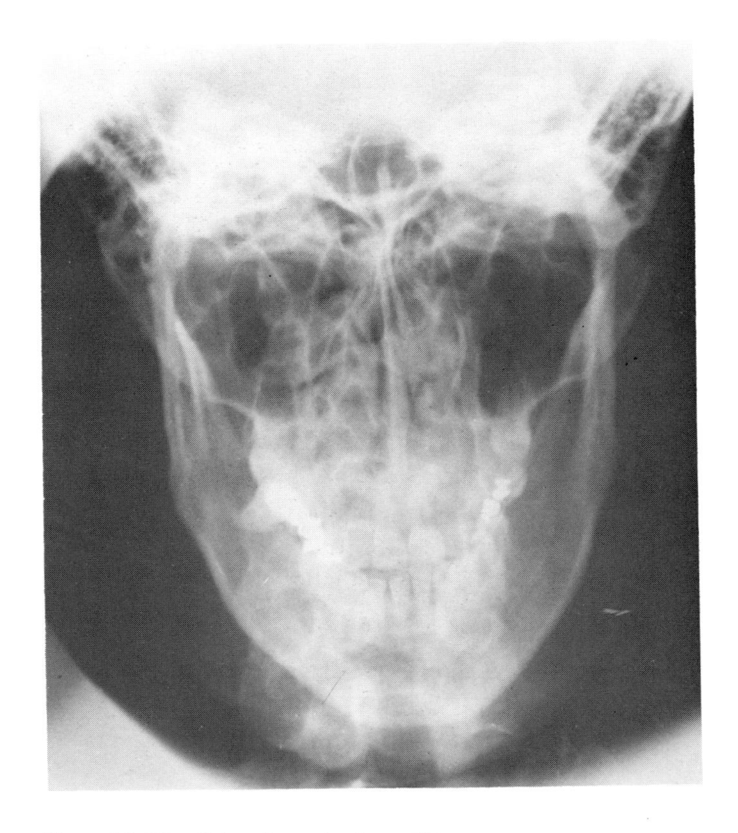

Figure 14–22. P-A radiograph of mandible.

The P-A skull radiograph is shown in Figure 14–20. The radiograph shows the superior-inferior and medial-lateral positions of objects or lesions affecting the skull. Together with the lateral skull radiograph, the P-A skull projection is very useful in localizing skull pathology.

Posteroanterior Mandible Radiograph

In the posteroanterior projection of the mandible (P-A mandible), the patient places the forehead on the cassette. The sagittal plane of the skull is positioned perpendicular to the cassette (Figure 14–21). The cassette may be held in a cassette holder with the patient seated or the cassette can be held against the wall by a standing patient who places the thumbs of both hands underneath the cassette and the forefingers on the sides of the cassette. The central ray is placed perpendicular to the film in both the vertical and horizontal planes. The central ray enters from the posterior of the skull in the sagittal plane at the level of the angle of the mandible. With the patient's forehead touching the cassette, the patient's head is tipped forward (or chin drawn backward) until the central ray bisects the angle of the mandible.

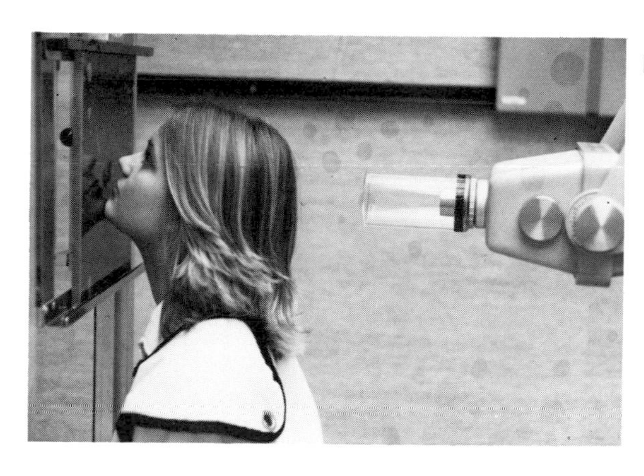

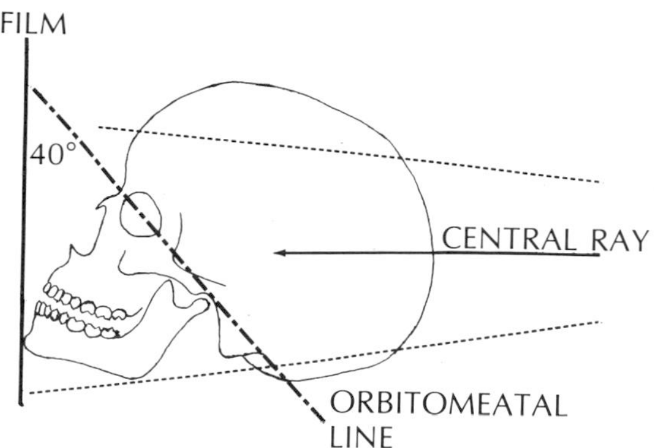

Figure 14–23. Technic for P-A sinus radiograph.

With the short cone, 24-inch tube-film distance, medium speed film and screen, 10 mA, and 65 kVp, the approximate exposure time is ½ second (30 impulses).

The P-A radiograph of the mandible is shown in Figure 14–22. This projection is valuable in surveying patients for any medial or lateral deviations of parts of the ramus, condyle, or coronoid processes. If this projection is made with the patient's mouth in an open position, it is possible for the head of the normal condyle to be seen outside of the glenoid fossa. Note that the vertebral column is superimposed upon the symphysis of the mandible and in this instance makes visualization of a fracture of the symphysis of the mandible difficult. Lesions in this anterior area of the mandible can be examined in a like manner without superimposition of the vertebral column by making two anterior lateral jaw radiographs.

The Posteroanterior Sinus Radiograph

In the P-A sinus radiograph the patient's chin is placed on the cassette with the sagittal plane of the skull perpendicular to the film (Figure 14–23). The head is so positioned that the orbitomeatal line makes an angle of 40 degrees with the film. The central ray is perpendicular to the film in both the horizontal and vertical planes. The central ray enters from the posterior of the skull in the sagittal plane at the level of the middle of the sinuses. Basically the projection is made in

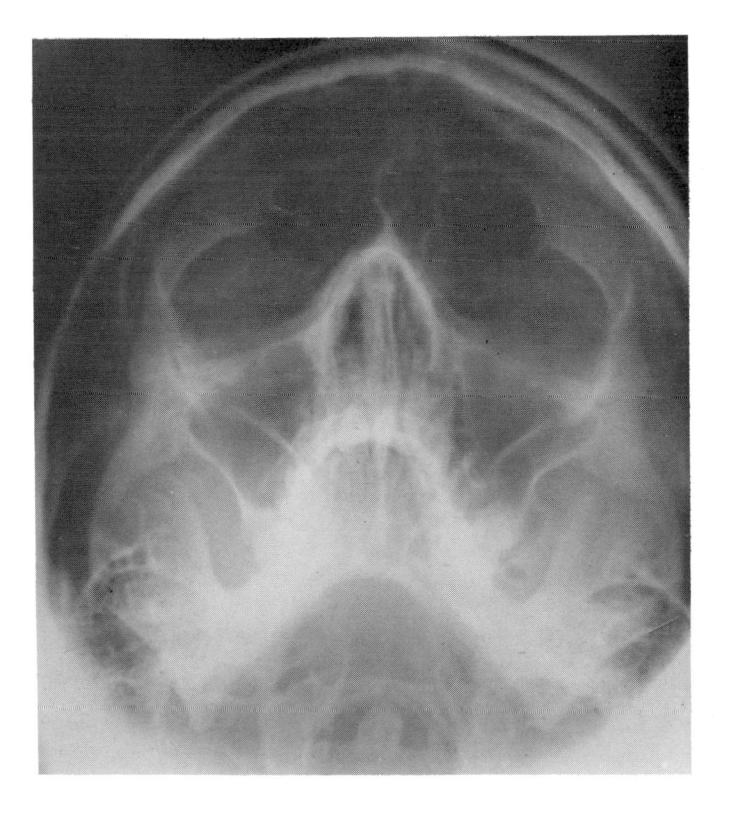

Figure 14–24. P-A sinus radiograph.

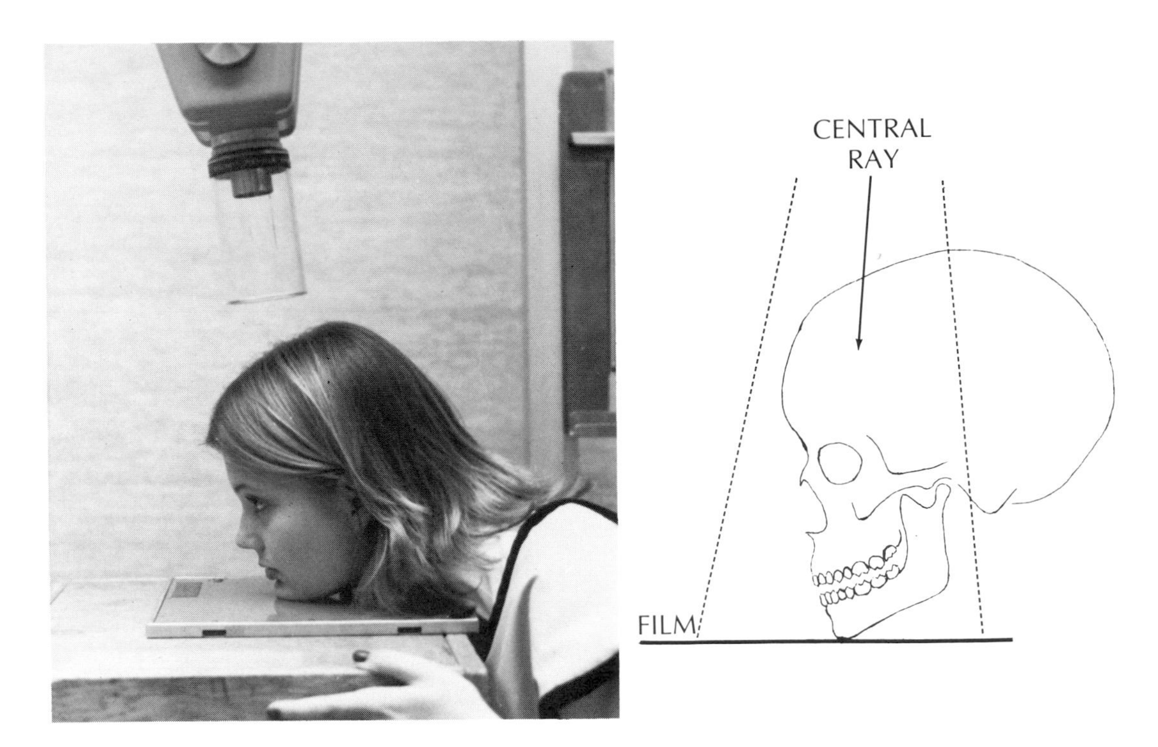

Figure 14–25. Technic for bregma-menton radiograph. The cassette is placed on a table top; a box or books can be used to further elevate the cassette for taller patients.

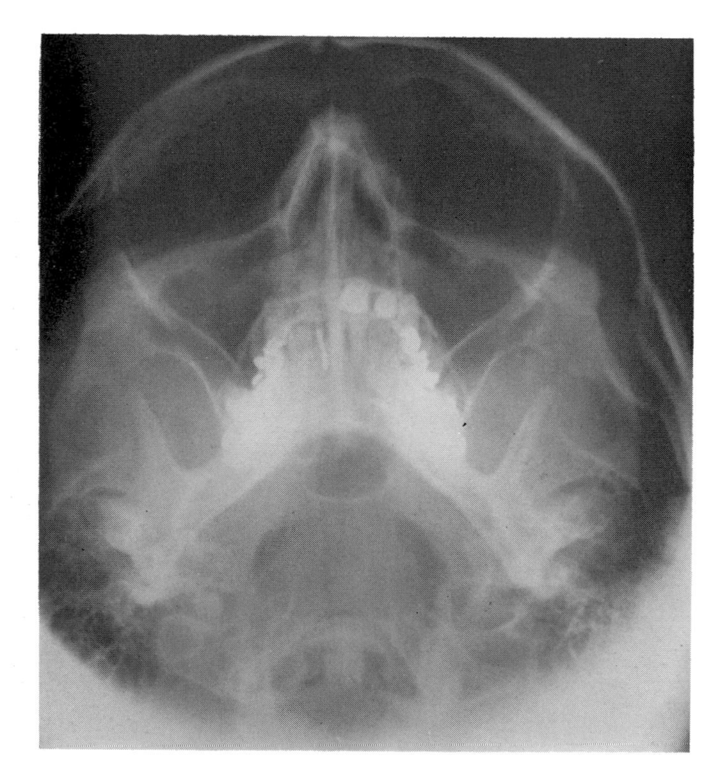

Figure 14–26. Bregma-menton radiograph.

this manner to avoid superimposing the shadows of the petrous portions of the temporal bones upon shadows of the maxillary sinuses. With the short cone, 20-inch tube-film distance, medium speed film and screens, 10 mA, and 65 kVp, the approximate exposure time is 1¼ seconds.

The P-A sinus radiograph is shown in Figure 14–24. The projection can also be made with the cassette in the horizontal plane on top of a metal table. This projection, or a modification of this technic, is often called Waters' view. The projection, made with the film in the upright position, is sometimes used to show the level or amount of fluid in the sinuses. If this projection is made with a slightly larger cone of radiation and with the mouth of the patient opened, it is possible to see the shadows of all the sinuses, the sphenoid sinus being superimposed upon the palate. The larger radiograph is sometimes called a general view of the sinuses.

The Bregma-Menton Radiograph

For the bregma-menton projection the film is placed in a horizontal position on top of

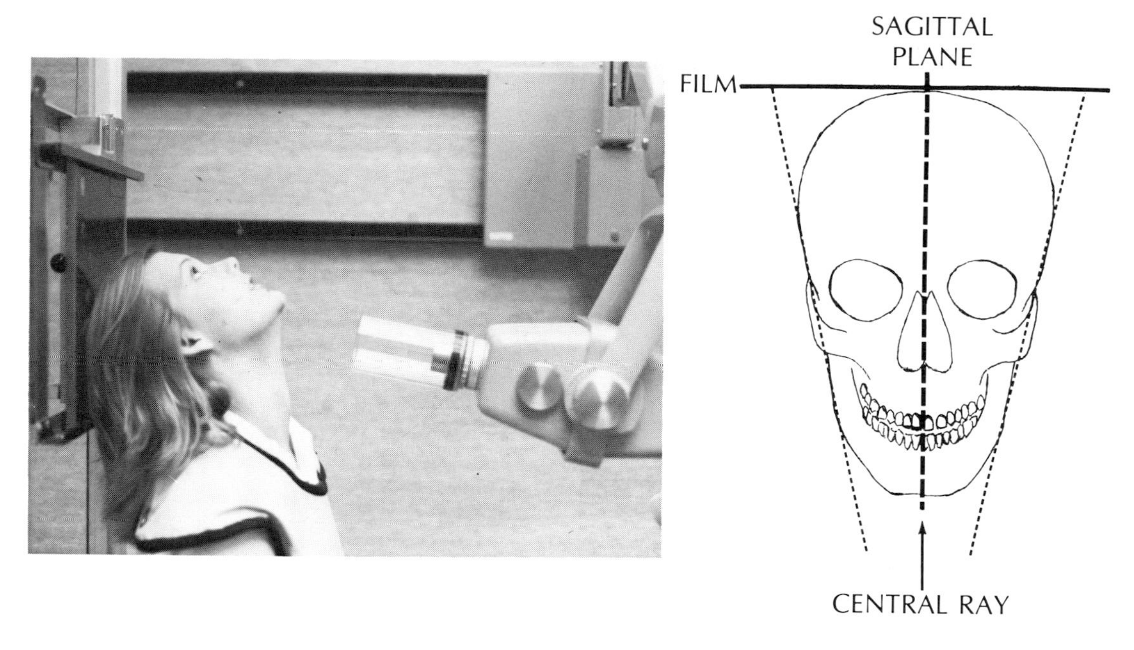

Figure 14–27. Technic for inferior-superior zygomatic arch radiograph.

a metal table. The film is tucked under the chin as far back as possible. The chin is extended as far forward as is comfortable. The sagittal plane of the skull is perpendicular to the film. The central ray enters at the bregma and exits at the menton (Figure 14–25). Using the short cone, a tube-film distance of 24 inches, medium speed film and screens, 10 mA, and 65kVp, the approximate exposure time is 1½ seconds.

The bregma-menton radiograph is shown in Figure 14–26. The radiograph is useful in the examination for medial or lateral deviations of any part of the mandible, the walls of the maxillary sinuses (especially in the posterior area), the orbits, the zygomatic arches, and the nasal septum.

The Inferior-Superior Zygomatic Arch Radiograph

The film for the inferior-superior zygomatic arch radiograph is exposed with the patient's head tilted backward in the dental chair. The cassette is placed on top of the patient's head as nearly perpendicular to the sagittal plane as possible (Figure 14–27). The cassette can be held in position by the pa-

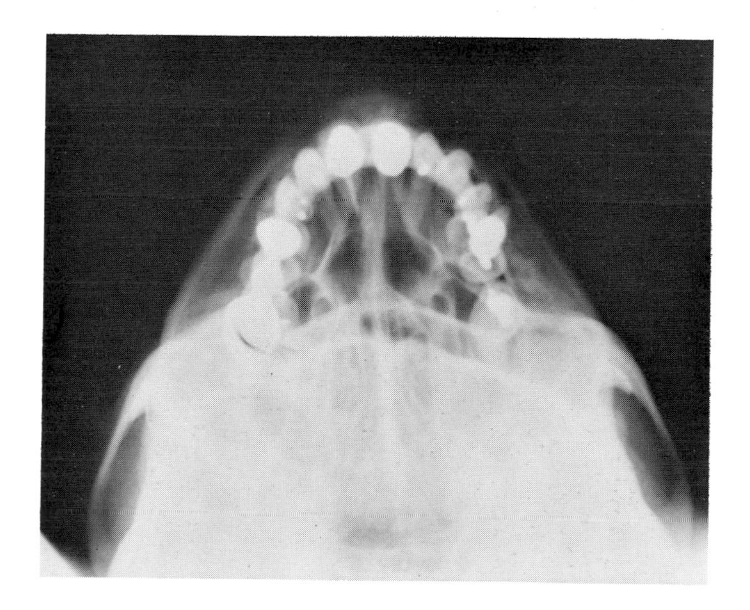

Figure 14–28. Inferior-superior zygomatic arch projection.

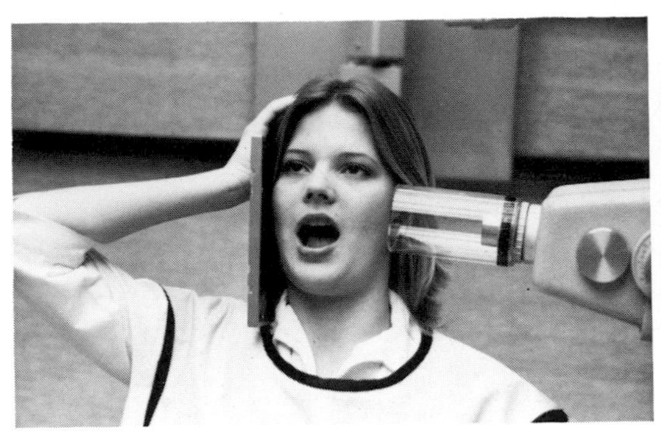

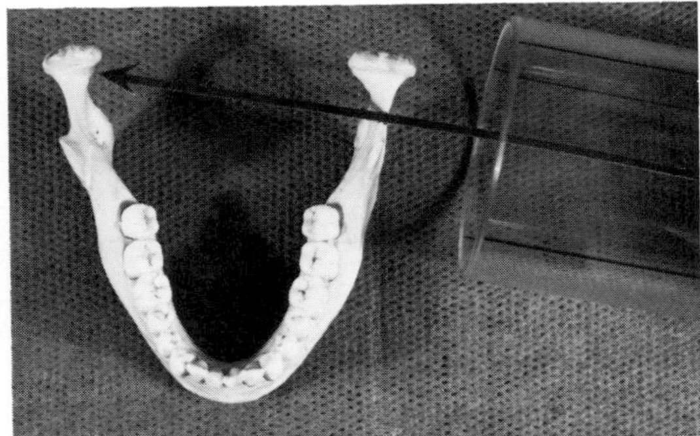

Figure 14–29. Technic for transpharyngeal TMJ radiograph.

tient. The x-ray tube is positioned to direct the central ray along the midsagittal plane, perpendicular to the film, and at the level of a point midway between the zygomatic arches. The x-ray tube is placed 22 inches from the zygomatic arches. Note that most extraoral radiographic technics use a tube-to-film distance; in this projection the tube-to-object distance is of importance. If the tube is placed too close to the patient's head, the image of the mandible will be superimposed upon the zygomatic arches; if the tube is placed too far from the patient's head, the shadows of the arches may be superimposed upon the cranium.

The short cone is used in the inferior-superior zygomatic arch projection. When medium speed film and screens are used with 10 mA and 65 kVp, the approximate exposure time is $\frac{1}{5}$ second (12 impulses). A relatively short exposure time is needed because the structures of interest are small bones and not heavier skull parts. Figure 14–28 shows an example of the inferior-superior zygomatic arch radiograph.

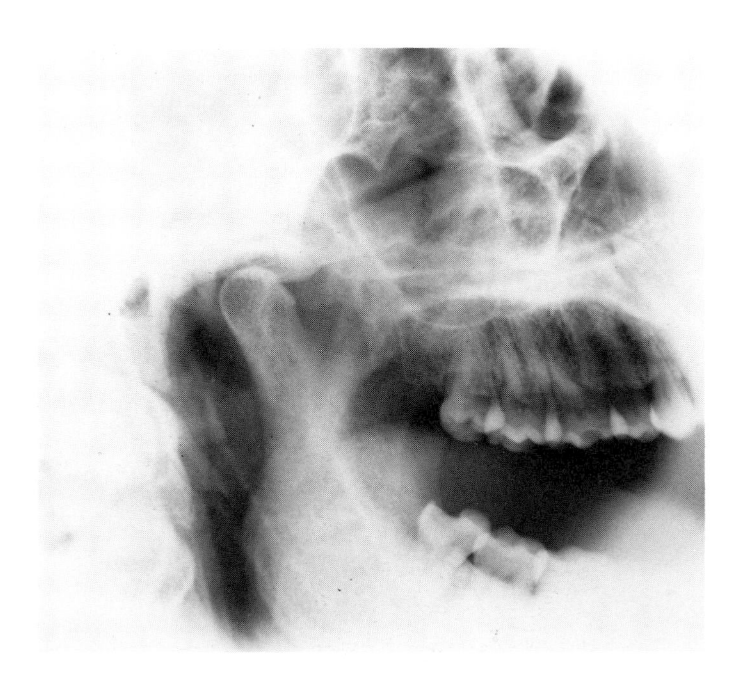

Figure 14–30. Transpharyngeal TMJ radiograph.

The Transpharyngeal Temporomandibular Joint Radiograph

A 5 × 7 inch film is used in the transpharyngeal TMJ projection with the cassette held against the side of the head by the patient (Figure 14–29). The central ray of the x-ray beam is directed through the sigmoid notch (between the condyle and coronoid process) of the mandible on the opposite side and aimed directly at the temporomandibular joint. The patient is asked to open the mouth; this action lowers the head of the condyle being examined out of its articular fossa and also lowers the coronoid process of the opposite side out of the path of the x-ray beam, thus lessening the chance of superimposing the coronoid process upon the TMJ under examination. With the short cone, medium speed film and screens, 10 mA, and 65 kVp, the approximate time is $^1/_{10}$ second (6 impulses).

Figure 14–30 shows the transpharyngeal TMJ radiograph. The projection surveys the head and neck of the condyle and the articular eminence; the articular fossa is less clearly seen; of particular importance is the unobstructed view of the superior surface of the condyle.

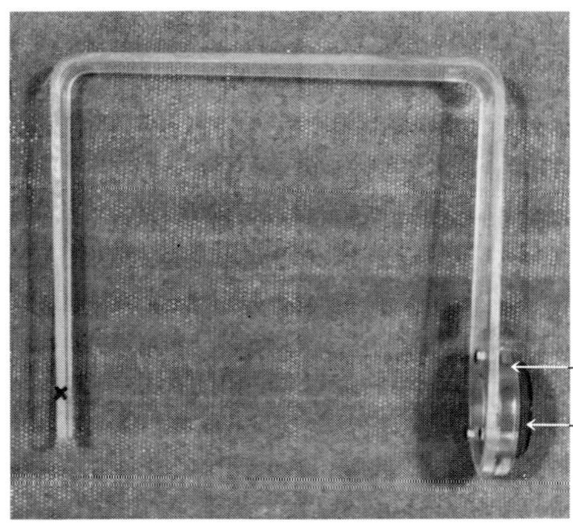

Figure 14–31. X-ray beam localizer made of Plexiglass attached to base of old tubehead cone. Position of central ray is located at X.

The Transcranial Temporomandibular Joint Radiograph

In the transcranial view of the TMJ the x-ray beam travels across the patient's cranium. The x-ray beam should not be more than 2½ inches in diameter at the joint being examined, and thus a collimator smaller than the one used in the short cone is needed. Usually an x-ray beam localizer is used to direct the narrow x-ray beam to the TMJ (Figure 14–31). The plastic localizer in Figure 14–31 is easily made by cutting ¼ (0.25)-inch thick plastic to the desired shape, bending the plastic over a flame, and attaching it to the threaded base of an x-ray machine cone. The distance across the localizer is 9 inches.

The patient holds a 5 × 7 inch cassette against the side of the head (Figure 14–32). The central ray's exit point located at X on the localizer is positioned behind the cassette adjacent to the TMJ being examined. The machine tubehead is positioned for the central ray to enter the opposite side of the patient's head at a point 2 inches above and 1 inch behind the external auditory meatus. With medium speed film and screens, 10 mA, and 65 kVp, the approximate exposure time is ½ second (30 impulses).

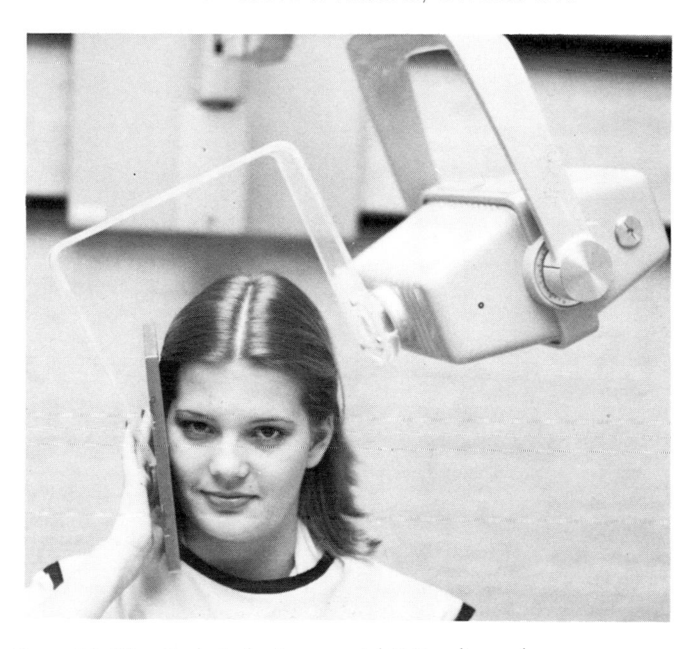

Figure 14–32. Technic for transcranial TMJ radiograph.

Figure 14–33 illustrates a transcranial TMJ radiograph. The projection shows an oblique lateral view of the condyle as seen from above the TMJ on the opposite side. The relationship of the condyle to the articulating surface (glenoid fossa and eminence) of the joint is seen in this radiograph. The projec-

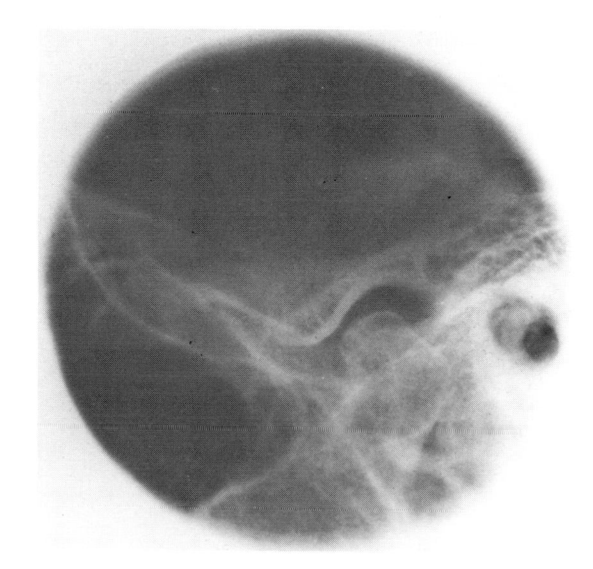

Figure 14–33. Transcranial TMJ radiograph.

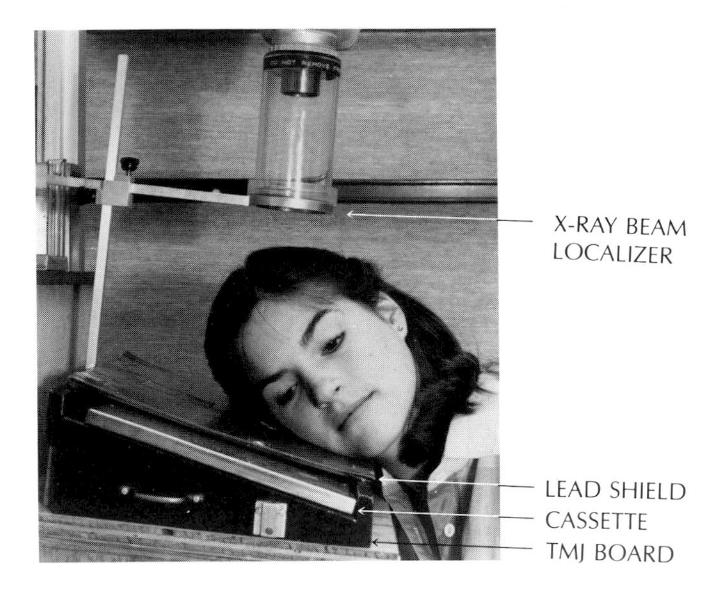

Figure 14–34. TMJ board with patient and x-ray tubehead positioned for transcranial series.

tion can be made with the jaws closed, at rest, or opened.

The Transcranial TMJ Series

Transcranial TMJ radiographs are often made in a series to show TMJ-condyle-fossa relationships with the mandible in different positions. The series of radiographs of a joint are made with the same film and positions of the patient and x-ray beam. To maintain the same tube-patient-film relationship between exposures, the patient and x-ray tube are placed in a device or TMJ board (Figure 14–34). The board assists the operator in placing the x-ray beam in the correct transcranial position. The cassette is moved between exposures, and 2 or 3 exposures are made of the joint. To examine the opposite TMJ the machine and patient are removed from the board, the cassette and patient are turned around, and the procedure is repeated for the opposite TMJ. Interpretation of the radiographic images is assisted by looking at the base of the cranium (Figure 14–35) and observing the direction of the x-ray beam. Figure 14–36 shows the transcranial TMJ series of radiographs.

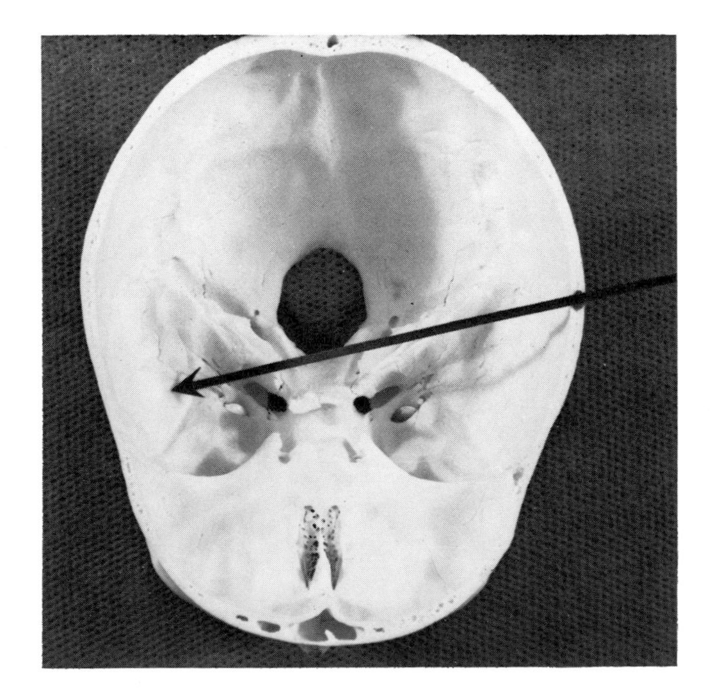

Figure 14–35. View of base of cranial vault and direction of transcranial x-ray beam.

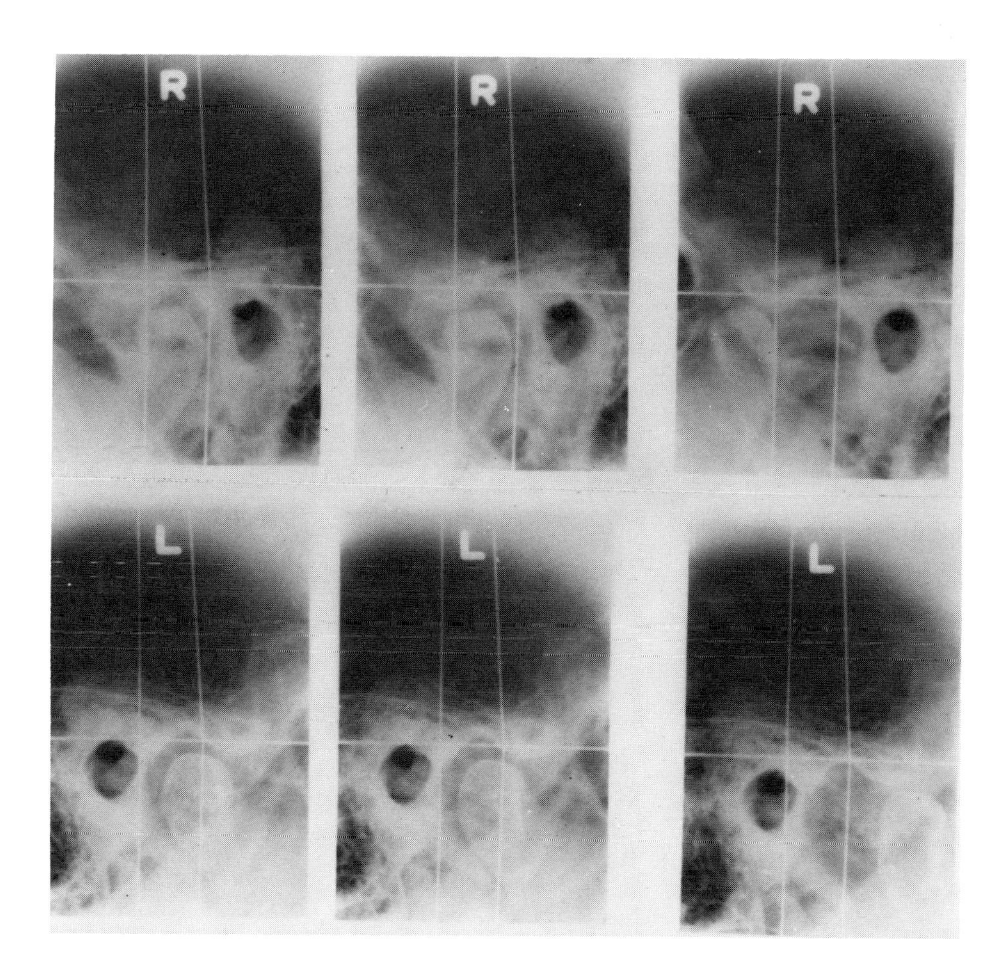

Figure 14–36. Transcranial TMJ radiographic series. These separate exposures are made for right (R) and left (L) temporomandibular joints. Three exposures are made with jaws closed, mandible in rest position (middle radiograph), and jaws open.

Chapter 15

Panoramic Radiography

A panoramic radiograph is a view of a large area of the mandible and/or maxilla as seen in a single large film. There are many different methods of obtaining a large area view of the jaws. Some methods are similar to the usual intraoral and extraoral radiographic technics in using a stationary x-ray source, patient, and film. Such methods can be called still-radiographic technics; these methods are not commonly used but will be briefly described in this text.

Panoramic radiographs can be made with the x-ray tube, patient, and film moving, relative to each other, during film exposure. This method is called *pantomography* and is by far the most common panoramic technic used in dentistry. Pantomography utilizes principles of slit-beam *scanography* and *tomography.* These principles must be understood by operators and diagnosticians using the pantomographic type of panoramic radiographic technic.

This chapter will present information on still-radiography panoramic technics, pantomographic theory, and pantomographic machines. Normal anatomic landmarks seen in panoramic radiographs are shown when individual machines are discussed. Artifacts and technic errors in pantomography radiographs are shown and their causes identified.

STILL RADIOGRAPHY TECHNICS

Relatively large areas of the jaws can be examined by a wide x-ray beam with the x-ray tube, patient, and film motionless or still. The x-ray source can be positioned intraorally or extraorally. Special machines have been developed to place the x-ray tube within the patient's mouth. Still-picture technics, with the x-ray tube outside the mouth, use the standard dental x-ray machine and devices to position the film, patient, and x-ray tubehead for a series of exposures similar to lateral jaw radiographs.

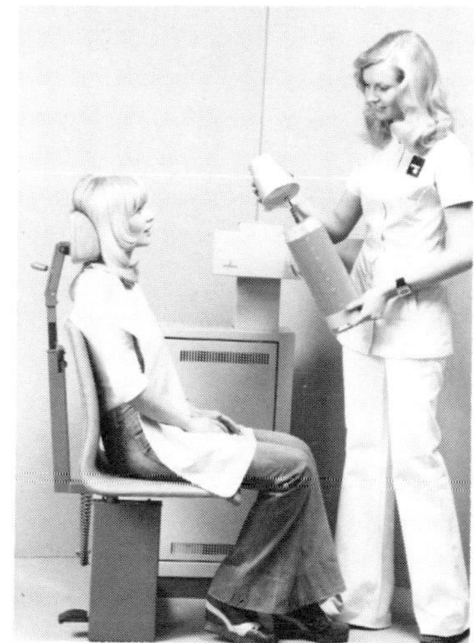

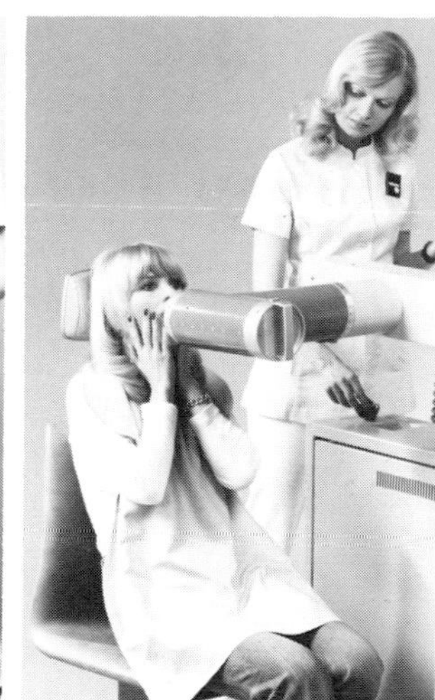

Figure 15–1. The Status-X intraoral source x-ray machine. (Courtesy of Siemens Corporation, Iselin, New Jersey.)

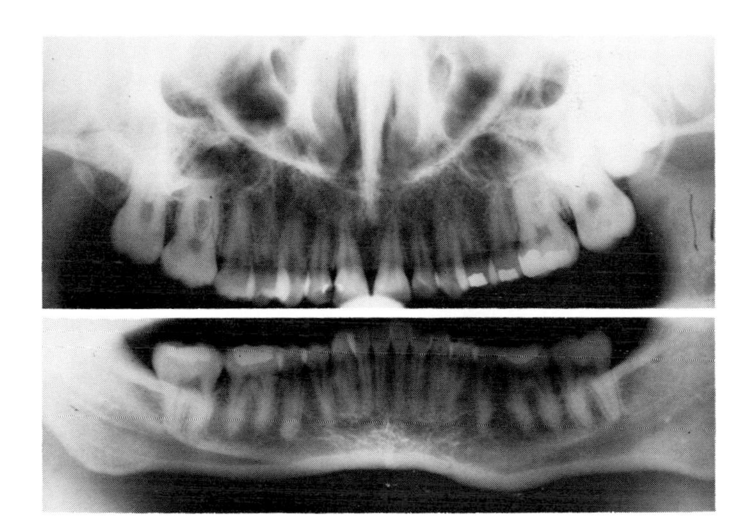

Figure 15–2. Separate radiographs made of maxilla and mandible with Status-X machine. (Courtesy of Siemens Corporation, Iselin, New Jersey.)

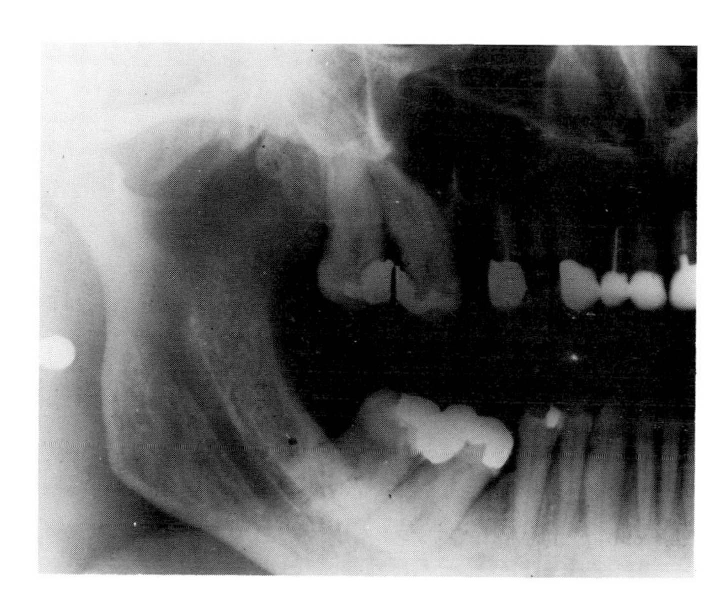

Figure 15–3. Intraoral source radiograph of ramus region.

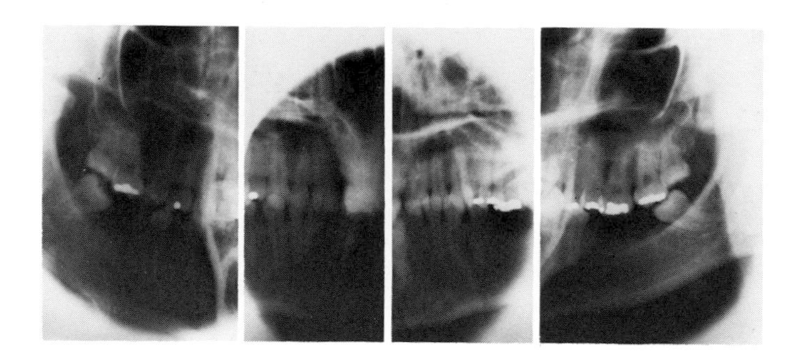

Figure 15–4. Lateral jaw radiographs on 5- × 12-inch film collectively showing panorama of dentition.

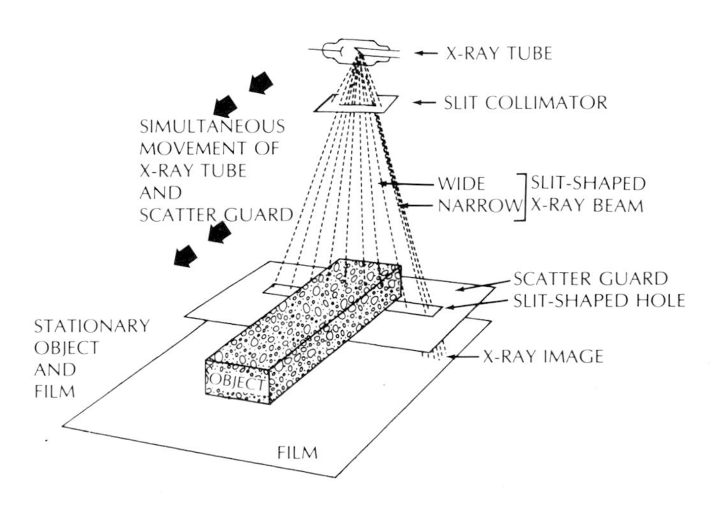

Figure 15–5. Diagram of x-ray beam collimation and movements of x-ray tube and scatter guard in scanography of an object.

Intraoral Source Radiography

Machines using an x-ray source positioned inside the patient's mouth have an x-ray tube with a cone-shaped anode mounted at the end of a rodlike extension (Figure 15–1). These machines are also referred to as rod anode x-ray machines. X rays are produced in all directions from the tip of the anode. A shield around the x-ray tube collimates the x-rays to a wide beam that examines the entire maxillary or mandibular dentition (Figure 15–2). A flexible cassette with screen film is used and the cassette is held by the patient. Separate radiographs are made for the maxillary and mandibular dental regions and for the ramus (Figure 15–3).

The radiographs are similar to intraoral radiographs in showing the teeth and bone, but the images are more magnified because of the short distance between the x-ray tube and the teeth. Image sharpness is quite good because these machines use a small focal spot and all radiopaque parts of the object appear in the radiograph.

Lateral Jaw Panoramic Series

Devices have been developed to place the patient, film, and regular dental x-ray machine in the positions for lateral jaw radiography. Separate exposures of different parts of a 5 × 12-inch screen film in a cassette are made for the molar and anterior regions of the patient's mouth (Figure 15–4). When all of the projections are observed collectively in the single film, a panoramic type of view of the dentition is obtained.

THEORY OF PANTOMOGRAPHY

A pantomogram is a panoramic radiograph made with tomographic principles. Dental pantomographic machines also utilize another radiographic system called scanography; this is not indicated in the term *pantomography*. A basic understanding of both scanography and tomography is necessary for the proper production and diagnosis of pantomograms.

Scanography

A radiograph can be made by scanning an object with a thin moving beam of x rays (Figure 15–5). A slit-shaped collimator is used to make a narrow (sheetlike) beam of x rays. The x-ray tube is moved to scan different parts of the object. Before reaching the film, the x-ray beam passes through a hole in a sheet of heavy metal that acts as a scatter guard; the hole is shaped to the size of the primary x-ray beam and the hole moves with the x-ray beam. The purpose of the scatter guard is to prevent scatter x rays from reaching parts of the film not being exposed by the primary x-ray beam.

Tomography

A tomogram is a radiograph that shows a sharp image of a layer of tissue with the layers above and below it being unsharp or blurred. The radiograph is made by moving the x-ray tube and film parallel to each other in opposite directions during film exposure. During movement of the tube and film the x-ray beam turns and is constantly directed at a point in the selected layer being examined (Figure 15–6).

A tomogram shows both sharp and blurred x-ray shadows. The width or thickness of the sharp layer (zone of sharpness or focal trough) seen in a tomogram varies with the angle of movement of the x-ray beam (Figure 15–7). A large angle during film exposure produces a narrow layer or focal trough; a small angle results in a thick layer of tissue being seen, i.e., a wide focal trough.

Tomography is used when objects cannot be seen in the usual diagnostic radiographs due to the superimposition of the images of other skull structures. The obstructing images of structures above or below the objects a dentist wishes to see can often be blurred or removed by tomography.

Curved Layer Tomography

A tomogram showing relatively sharp images of a curved layer of tissue can be produced by combining tomography and slit beam scanography. The basic factors in curved layer tomography are shown in Figure 15–8. A narrow beam of x rays is used to scan a stationary object. The x-ray tubehead and film carrier are connected to each other; they circle around the object so that the x-ray beam turns around a pivotal point (x-ray

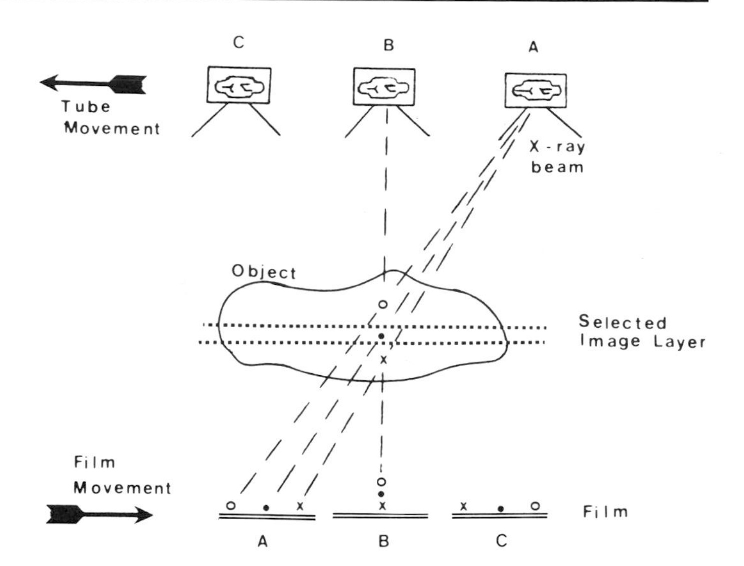

Figure 15–6. Diagram of basic tomographic movements. X-ray source and film move during exposure (A to B to C). The movement is synchronized so that turning point of x-ray beam is situated at tissue layer selected to appear sharp in radiograph. Note that dot situated in selected layer casts its x-ray image on same area of film during film exposure while parts above and below (represented by O and X) have their images smeared across film and thus appear blurred in the radiograph. (From Manson-Hing, L.R.: Panoramic Dental Radiography, 1976. Courtesy of Charles C Thomas, Publisher, Springfield, Illinois.)

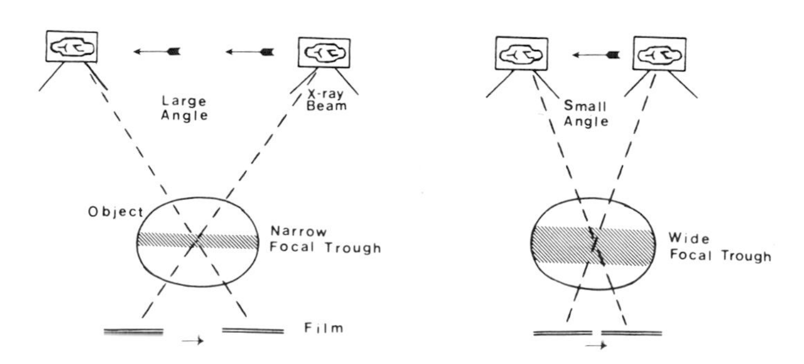

Figure 15–7. Diagram showing large and small angles traversed by x-ray beam during film exposure in tomography and their effect on width of focal trough. (From Manson-Hing, L.R.: Panoramic Dental Radiography, 1976. Courtesy of Charles C Thomas Publisher, Springfield, Illinois.)

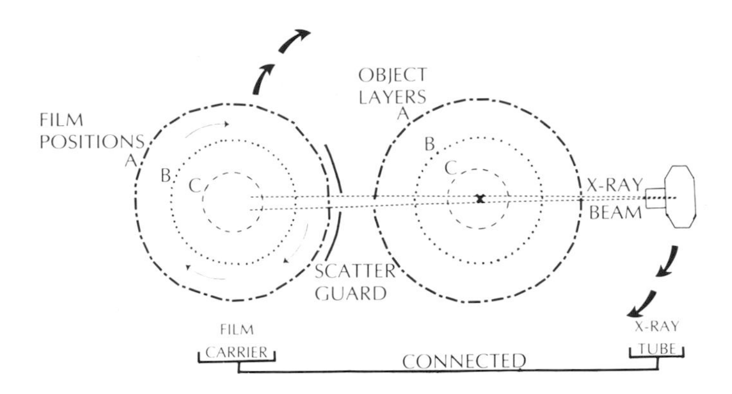

Figure 15–8. Diagram showing basic factors in curved layer tomography. X-ray tubehead is connected to film carrier; they move around object. X-ray beam turns around pivot or axis X and scans the stationary object. Films positioned at A, B, or C will image object layers A, B, or C.

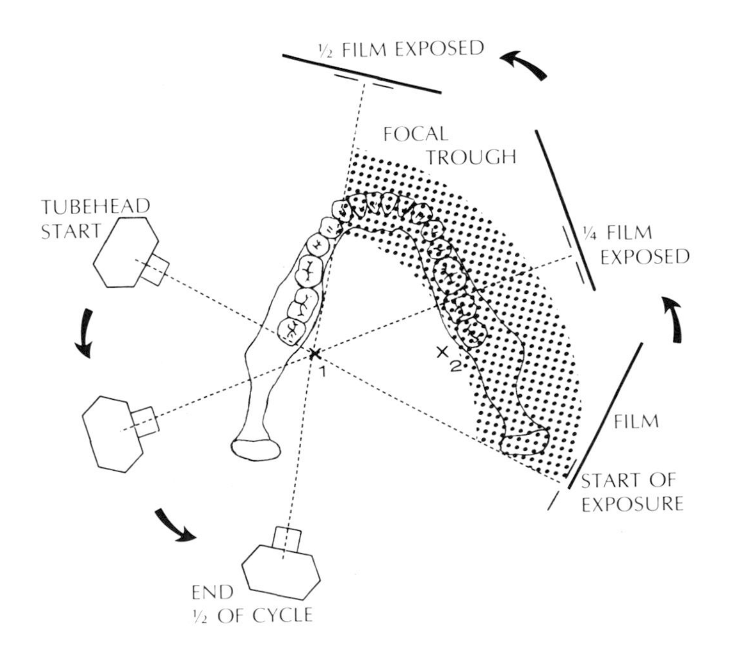

Figure 15–9. Diagram of two-center (X_1, X_2) curved layer pantomographic system using flat film. Dotted area indicates focal trough or zone of sharpness in projection of one side of patient.

beam axis or rotation center) in the object. While the tube and film carrier are moving, the film moves behind a scatter guard. The scatter guard prevents scattered x rays from reaching parts of the film not being exposed by the x-ray beam. The film moves through the x-ray beam at the same rate as the layer being imaged in the object. In other words, when one inch of film moves through the x-ray beam, the layer in the object where one inch has been scanned by the beam appears sharp in the radiograph. Other layers are blurred.

A patient's jaw can be examined with the x-ray beam rotating around two axes, centers, or pivots (Figure 15–9). The center of rotation is located on the side opposite to the jaw side being examined. Two individual exposures must be made, one for each side. The single film thus contains two separate radiographic views. The x-ray beam is turned off during the machine's shifting from one center of rotation to the other center on the opposite side. A flat film can be used; the film has to pass through the x-ray beam at the same speed as the tooth layer being scanned by the x-ray beam. A curved film is not necessary to satisfy this requirement. The width of the tomographic layer (focal trough or zone of sharpness) is affected by the changing angle formed by the x-ray beam and the determined curved layer as the beam scans the layer. The greater the angular change the thinner or narrower is the focal trough. In the two rotational center system shown in Figure 15–9 the angular changes of the x-ray beam in the posterior and anterior jaw areas are similar and thus the width of the focal trough is similar in both of these jaw areas.

Three centers of x-ray beam rotation can be used to make a single continuous radiographic image of the jaws. Two lateral centers are located posteriorly and one midline center is in the anterior region of the jaws (Figure 15–10). The x-ray beam starts its scan of the jaws at one lateral center by examining the TMJ of the opposite side. When one side of the patient has been scanned to the cuspid region, the x-ray beam is shifted from the lateral rotational center to the midline anterior center. The incisor region of the patient is now scanned by the x-ray beam. The x-ray beam is then shifted to the third or opposite lateral rotation center to scan the remaining jaw areas of the patient.

The angular change of the x-ray beam during scanning of the posterior jaw areas, with the beam rotating around a lateral pivot, is much less than the angular change of the beam when scanning the incisor area with the beam rotating around the middle rotational center or pivot. Note that the middle center is closer to the tooth layer. This results in the focal trough or zone of sharpness being wide in the posterior areas of the jaws and narrow in the anterior region (Figure 15–10).

A single unbroken pantomographic exposure of the jaws can also be made with the rotational center of the x-ray beam moving during film exposure. This results in an x-ray beam that is continuously shifting or sliding (Figure 15–11). Like the zone of sharpness in the system with three rotational centers the zone of sharpness is wide in the posterior jaw areas and narrow in the incisor region of the jaws.

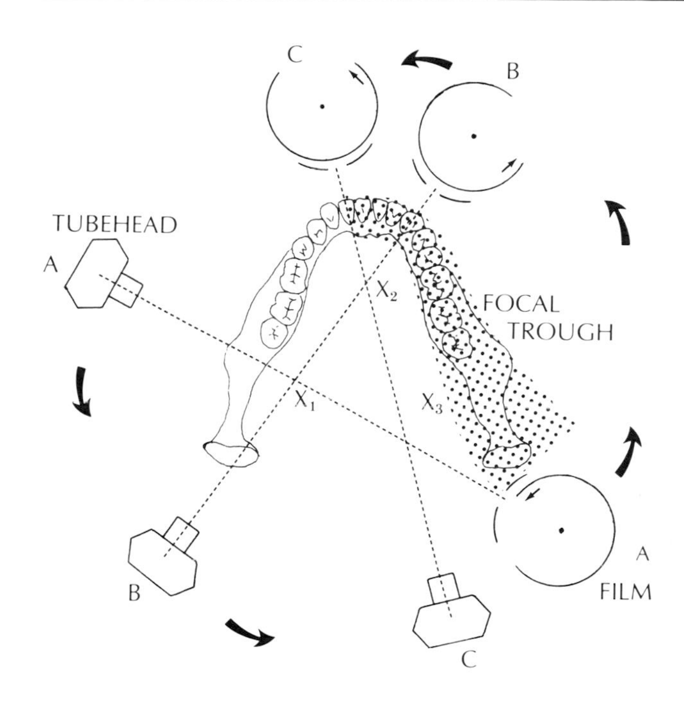

Figure 15–10. Diagram of three-center (X_1, X_2, X_3) curved layer pantomographic system using film on curved film carrier. At position B, x-ray beam shifts from rotation center X_1 to X_2. Dotted area shows focal trough or zone of sharpness seen in the radiograph.

PANTOMOGRAPHY MACHINES

Many different pantomographic machines are manufactured. Not all of these machines are sold in the U.S.A.; of those sold in America only some are sold nationwide. Major differences between machines are in the location of beam rotation centers, fixed or adjustable focal troughs, split or continuous images, type and shape of film transport systems, electrical supply to the x-ray tubes, head positioning devices, sitting or standing patients and wall mounted or free standing installation. This chapter will discuss mainly the Panorex, Orthopantomograph, Panelipse, and Panex (Panoral) panoramic machines. These machines are examples of the different types of beam rotation not visible to the operator. The machines also demonstrate the great differences among pantomographic x-ray machines that are more obvious to the radiographer.

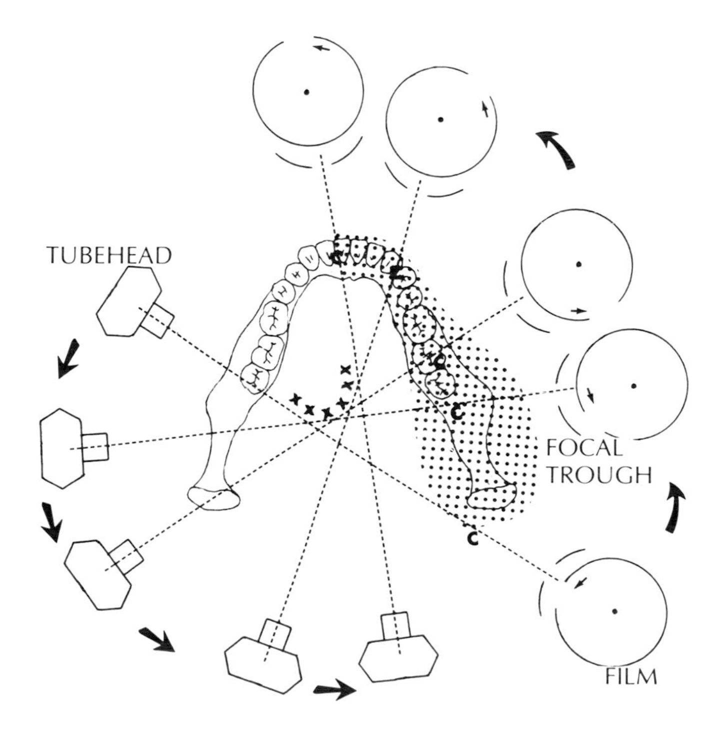

Figure 15–11. Diagram of pantomographic system using moving rotational center (C) of x-ray beam. Dotted area shows zone of sharpness or focal trough seen in entire radiograph. The real center of rotation of the x-ray beam is at X.

The Panorex I

The Panorex I machine (S.S. White Dental Products International) uses an x-ray beam with two centers of rotation (Figure 15–12).

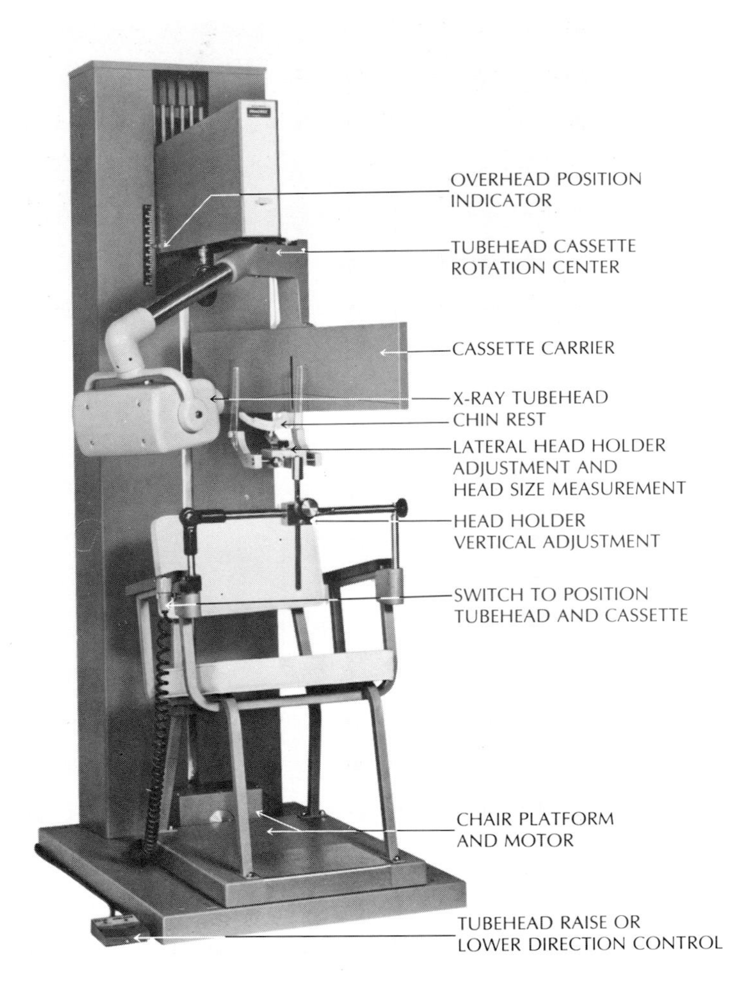

Figure 15–12. Panorex I panoramic x-ray unit. (Photograph courtesy of S.S. White Dental Products International, Pennwalt Corporation, Philadelphia, Pa.)

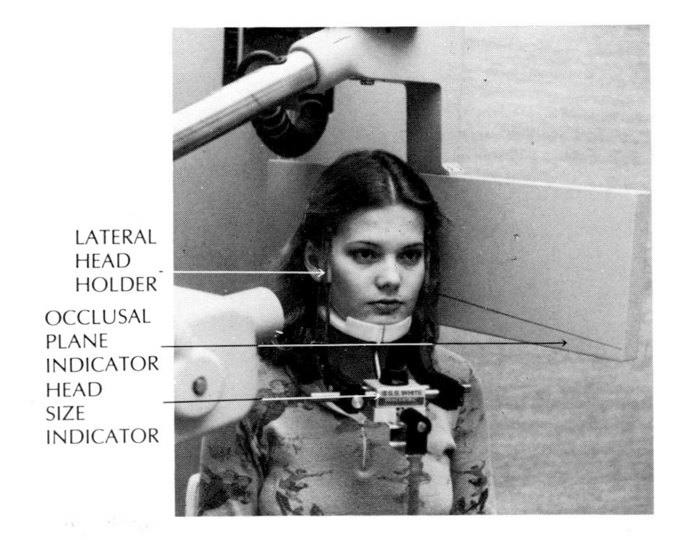

Figure 15–13. Patient's head positioned in Panorex I head holder.

The patient is seated in the chair facing the operator and told to keep his elbows off the arms of the chair. The machine's head positioner, on a horizontal bar, is placed in front of the patient and locked in position. The patient's head is placed in the head positioner with the patient's back in an erect position; this is done by supporting the patient's back with the wedge-shaped cushion. The x-ray tubehead-cassette assembly is lowered into position by reading the head position scale, activating the foot and hand switches simultaneously, and lowering the overhead assembly until the tubehead pointer is at the same number as the head position scale. The patient's head is positioned with the occlusal plane slightly downward in the incisor region; a line on the cassette holder indicates the correct position (Figure 15–13). The lateral head holders are brought inward until they touch the patient's head; the operator notes the width of the patient's head indicated on a scale on the head positioner. The patient's incisor teeth are placed edge to edge; a cotton roll can be placed between the teeth.

The patient is then told (1) that the tubehead cassette assembly will circle around his/her head, (2) that he/she must not follow the cassette carrier with the eyes as it moves around the head, (3) that when the cassette carrier is in front of the face the chair will shift to the side about 3 inches, (4) that he/she must hold still, (5) that he/she will feel nothing, and (6) that the procedure will take about 20 seconds.

The operator must check the milliamperage, read from a chart the kilovoltage needed for the head width of the patient, and set the kVp selector. The operator then tells the patient to hold still and activates the exposure switch. During film exposure the operator must always watch the patient. After film exposure the patient and cassette are removed from the machine.

A Panorex I panoramic radiograph is shown in Figure 15–14. Two separate radiographic images are recorded on a 5 × 12 inch film. The unexposed film area separating the images of the right and left sides of the jaws is a result of the x-ray beam being turned off during the chair shift when the machine changes the x-ray beam rotational center; during the chair shift the cassette continues to move behind the opening in the scatter guard of the cassette holder.

The panoramic radiograph shows the patient's jaws from TM joint to TM joint with some duplication of the anterior midline region. Vertically the region examined is from the level of the chin to 5 inches above. The basic anatomic landmarks seen in this area are shown in Figure 15–15.

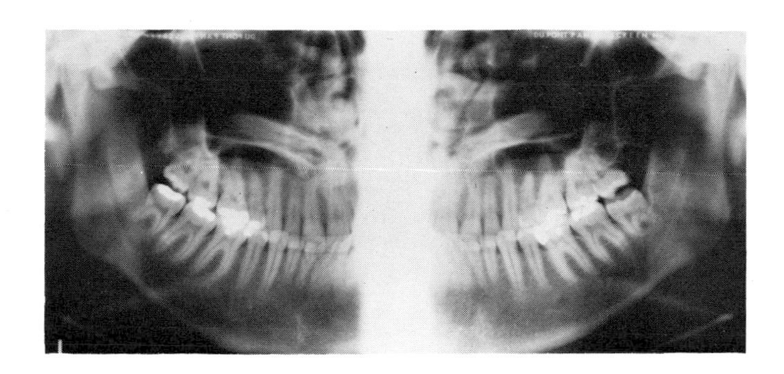

Figure 15–14. Panoramic radiograph made with Panorex I x-ray machine.

The Orthopantomograph-3

The Orthopantomograph-3 (Siemens Corporation) uses an x-ray beam which moves around three centers of rotation (Figure 15–16). Also, in contrast to the Panorex, the machine places the patient in a standing position. The machine is attached to a wall and the patient stands in the machine, facing the wall. Handrails are provided for the patient to hold while in the machine. The machine is raised or lowered manually and is locked into position with electric locks that are easily operated by pressing a button. The machine is placed at a height where the patient's chin is on the chin rest and the spine is erect (Figure 15–17).

The maxillary and mandibular central incisors are placed edge to edge in the grooves of a bite block. The bite block places the crowns of the teeth in the focal trough of the machine. The operator locates the focal trough of the incisor region by looking from the side of the machine at the trough-locating lines marked on both sides of the transparent plastic hood that partially surrounds the patient's head. The apices of the incisor teeth are placed in the focal trough by adjusting the forehead positioner to tip the head forward or backward (Figure 15–17).

The lateral head holders are activated to place the sagittal plane of the head in the middle of the machine. The machine uses a rigid curved cassette. Before film exposure the patient should be told that the tubehead cassette carrier will circle around the head, that he/she must hold still, that he/she will feel nothing, and that the procedure will take about 15 seconds.

The Orthopantomograph has a fixed milliamperage of 15 mA and variable kilovotage. Kilovoltage is adjusted to the size of the patient's head. The machine exposes the film with the tubehead-cassette assembly moving

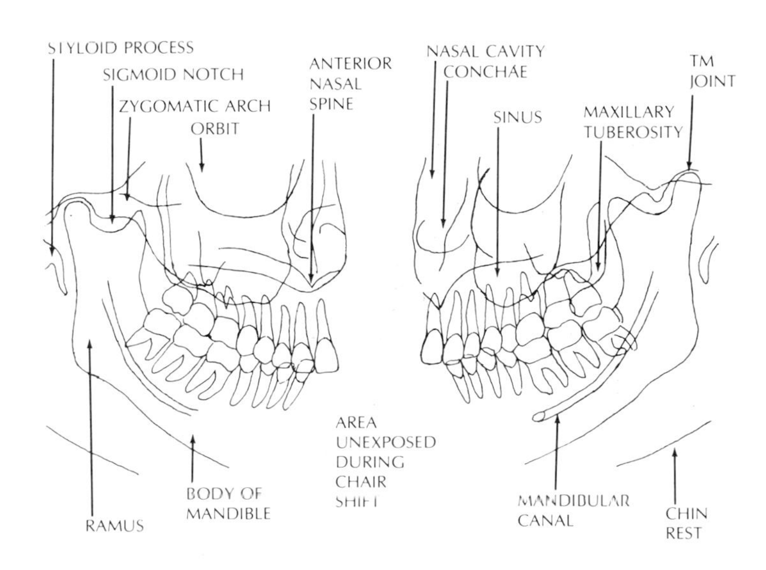

Figure 15–15. Diagram of anatomic landmarks seen in Panorex I panoramic radiograph.

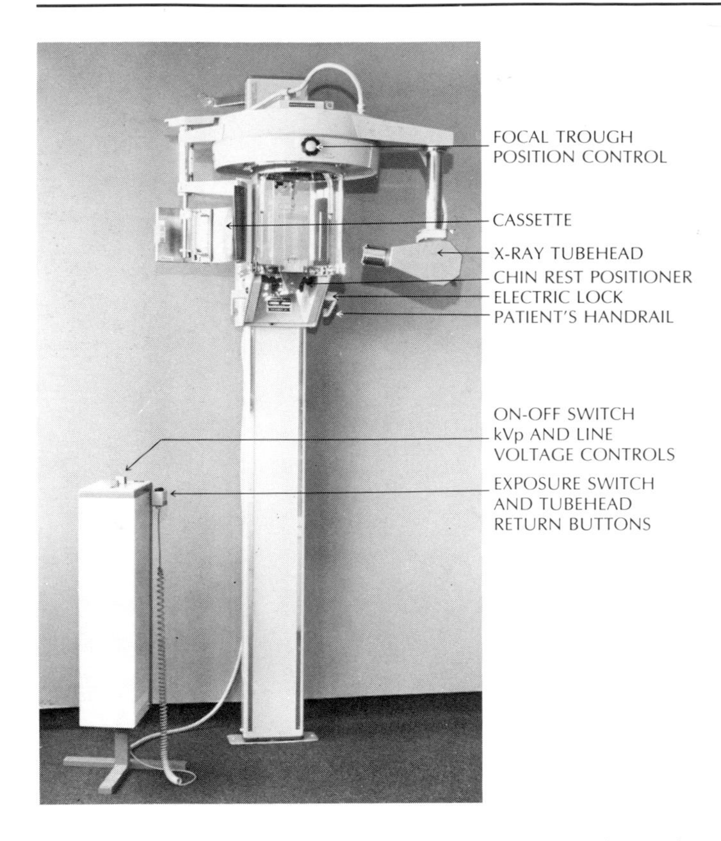

Figure 15–16. Orthopantomograph-3 panoramic x-ray machine. (Photograph courtesy of Siemens Corporation, Iselin, New Jersey.)

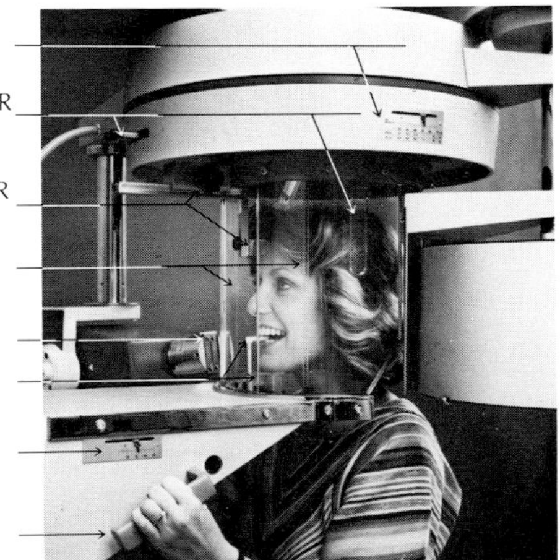

Figure 15–17. Patient positioned in Orthopantomograph-3. (Photograph courtesy of Siemens Corporation, Iselin, New Jersey.)

in only one direction. After a film has been exposed, the tubehead-cassette assembly must be returned to its starting position by pressing a button situated next to the film exposure button. The machine has additional movements to place the patient's chin in other positions or move the focal trough. Only the technic for the regular diagnostic radiograph has been described.

An Orthopantomograph panoramic radiograph is shown in Figure 15–18. The radiographic image is continuous from TM joint to TM joint on a 5 × 12 inch film. The basic anatomic landmarks seen in an orthopantomogram are shown in Figure 15–19.

The Panelipse

The Panelipse (Gendex, formerly of General Electric Corp) uses an x-ray beam with a continuously moving rotational axis that follows the arc of the mandible and maxilla. The object-to-film and object-to-radiation-source distances are kept constant, and vertical magnification is uniform between the anterior and posterior regions of the radiographic image. The magnification is approximately 19%. The arc is not of fixed size but can be adjusted for different-sized jaws (Figure 15–20). The shape of the arc is essentially one half of a 2.5 to 1 ellipse. The ability to change the x-ray beam rotational axis path permits the operator to select the layer for tomographic examination. Such layers can be different from the normal layer through the dentition.

The machine uses a screen film in a flexible cassette. The cassette is placed on a rotating drum and the movement is adjusted for the different sizes of dental arches; thus the length of the radiographic image varies with the jaw size of the patient.

The patient enters from the front of the machine and is seated facing the operator in a chair that can be removed; this feature is desirable for wheelchair patients (Figure 15–21). The backrest of the chair can move forward or backward for different-sized patients after being released by a lever located at the side of the chair. The patient's head is placed in a head holder that swings inward or outward about its attachment to a vertical bar located on one side of the machine. The head holder arm is automatically locked into

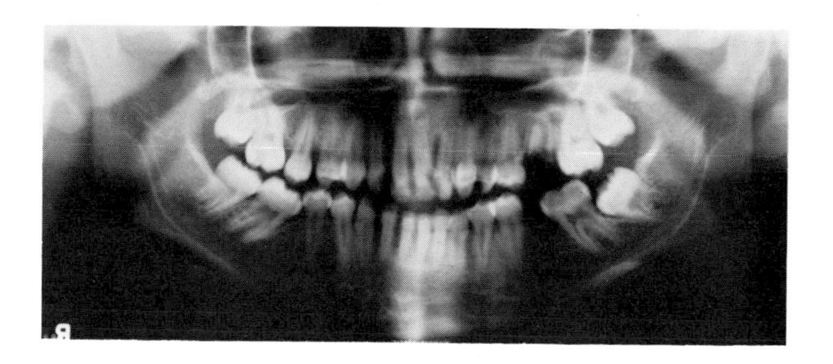

Figure 15–18. Panoramic radiograph made with Orthopantomograph.

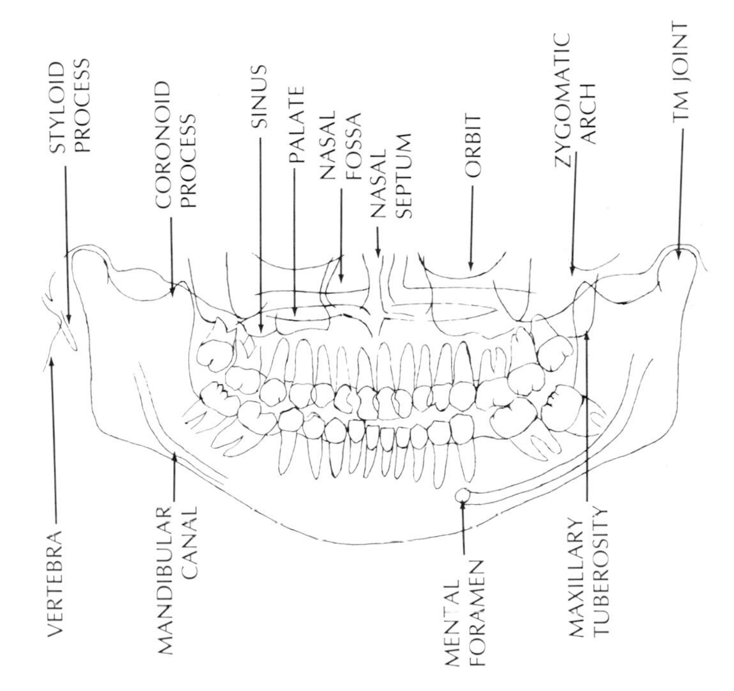

Figure 15–19. Diagram of anatomic landmarks seen in Orthopantomograph.

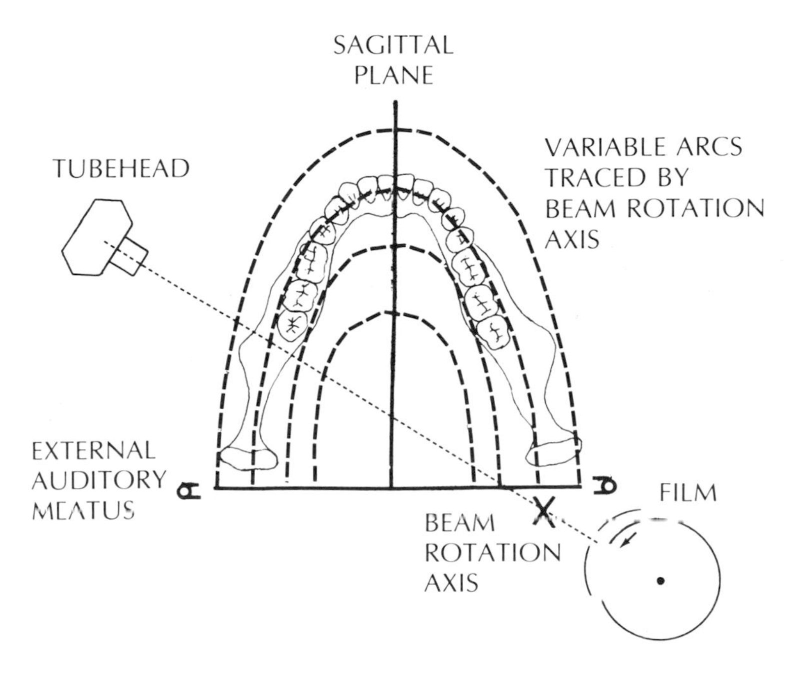

Figure 15–20. Diagram showing variable arcs traced by x-ray beam rotational axis of Panelipse.

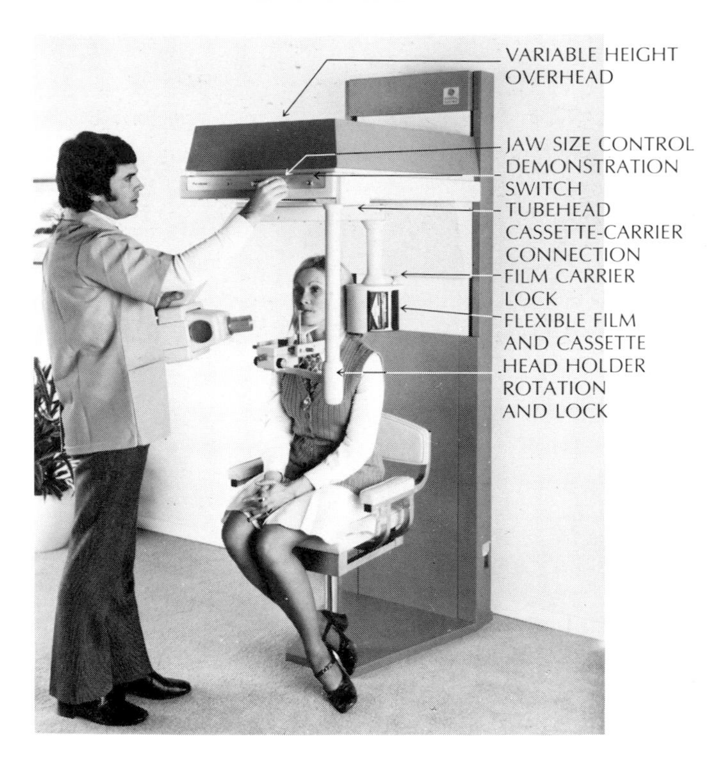

Figure 15–21. Panelipse panoramic x-ray unit. (Photograph courtesy of General Electric Co. Dental Division, Milwaukee, Wisconsin.)

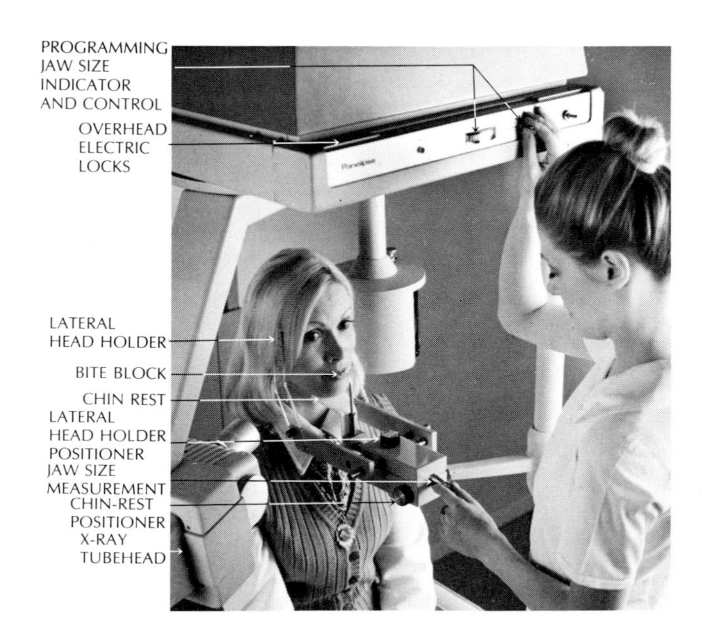

Figure 15–22. Patient positioned in Panelipse with operator positioning x-ray beam axis for jaw size of patient. (Photograph courtesy of General Electric Co. Dental Division, Milwaukee, Wisconsin.)

a fixed position and is attached to a canopy-like section. The overhead section is counterbalanced and is manually raised or lowered along with the attached tubehead film holder assembly to position the patient's occlusal plane. Lines on the lateral head positioners assist in positioning the occlusal plane. The locking mechanism of the overhead section is released or activated through one of two touch bars located above the front of the section.

The patient is asked to place the incisal edges of the teeth in the grooves of the bite block. The anteroposterior position of the patient's head is established by moving the bite block with the chin position control to place the external auditory meatus at the posterior border of the lateral head holder; this is at the posterior limit of the machine's focal trough. The occlusal plane is positioned slightly downward in the incisor regions; this places the apices of the incisors in the same vertical plane. The lateral head holders are positioned. The operator reads the size of the patient's jaw on the indicator on the head holder and sets the beam rotation axis at the correct arch-size starting position by moving the tubehead-cassette arm with the arch-size control on the overhead assembly until the indicator shows the same number as the patient's jaw size number (Figure 15–22).

The remote control box has a variable kVp control and 8, 10, 12, and 15 mA controls. The exposure time necessary to complete the examination of the jaws is 20 seconds. The exposure can be made with the tubehead starting from either side of the patient.

Radiography with the Panelipse is accomplished by seating the patient in the chair, positioning the overhead assembly and the head holder, having the patient place the incisor teeth in the grooves of the bite block, moving the patient's head so that the external auditory meatus is at the posterior border of the lateral head holder, positioning the occlusal plane slightly downward, measuring the jaw size, positioning the beam rotational axis at the correct starting position, setting the kVp and mA needed for the size of the patient's head, and making the exposure.

A Panelipse panoramic radiograph is shown in Figure 15–23. The single continuous image on a 5 × 12 inch film shows a vertical dimension similar to that of other machines; the horizontal dimension varies with the jaw size of the patient. Basic anatomic landmarks seen in the Panelipse panoramic radiograph are shown in Figure 15–24.

The Panex

The Panex-E (also called Panoral) is attached to a base (Figure 15–25). The x-ray beam has a moving center of rotation that traces an elliptical arc. Unlike the Panelipse the arc traced by the moving center is not variable. The patient stands facing the wall and the machine is positioned vertically for the individual's height. Handrails are provided for the patient to hold while in the machine (Figure 15–25). The patient's chin is placed in the chin rest with the spine erect (Figure 15–26). The incisor teeth are placed edge to edge in a bite block. The forehead positioner is placed touching the patient's head with the patient's occlusal plane slightly downward in the incisor region; this places the apices of the incisor teeth in the same vertical plane. The lateral head positioners are brought inward to touch the sides of the patient's head and position the sagittal plane in the middle of the machine. The mA and kVp are adjusted for the patient's head size. The machine uses a flexible cassette held by a spring-tensed sheet of plastic against a curved metal cassette holder. The exposure can be made with the tubehead starting from either side of the patient.

A Panex panoramic radiograph is shown in Figure 15–27. The vertical and horizontal dimensions of the exposed film area are constant.

The Panorex 2

Many differences exist between the two Panorex models. The new machine, since 1982, places the patient in a chair on a raised platform (Figure 15–28). The tubehead cassette carrier is rigidly attached to the vertical column; the x-ray beam scans the patient by moving the entire vertical column around the raised platform. The machine can produce a split image radiograph, like the Panorex 1, or a continuous image radiograph. The split mode is achieved with a chair shift between two fixed centers of beam rotation like the

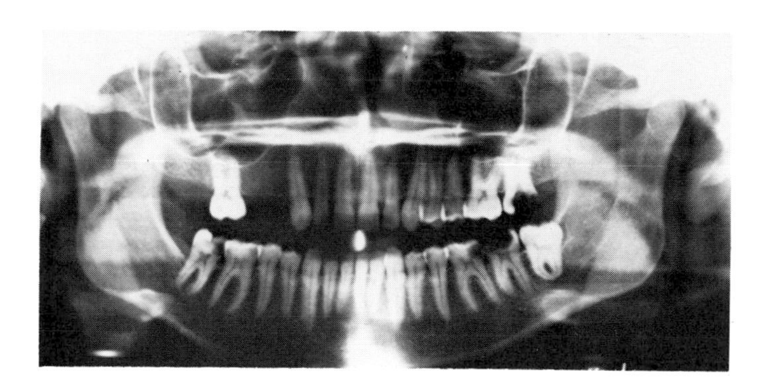

Figure 15–23. Panoramic radiograph made with Panelipse.

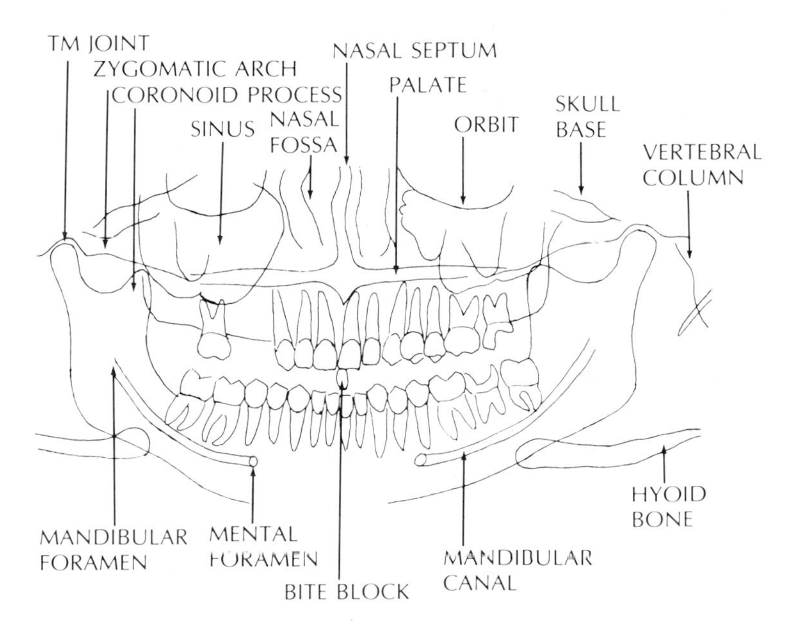

Figure 15–24. Diagram of anatomic landmarks seen in Panelipse panoramic radiograph.

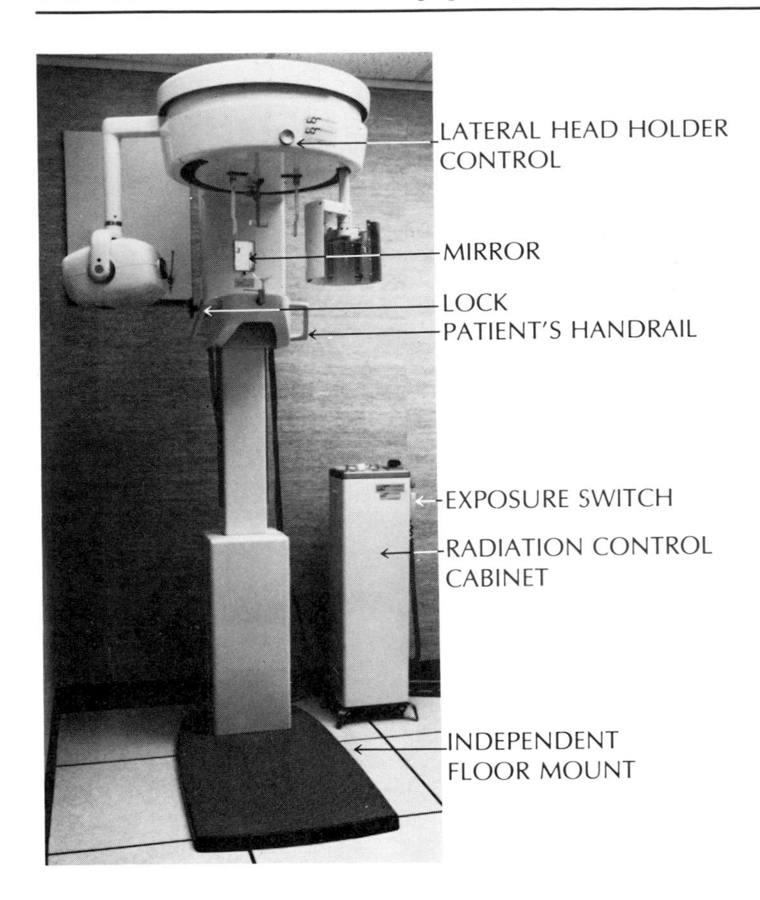

Figure 15–25. Panex (Panoral) panoramic x-ray unit.

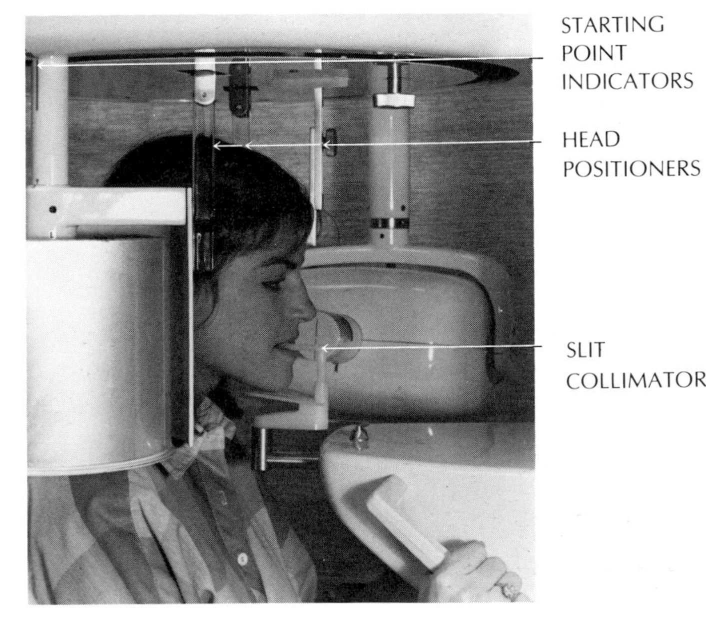

Figure 15–26. Patient positioned in Panex (Panoral).

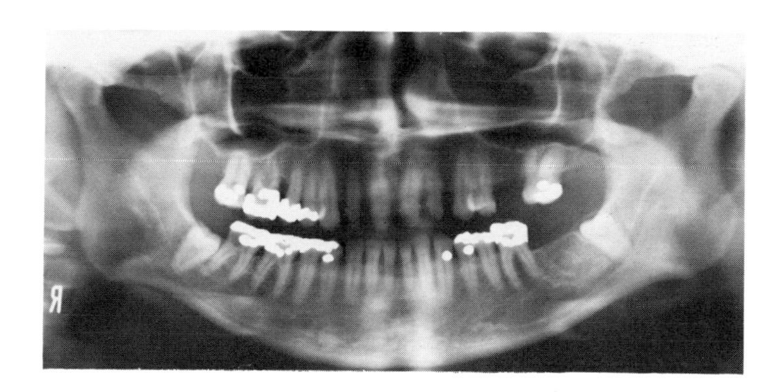

Figure 15–27. Panoramic radiograph made with Panex.

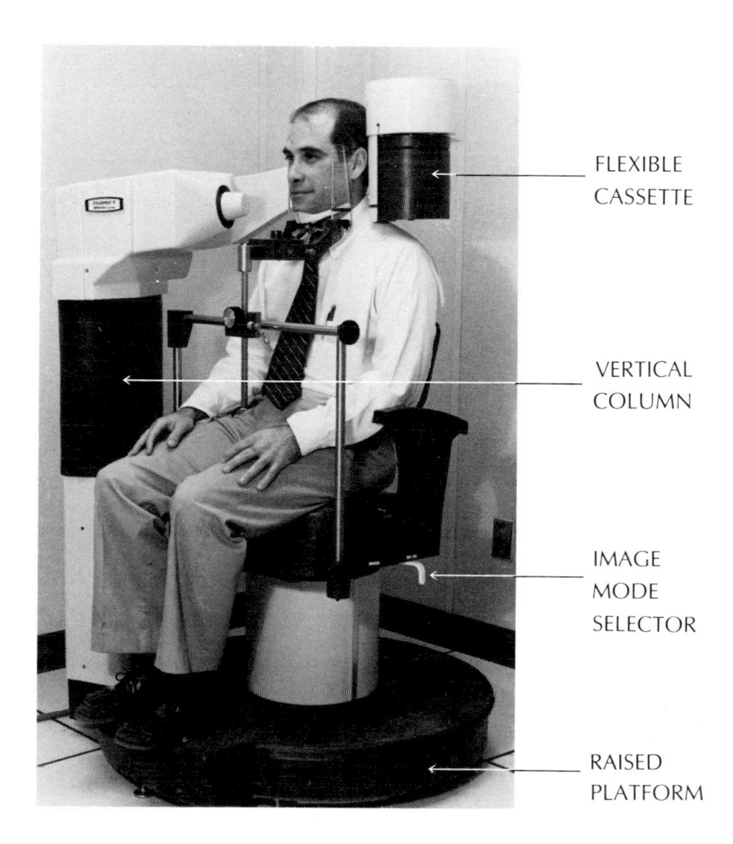

Figure 15–28. The Panorex II panoramic x-ray machine.

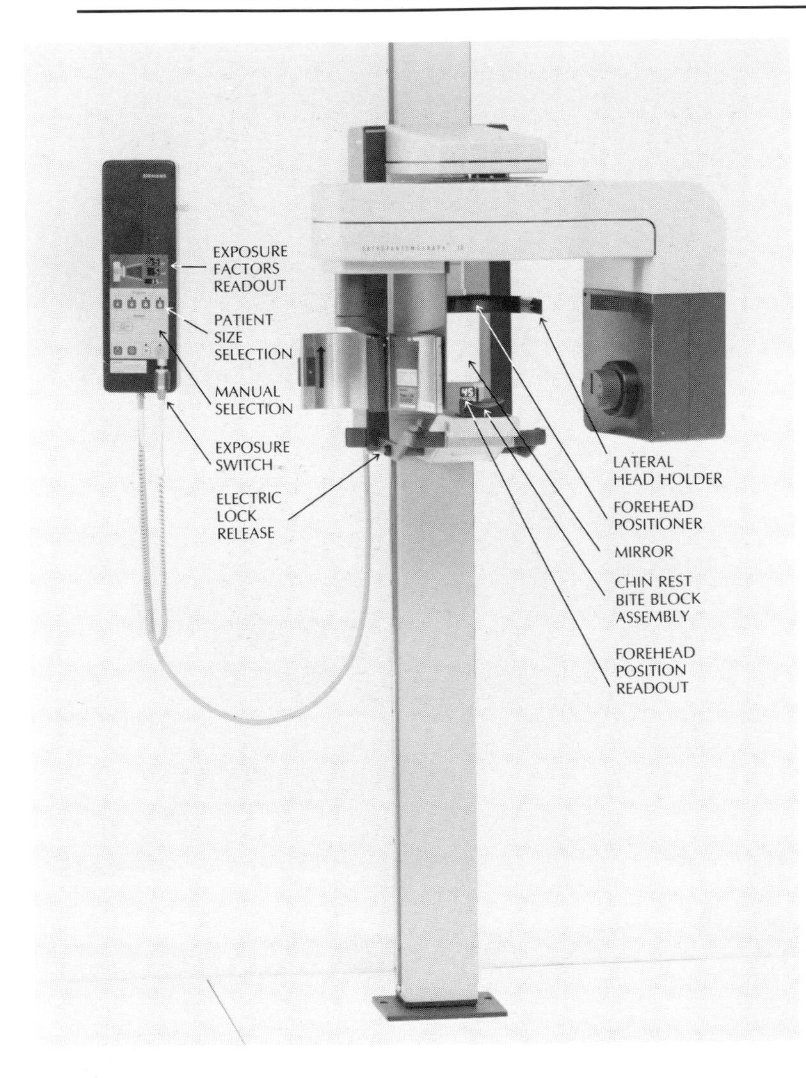

Figure 15–29. The Orthopantomograph 10 panoramic x-ray unit. (Courtesy of Siemens Medical Systems Inc.)

Panorex 1. When the continuous mode is selected, by moving a lever at the side of the chair, the chair and patient slowly move laterally during the x-ray exposure cycle. The height adjustment of the tubehead cassette carrier is similar to the Panorex 1. The machines use a flexible cassette on a circular drum. The patient head positioning for the split mode is similar to the Panorex 1; however, for the continuous mode, the chin guard (anterior stop) is moved forward and a bite block used to accurately position the incisor teeth. Instead of a cushion, a moveable back rest is used to straighten the patient's neck. Patient instructions are similar to instructions provided for the Panorex 1.

The Orthopantomograph-10

There have been many improvements between the OP-3 (1970) and OP-10 (1984) models. The OP-10 (Figure 15–29) uses an x-ray beam that rotates with a continuous moving center of rotation. The film, object and x-ray tube distances produce an image size that is less than 5 x 12 inches and thus allows space on a film to print patient information on the radiograph. There is no plastic shield between the operator and the patient's head permitting easy patient access for the operator. The forehead positioner and lateral head holders are incorporated into a single unit above the patient (Figure 15–30). Anteroposterior movement of the forehead positioner is by an electric switch and the position is recorded in a visible digital display. Anterior tilting of the patient's head is accomplished with an adjustable light beam that positions the Frankfort Horizontal Plane (ear to lower border of orbit). A large mirror on the machine column assists patients to position themselves. The mirror can be tilted to give the operator a frontal view of the patient's face. A vertical light line indicates the proper position for the mid sagittal plane of the patient's head (Figure 15–31). The patient positions the incisal edges of the central teeth in a bite block attached to a chin rest. A vertical light line locates the position of the zone of sharpness in the anterior region. Minor anterior posterior head movement for positioning of the apices of the incisor teeth precisely in the zone of sharpness is accomplished with a switch that simultaneously moves the chin rest and forehead positioner as a unit. After every exposure the chin rest returns automatically to the standard position. The control panel is activated by touch. Pre-selected exposure factors for average patient size can be activated by touching the desired patient size on the panel. These factors can be increased or decreased as desired for patients of unusual size by touching the manual indicators on the panel. The electric supply to the x-ray tube produces a large number of x-ray pulses per second. The multi-pulse system produces x-ray beam similar to the beam produced by a direct electric current. The electric circuit is programmed to use an increased x-ray beam intensity in the anterior teeth region to compensate for the spine shadow and produce a more uniform image density between anterior and posterior teeth. Patient head positioning in the zone of sharpness, patient erect standing posture and patient instructions are similar to the OP-3.

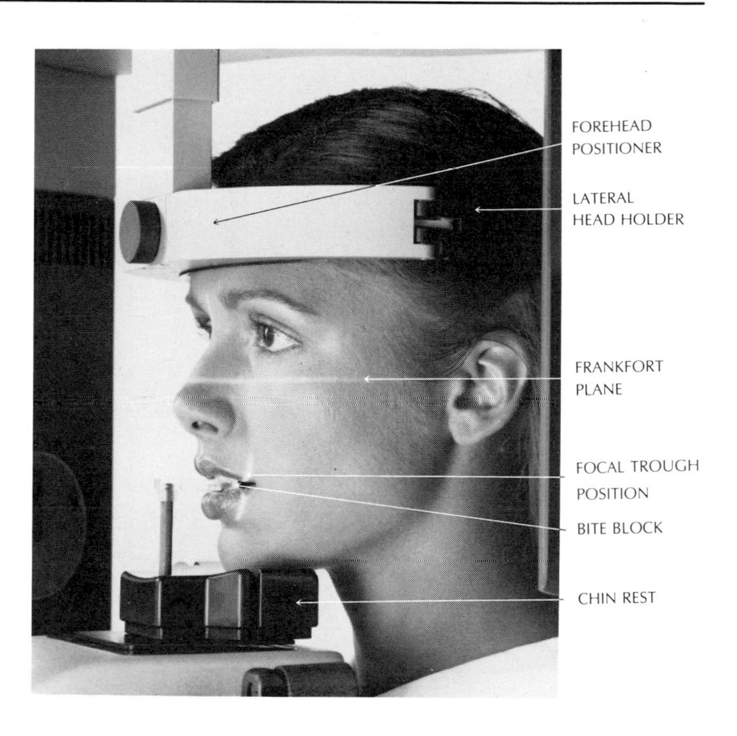

Figure 15–30. Head positioning system of the Orthopantomograph 10.

The Planmeca

The machine places the patient in a standing position (Figure 15–32). The support column is at the side of the patient and the operator can view the patient from in front of or behind the patient. The controls are located on the machine in front of the patient. Patient positioning by the operator is assisted by three light beams and a digital display of the position of the focal trough and the patient's head. Machine adjustments for patient positioning are motorized. A microprocessor gives the machine additional functions such as an adjustable focal trough form which can be selected to conform to the patient's anatomy, self monitoring of machine functions with displays of abnormal use conditions, and in addition to the usual panoramic projection, selection of segmented exposures of a specific dental area without exposing the entire film. An example of four segmented views of the temporomandibular joints is shown in Figure 15–33.

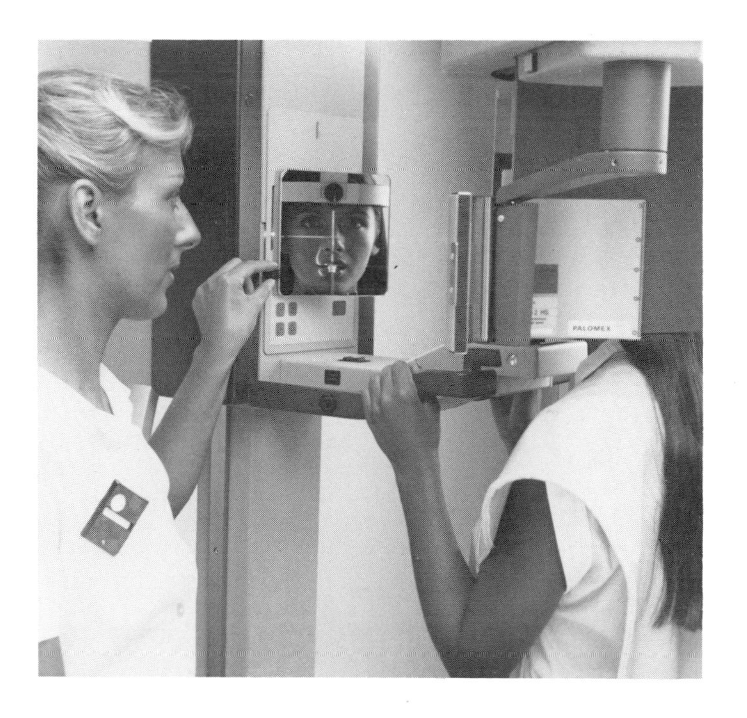

Figure 15–31. Operator adjusting the vertical position of the Frankfort horizontal light line. All three patient positioning light lines can be seen in the tilted mirror.

TECHNIC ERRORS AND ARTIFACTS

Panoramic radiographs of good quality can only be produced when the patient is properly positioned in the focal trough of the ma-

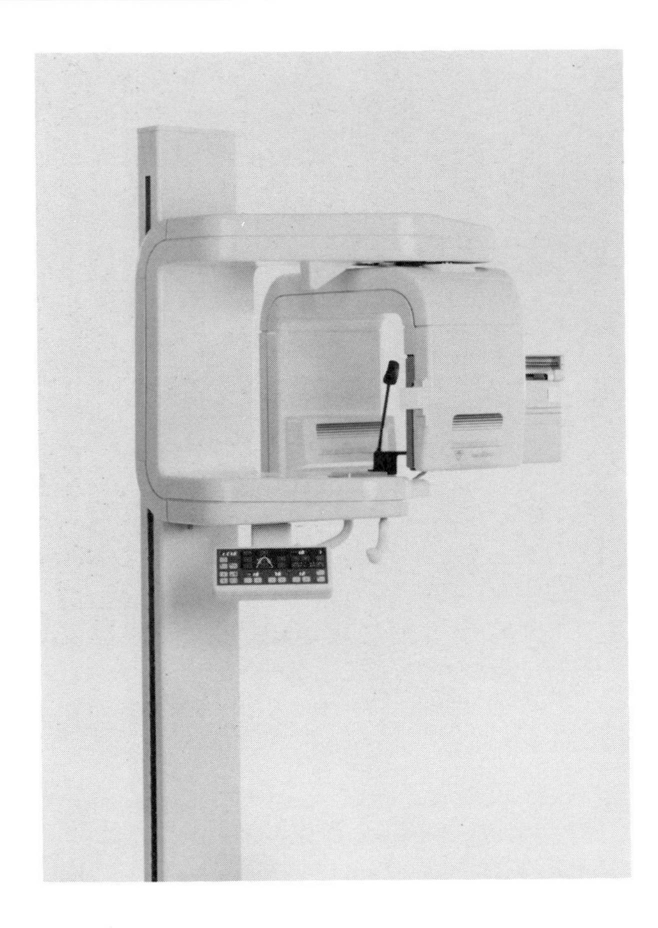

Figure 15–32. The Planmeca Panoramic Machine.

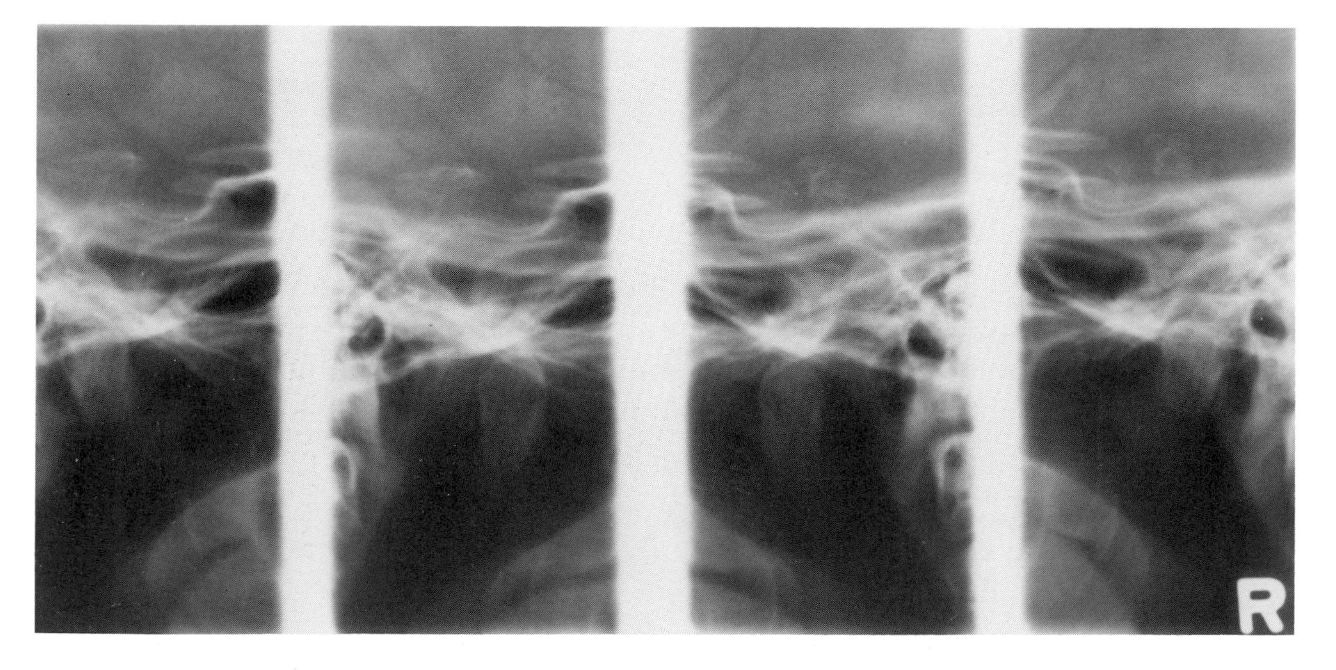

Figure 15–33. Four segmented views of the temporomandibular joints in open and closed positions made with the Planmeca Panoramic Machine.

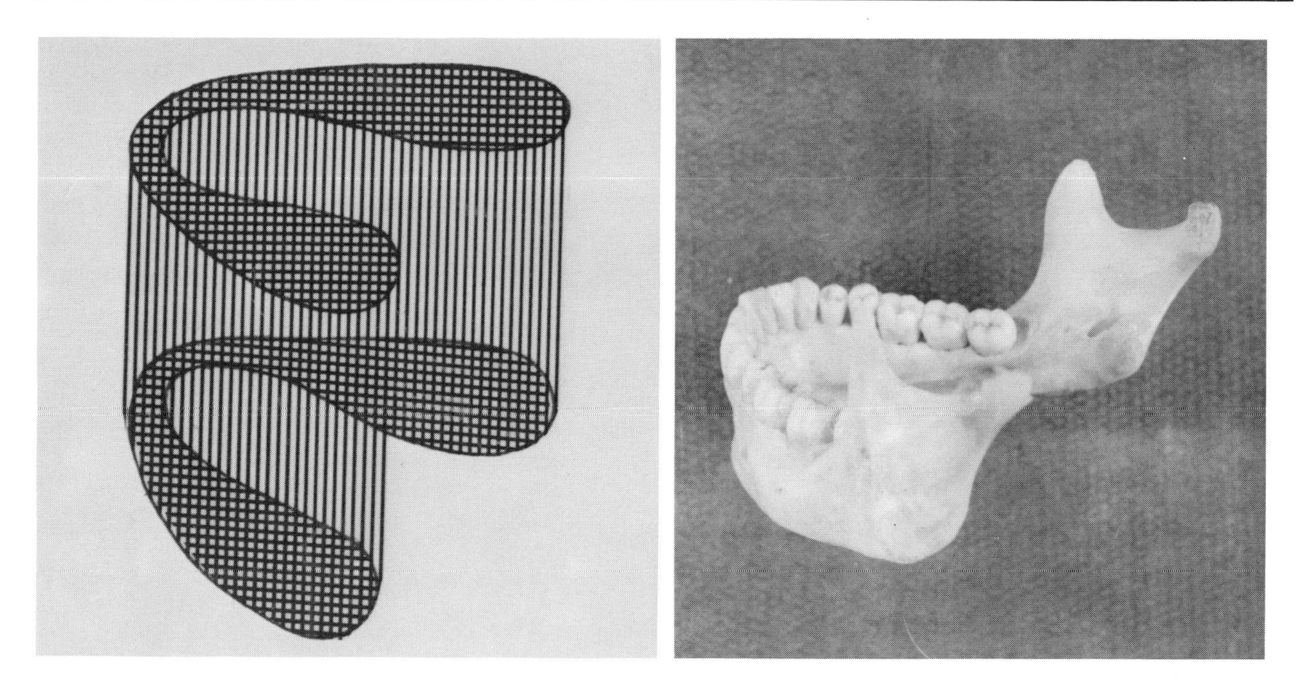

Figure 15–34. Diagram showing the three dimensional aspect of a focal trough and photograph of a mandible demonstrating the shape of the dental arch. (From Manson-Hing, L.R.: Panoramic Dental Radiography, 2nd Ed, 1980. Courtesy of Charles C Thomas, Publisher.)

chine and artifacts are avoided. The focal trough or zone of sharpness is three dimensional and lies in a curved vertical plane. This is mainly because all panoramic machines use a film that has its flat surface in the vertical plane. Machines are designed to have the zone shaped like the dental arch. This relationship is shown in Figure 15–34. The patient's teeth must be placed in the middle of the focal trough. This is most critical in the anterior or incisor region where the zone of most machines is very narrow. There is little error for patient positioning as is shown in Figure 15–35. A good panoramic radiograph will show the images of teeth and jaw structures that are sharp and well proportioned (Figure 15–36).

When the patient's chin is positioned too superiorly with the occlusal plane tipped upward, as shown in Figure 15–37, the mandibular incisor apices will be placed in a more favorable position in the focal trough; however, the palate is often superimposed on the apices of the maxillary incisors. The radiograph will also show the occlusal plane going straight across the radiograph and with the mandibular condyles tipped backward

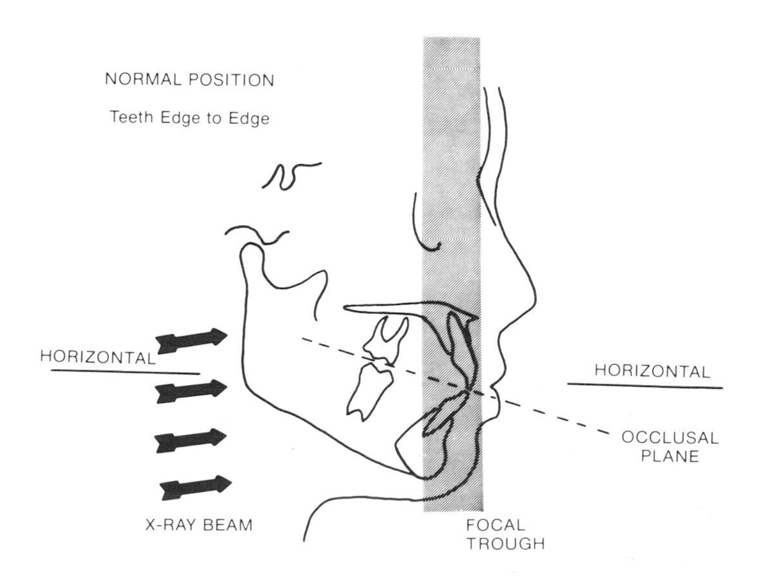

Figure 15–35. Diagram showing the patient to focal trough relationship in the incisor region. The incisors are best placed in an edge-to-edge position. (From Manson-Hing, L.R.: Panoramic Dental Radiography, 2nd Ed, 1980. Courtesy of Charles C Thomas, Publisher.)

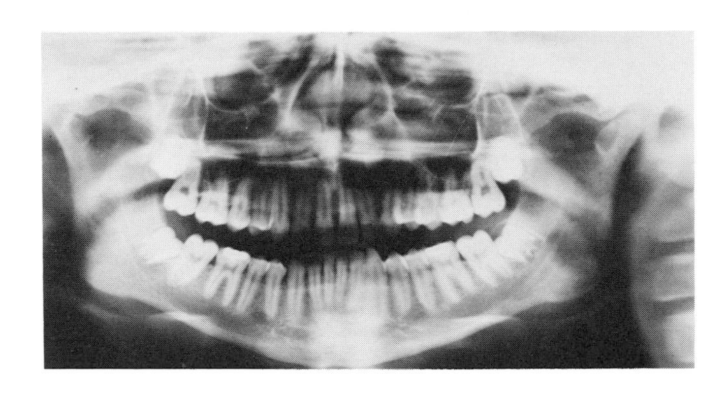

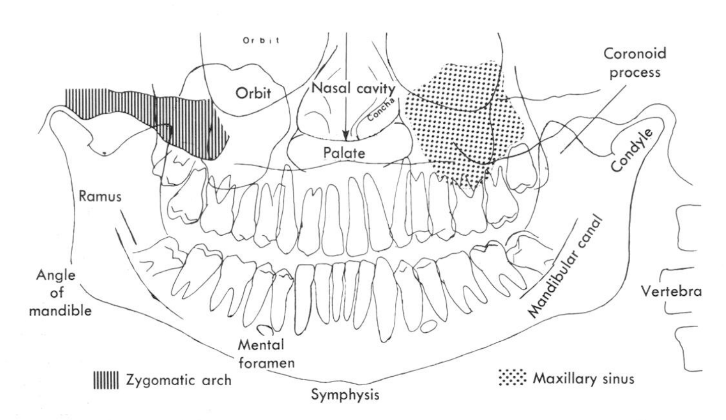

Figure 15–36. Panoramic radiograph and diagram showing well proportioned teeth and jaws. (From Manson-Hing, L.R.: Panoramic Dental Radiography, 2nd Ed, 1980. Courtesy of Charles C Thomas, Publisher.)

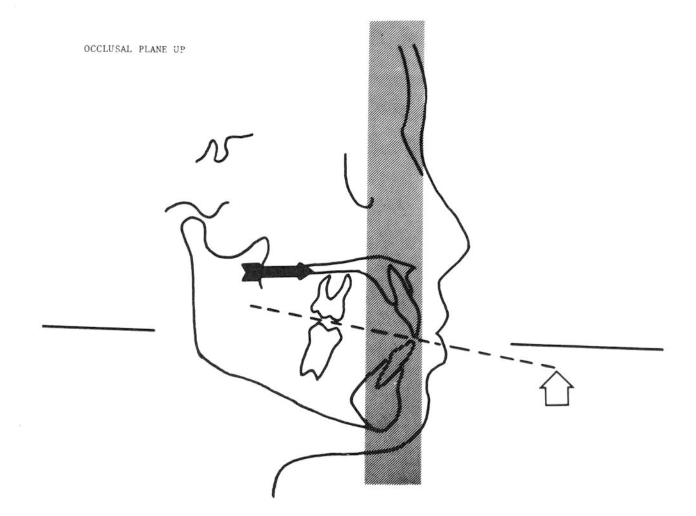

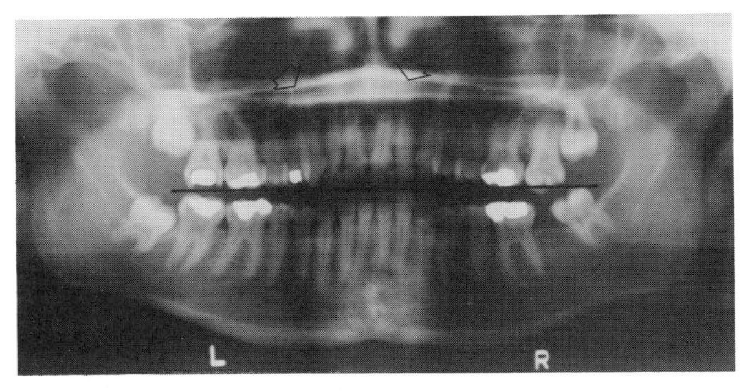

Figure 15–37. Diagram showing the patient's chin positioned too high in the machine during radiography and the resultant panoramic radiograph. (From Manson-Hing, L.R.: Panoramic Dental Radiography, 2nd Ed, 1980. Courtesy of Charles C Thomas, Publisher.)

the condyle images appear closer to the lateral borders of the radiograph. If the patient's chin is positioned too low with the occlusal plane tipped downward, the mandibular incisor apices are positioned out of the focal trough (Figure 15–38). The resultant radiograph shows the occlusal plane curving downward in the middle, the apices of the mandibular incisors are unsharp, the apices of the maxillary incisors are much below the image of the palate and the condyles are positioned farther from the lateral borders and more towards the midline of the radiograph.

When the patient is positioned in the x-ray machine anterior to the tomographic layer or focal trough, only the incisor teeth are placed out of the zone of sharpness (Figure 15–39). The radiograph shows abnormally slender maxillary and mandibular teeth and the condyles are positioned more medially from the lateral borders of the radiograph. In addition, there is greater overlapping of the proximal areas of the posterior teeth. While the incisor teeth are distorted and made much smaller horizontally, they do not become greatly unsharp as might be expected of teeth being placed out of the sharpness zone. This is because the teeth are now being placed closer to the film and are gaining image sharpness from this movement while losing sharpness from being placed out of the sharpness zone. When the patient is positioned in the machine posterior to the tomographic layer, only the incisor teeth are placed out of the zone of sharpness (Figure 15–40). The radiograph shows greatly wider maxillary and mandibular incisor teeth with unrecognizable apices due to great unsharpness and magnification. The loss of sharpness is particularly great when teeth are positioned posterior to the focal trough because the teeth are not only moved out of the focal trough, but also farther from the film; both of these movements increase image unsharpness. The incisor teeth apices are affected more than the crowns because the apices are located slightly posterior to the crowns.

When the patient's head is not placed in the middle of the machine's head positioner, one side of the dental arch is moved closer to the film and the other moved farther from the film. The posterior teeth on both sides can still be seen because the focal trough is wider in the posterior region (Figure 15–41).

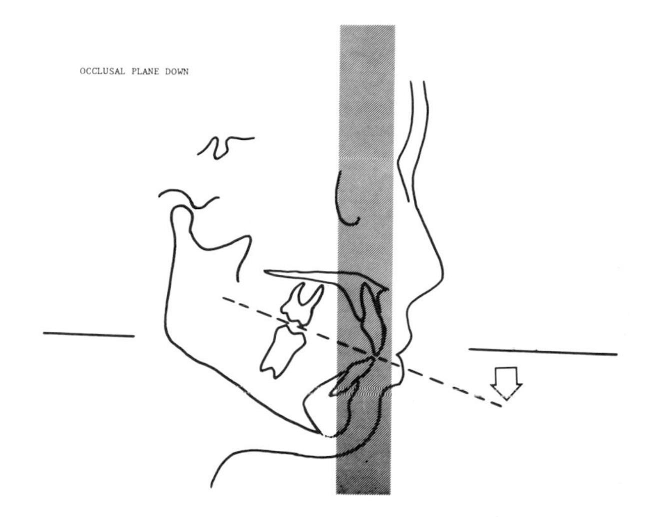

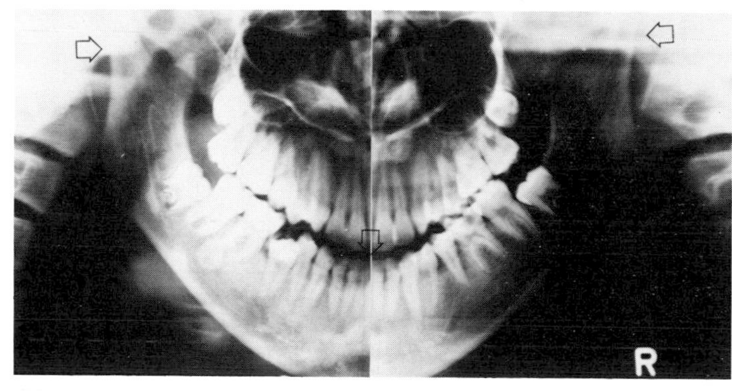

Figure 15–38. Diagram showing the patient's chin positioned too low during radiography and the resultant radiograph. (From Manson-Hing, L.R.: Panoramic Dental Radiography, 2nd Ed, 1980. Courtesy of Charles C Thomas, Publisher.)

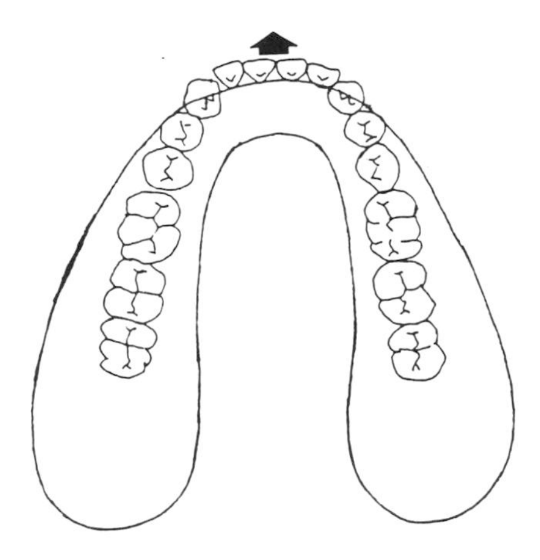

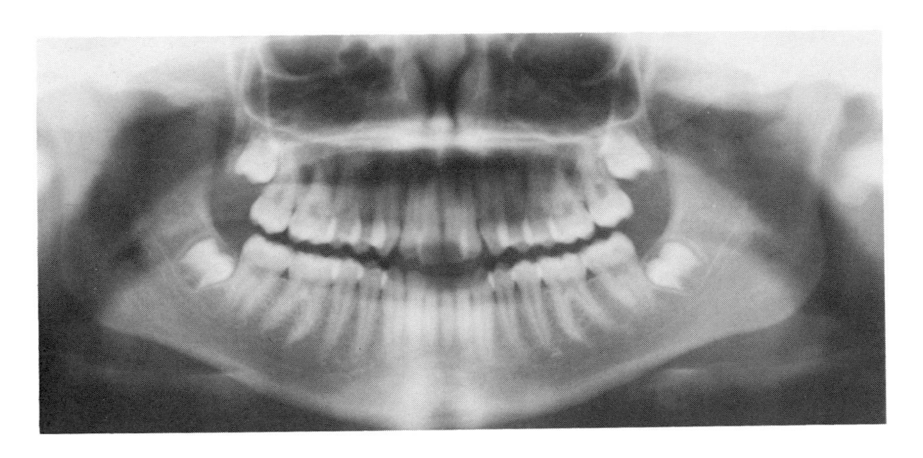

Figure 15–39. Diagram showing the patient positioned anterior to the focal trough of the x-ray machine and the resultant radiograph. (From Manson-Hing, L.R.: Panoramic Dental Radiography, 2nd Ed, 1980. Courtesy of Charles C Thomas, Publisher.)

The resultant radiograph shows demagnified teeth and jaws that are darker or of increased radiographic density on the patient's side that is placed closer to the film. The side moved farther from the film shows enlarged teeth and jaw images with less film density.

Air spaces appear as indistinct dark images in panoramic radiographs and should be avoided whenever possible. Good technic requires the patient to place the tongue on the palate during radiography to avoid formation of an air space in this region. Failure to do this procedure produces a radiograph with a dark band between the tongue and palate images. This dark band is superimposed upon the apices of the maxillary incisor teeth and interferes with the visualization of these structures (Figure 15–42).

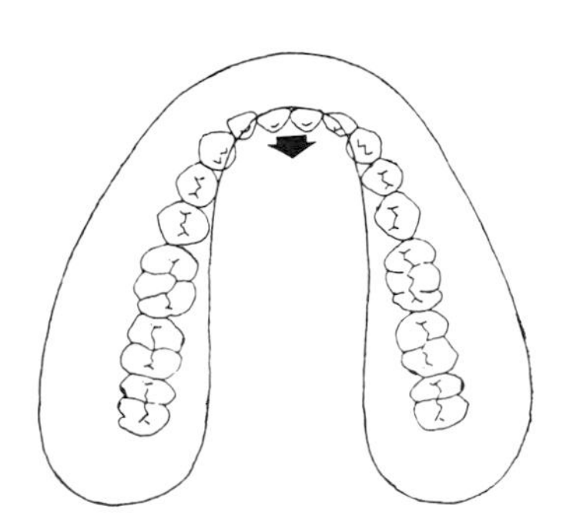

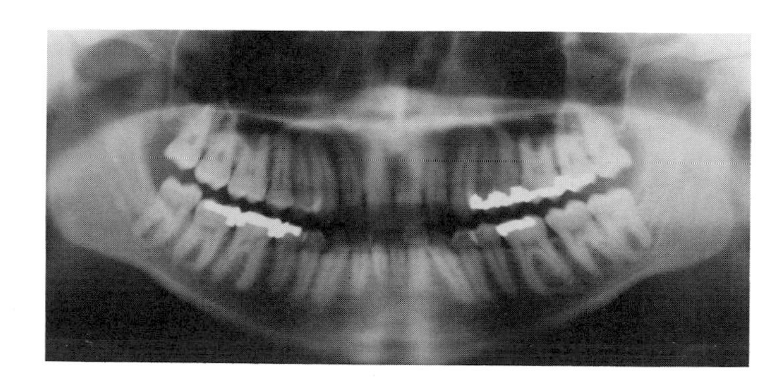

Figure 15–40. Diagram showing the patient positioned posterior to the focal trough of the x-ray machine and the resultant radiograph. (From Manson-Hing, L.R.: Panoramic Dental Radiography. 2nd Ed, 1980. Courtesy of Charles C Thomas, Publisher.)

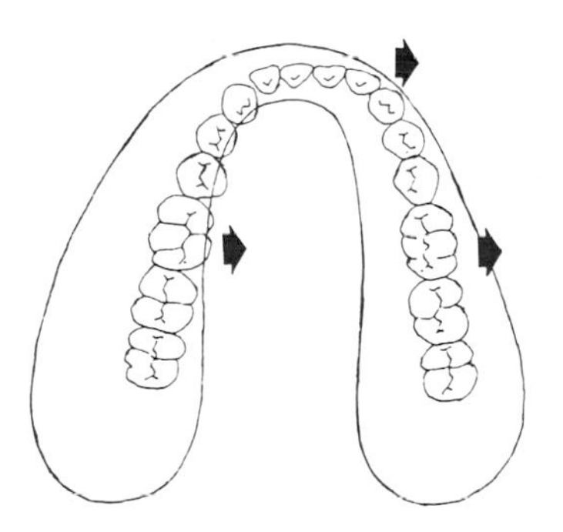

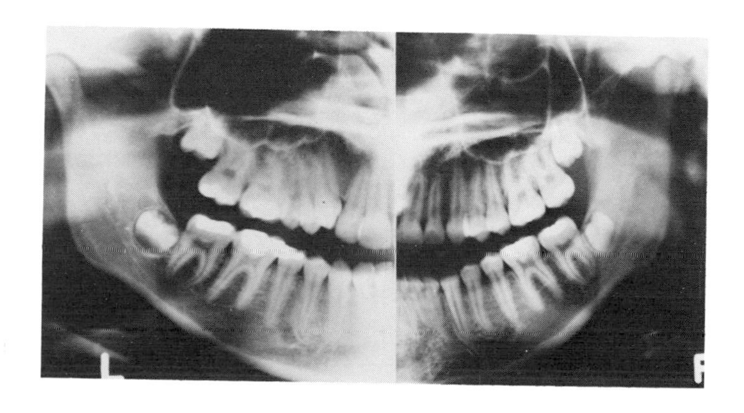

Figure 15–41. Diagram showing the patient's dental arch positioned to the right of the midline of the focal trough and the resultant radiograph. (From Manson-Hing, L.R.: Panoramic Dental Radiography, 2nd Ed, 1980. Courtesy of Charles C Thomas, Publisher.)

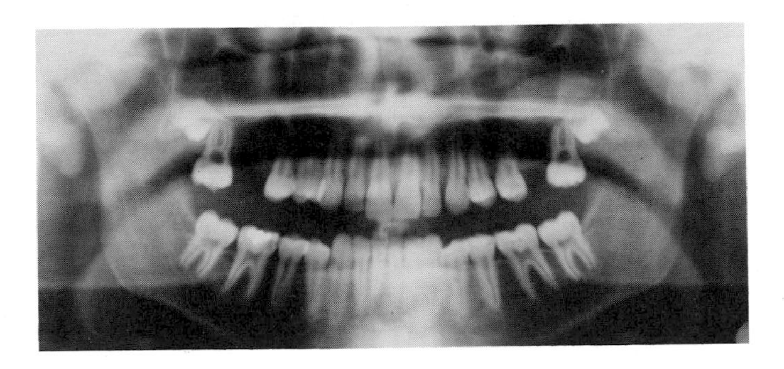

Figure 15–42. Panoramic radiograph made with the patient's tongue not placed on the palate during film exposure.

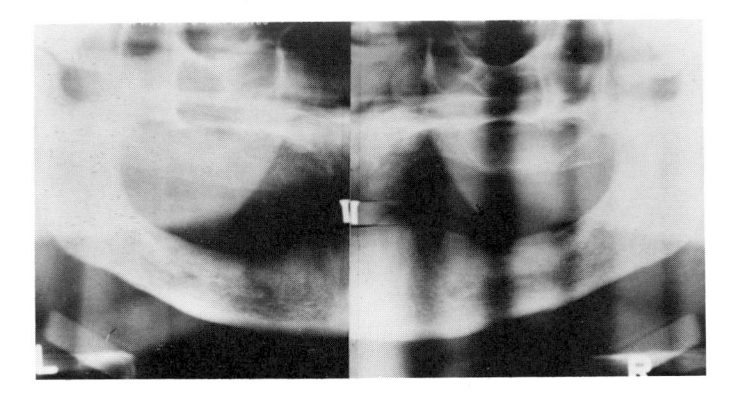

Figure 15–43. Panoramic radiograph made with the patient's shoulder touching the cassette carrier during exposure of the right side of the patient. (From Manson-Hing, L.R.: Panoramic Dental Radiography, 2nd Ed, 1980. Courtesy of Charles C Thomas, Publisher.)

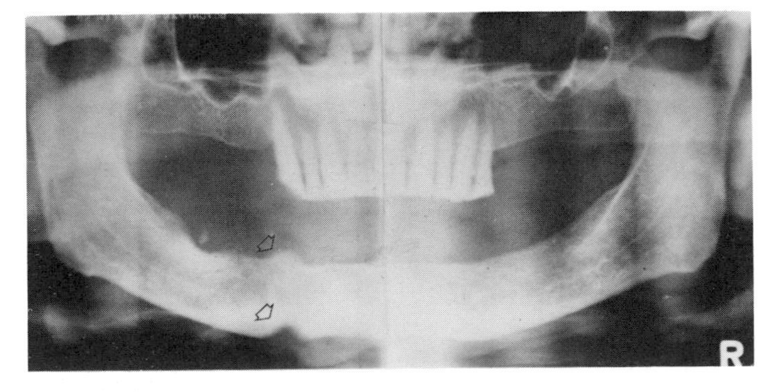

Figure 15–44. Panoramic radiograph made with the patient making a quick temporary upward movement (arrows) when the left cuspid region was being exposed. (From Manson-Hing, L.R.: Panoramic Dental Radiography, 2nd Ed, 1980. Courtesy of Charles C Thomas, Publisher.)

When the film cassette does not move smoothly behind the slit opening in the x-ray shield or scatter guard, dark or light vertical bands appear in the radiograph (Figure 15–43). A common cause is when the film carrier touches the patient's shoulder during the exposure cycle. Film carriers driven by belts or friction wheels may have the belt or wheels slipping. The patient touching the cassette carrier is likely to occur with uncooperative patients.

Patient movement during the film exposure cycle can produce unusual images. Figure 15–44 shows a radiograph made with the patient quickly moving the chin upward for a short time and then returning to the proper position. This produced a temporary elevation of all the images in the vertical plane during the movement because all parts of a vertical section of the patient are exposed at any point in time during the exposure cycle. The end result in this case is seen as a notch in the lower border of the mandible, a bump on the mandibular alveolar ridge, a distal sloping of the incisal of the maxillary cuspid tooth and a bump on the floor of the maxillary sinus, all at the same horizontal position of the radiograph. A similar quick temporary movement of the patient in the horizontal or sideways direction can produce blurred double images. Figure 15–45 shows such a case where the movement creates a double image of an unerupted mandibular third molar that resembles an odontoma. The periapical radiograph confirms that the double image is an artifact. Note that the panoramic radiograph will not show a broken mandibular cortical plate because the bone is in the x-ray beam at all times during the patient's movement and will cast a continuous image. The operator should always remake the radiograph when such artifacts appear to avoid possible misrepresentation. Patients should be watched carefully during film exposure.

When the patient is positioned with the cervical spine in the neck not erect and the head not placed in the most superior position, the cervical spine will be curved. The curvature is greater in the lower part of the spine and can cast a triangular, pyramid shaped, opaque shadow on the radiograph. Figure 15–46 shows such a spine image that is outlined by the image of a metal chain around the patient's neck. Such radiopaque

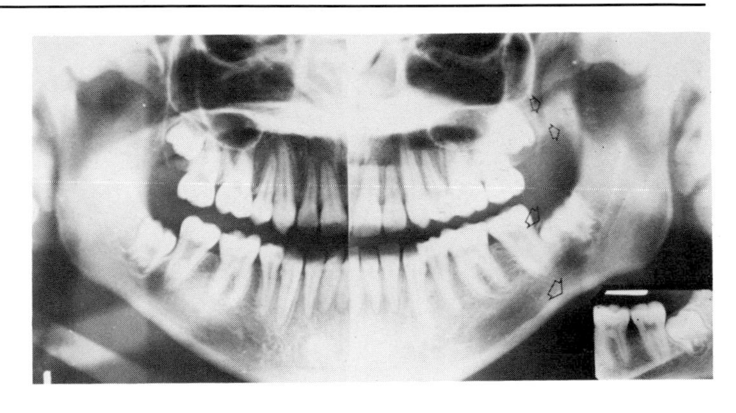

Figure 15–45. Panoramic radiograph made with the patient making a quick temporary movement in the horizontal plane during film exposure (arrows). The double image of the mandibular third molar is identified as an artifact in the periapical radiograph of the same area. (From Manson-Hing, L.R.: Panoramic Dental Radiography, 2nd Ed, 1980. Courtesy of Charles C Thomas, Publisher.)

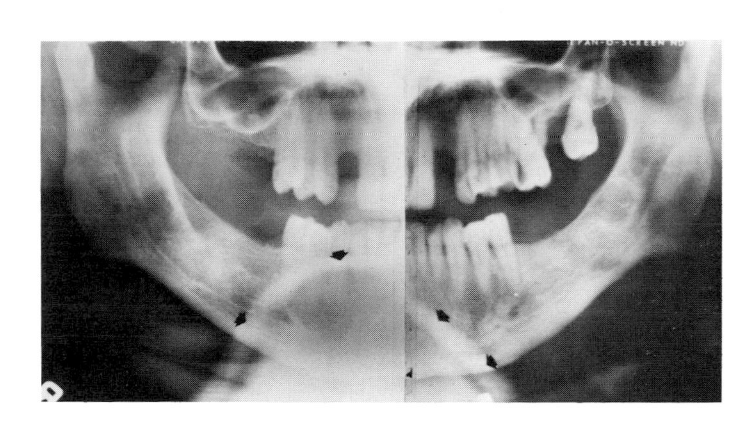

Figure 15–46. Radiograph made with the patient's cervical spine in a curved position. A metal chain around the patient's neck (arrows) outlines the cervical spine image. (From Manson-Hing, L.R.: Panoramic Dental Radiography, 2nd Ed, 1980. Courtesy of Charles C Thomas, Publisher.)

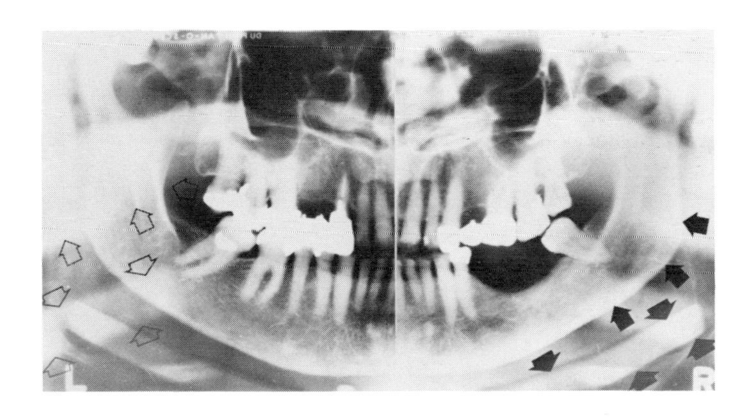

Figure 15–47. Radiograph demonstrating reversed or ghost images. The ramus and plastic chin rest on the right side (long and short solid arrows respectively) cast reverse images on the opposite side (long and short outlined arrows). (From Manson-Hing, L.R.: Panoramic Dental Radiography, 2nd Ed, 1980. Courtesy of Charles C Thomas, Publisher.)

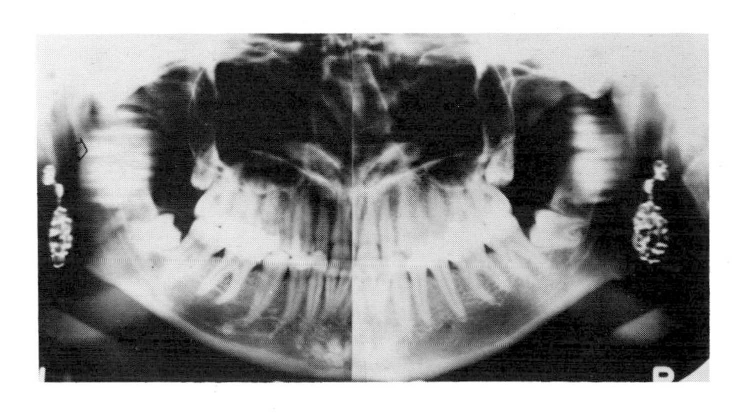

Figure 15–48. Radiograph of a patient with metal earrings. The radiopaque earring on the right side produces the reversed shadow on the left side (arrow). A similar shadow is produced by the left earring on the right side. (From Manson-Hing, L.R.: Panoramic Dental Radiography, 2nd Ed, 1980. Courtesy of Charles C Thomas, Publisher.)

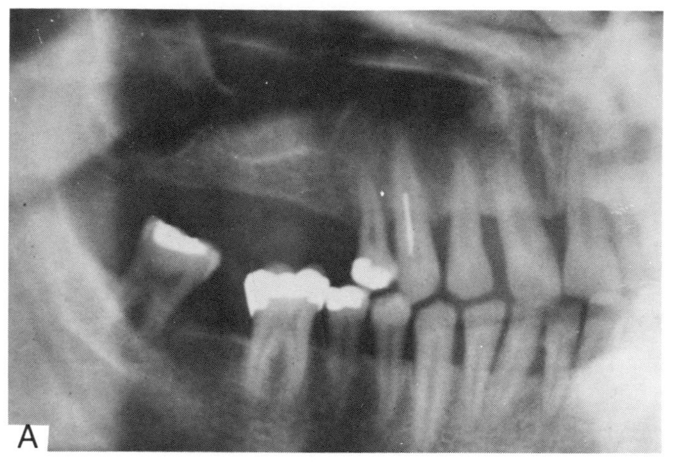

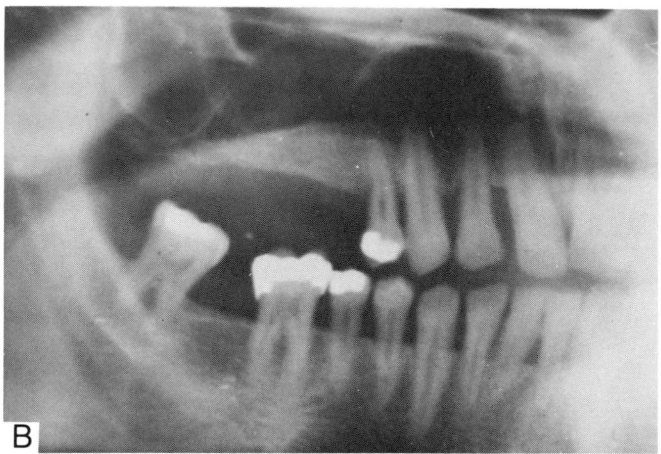

Figure 15–49. A routine panoramic radiograph (A) shows an apparent incomplete root canal filling on the maxillary cuspid tooth. A follow up radiograph (B) shows no sign of the radiopaque restoration. The artifact was caused by a piece of loose felt in the cassette (C).

objects in this area should be removed before the patient is placed in the machine. In machines where the patient is seated, the operator must place the patient's back in an anterior erect position; this is accomplished by moving the back rest as far forward as possible. In machines where the patient is standing, the patient must be made to place the feet anteriorly on the floor or machine platform and use the hand grips provided to avoid tipping backward. Keeping the patient's back forward, the neck extended and the head in a superior position, prevents curving of the cervical spine.

Reverse images (sometimes called ghost images) of the ramus area are cast on the ramus area of the opposite side during pantomography. The reversed shadows are faintly radiopaque, magnified, blurred and positioned more superiorly on the opposite side of the patient where the objects are located. Figure 15–47 shows reversed ramus and plastic chin support images. These images appear because the slit x-ray beam must pass through the lower ramus areas of the side opposite the ramus region being examined during panoramic radiography. The non-examined side is scanned in an anterior-to-posterior direction, while the side being examined is scanned in a posterior-to-anterior direction; this produces the reversed images of the non-examined side. Metal objects (whether in or out of the patient's tissues) in the lower ramus area will cast reverse or ghost images in panoramic radiographs. All such objects should be removed, whenever feasible, prior to panoramic radiography. Figure 15–48 shows a radiograph made of a patient with metal earrings.

While radiopaque objects in the x-ray beam will cast radiopaque shadows on the radiograph, a similar image can be produced if light-opaque material is located between the cassette screen and the film. Figure 15–49 shows such a case where a loose piece of black felt in the cassette creates an artifact resembling an incomplete root canal in an otherwise normal tooth. The light-opaque felt prevented the light, created in the fluorescent screen by the x rays, from reaching the film.

A multitude of artifacts, similar to those seen in intraoral radiography, can also be produced in panoramic radiographs during film developing and processing. These artifacts will not be repeated in this chapter; however, the static electricity artifact should be reemphasized because it is rare in intraoral radiography and can be common in screen film radiography (Figure 15–50). The electric discharge is created by forceful opening or closing of the cassette or screens onto the film. The artifacts tend to occur more often in a room with low humidity. Anti-static sprays are available for areas where this problem is difficult to control.

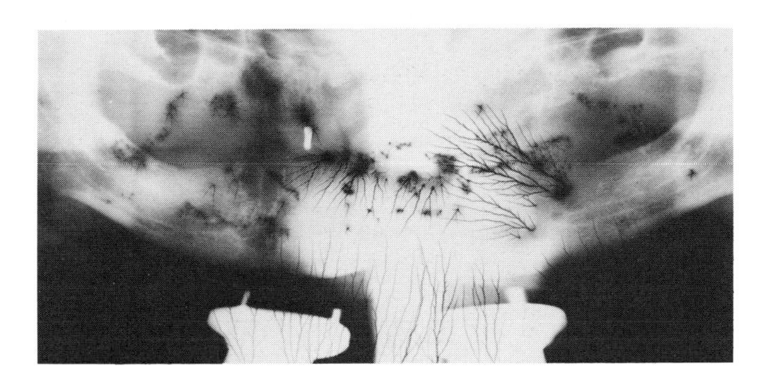

Figure 15–50. Lightning-like dark streaks produced by static electricity. (From Manson-Hing, L.R.: Panoramic Dental Radiography, 2nd Ed, 1980. Courtesy of Charles C Thomas, Publisher.)

Chapter 16

Radiography of Special Patients

Dental radiographic technics cannot be standardized for all patients. In intraoral radiography, the positions of the patient's teeth and shape of the arch often require the operator to use unusual film positions and different vertical and horizontal x-ray beam angles. Likewise, the diagnostic needs of the special patient such as a gagger, a child, or an endodontic patient will require the x-ray operator to modify radiographic technics and radiographic surveys. Flexibility and patience are necessary qualities the radiographer must possess if he or she is to obtain good radiographs of these more difficult patients.

THE HANDICAPPED RADIOGRAPHY PATIENT

Many patients find it difficult to place and maintain a dental film in position in the mouth for dental radiography because of an accentuated gag reflex, unsteady hands, limited mouth opening, or any other condition that interferes with normal intraoral radiographic procedures. These patients are actually handicapped in their ability to achieve and maintain a position conducive to obtaining proper intraoral radiographs. Technics can be modified by the operator to obtain intraoral radiographs in most cases. However, some patients may be unable to give the minimum required cooperation and extraoral radiographic technics must be used. When extraoral technics cannot be used, the patient may have to be placed under general anesthesia.

The Gagging Patient

The maxillary posterior region is the area most difficult for the gagging patient to tolerate dental radiography. If the patient is being radiographed for a complete mouth survey, the operator should alter the routine radiographic sequence to obtain film exposures of all other areas before radiographing the sensitive region. The sequence is altered because stimulation of the gag reflex area often results in the patient gagging in other areas where he would not normally gag. Before modifying radiographic technic for such patients, the operator must evaluate the type and severity of the patient's gag reflex. One must remember that there are both psychologic and physiologic aspects to any gag reflex. Evidence of the psychologic component is seen when a patient starts to gag as the operator approaches the patient with the film without the film touching the patient. The physiologic component is best seen when the patient gags only when the film touches the palate. The individual gagger will have varying amounts of each component and the operator must evaluate each patient to find the most appropriate radiographic technic.

When the gag reflex is due mainly to a psychologic problem, the patient needs to be educated about the condition. The reflex should be demonstrated and explained to the patient. Such patients are often able to touch the palate with the film themselves without gagging. In many cases patients can be trained, with the use of models, to position the film themselves; often in subsequent visits to the dental office patients will permit the operator to position the film and will not gag.

Patients who gag when the film touches the palate react in different degrees. Some patients can hold the film in position but will be slightly shaking or moving; others may be able to hold the film steady for varying amounts of time.

When the patient tolerates film placement in the bicuspid area but not in the molar area, the operator can make a distal-oblique projection of the molar teeth using the paralleling technic; the film is kept in the anterior region of the palate. The distal-oblique molar projection adequately shows the periapical tissues but overlaps the images of the proximal surfaces of the teeth. However, the interproximal area is seen in the molar bitewing radiograph.

In all gagging patients it is advantageous to use a fast exposure technic. The operator must be able to preset the patient and the machine, use quick angulation procedures, and adjust the machine for a short film-exposure time. The operator must be constantly

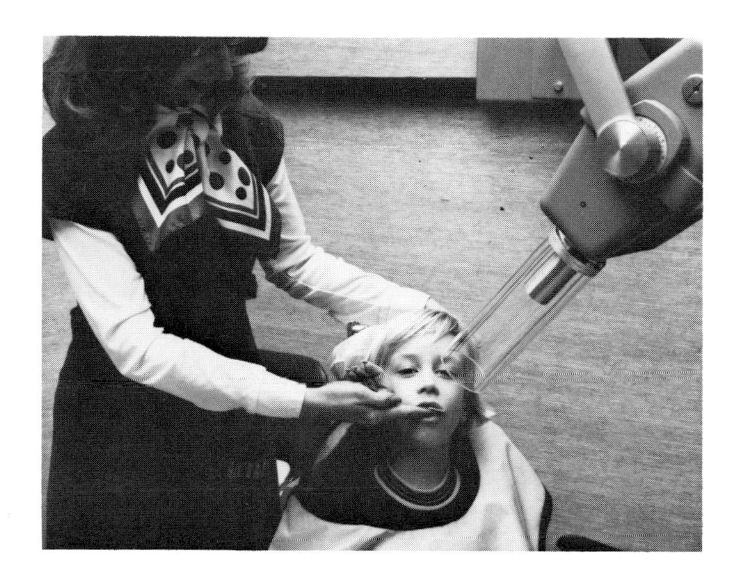

Figure 16–1. Parent of hyperactive child holding film in position.

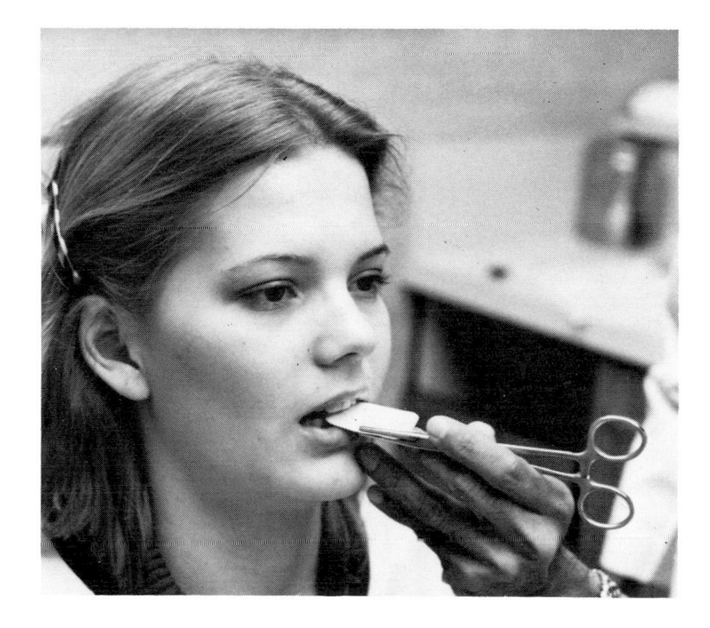

Figure 16–2. Hemostat film holder, with bite block removed, being used to insert film into mouth of patient with little intermaxillary separation.

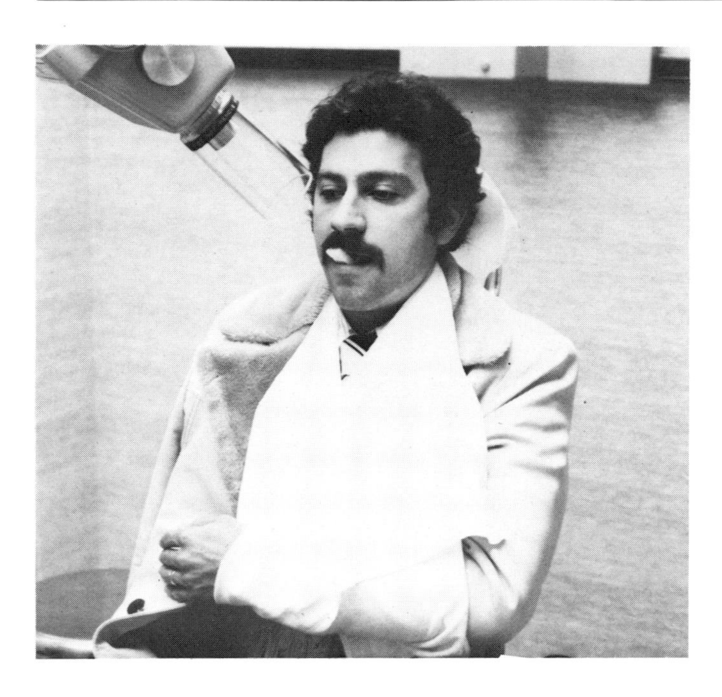

Figure 16–3. Patient with temporarily useless hands using bite block to maintain film in position in mouth.

aware, and indicate to the patient, that the only important time for the patient to be still is during x-ray exposure of the film.

In some gagging patients the removal of film holders or the patient's own finger from the mouth is beneficial. The technic of bending the film and using the bent part like a bitewing tab to hold the film in position is useful in these cases. The technic is most often used in children with small mouths and is described on pages 195–196 and in Figure 16–16.

Suppressing the gag reflex is sometimes necessary. The method used depends upon the severity of the reflex. Deep breathing by the patient, having the patient observe and concentrate on a spot on the wall or keeping one foot elevated off the floor is useful in some patients with a slight gag reflex. Having the patient rinse the mouth with cold water will slightly reduce the reflex. Increasingly greater suppression can be obtained with the application of a topical anesthetic, the injection of a local anesthetic, or the use of general anesthesia.

When the operator is unable to make an intraoral radiograph of the molar region, an extraoral technic is used. A lateral-jaw or panoramic radiograph using screen film will provide most of the information needed; however, extraoral radiographs lack some of the fine details seen only in films placed intraorally and exposed directly to the x-rays.

The Hyperactive Patient

Many patients cannot keep their bodies motionless. Such is the case with the very young, the spastic, the mentally retarded, and the hyperactive patient. A fast exposure technic is used for such patients. In addition it may be necessary to have someone other than the operator assist the patient in holding the film in the mouth or keep the patient's head motionless (Figure 16–1). This person should be an adult, preferably a relative or guardian of the patient, and should be a person not occupationally involved with x rays.

The Patient with Trismus

A patient may be unable to open the mouth or have limited opening of the mouth due to trauma, infection, ankylosis, or other causes.

When the mandibular and maxillary teeth are in contact and there is no space between them to place the film in the mouth, intraoral radiography is not possible. Extraoral lateral jaw and panoramic radiographs are the only radiographic surveys of the teeth possible. When a small separation of maxillary and mandibular teeth exists or is obtainable, the operator can maneuver the film into the patient's mouth by holding the film with a hemostat without a bite block (Figure 16–2). The patient must cooperate by moving the tongue around the palate to allow the film to be slipped into position. The film can be positioned in this manner only for the bisecting-angle technic. Since the operator is unable to see the film in the patient's mouth, external anatomic landmarks are used to achieve average vertical x-ray beam angulation. Horizontal angulation is achieved by observing the plane of the buccal or labial surfaces of the teeth being examined. With a cooperative patient intraoral radiographs can be obtained of any area of the dentition if the film and hemostat can pass between the teeth.

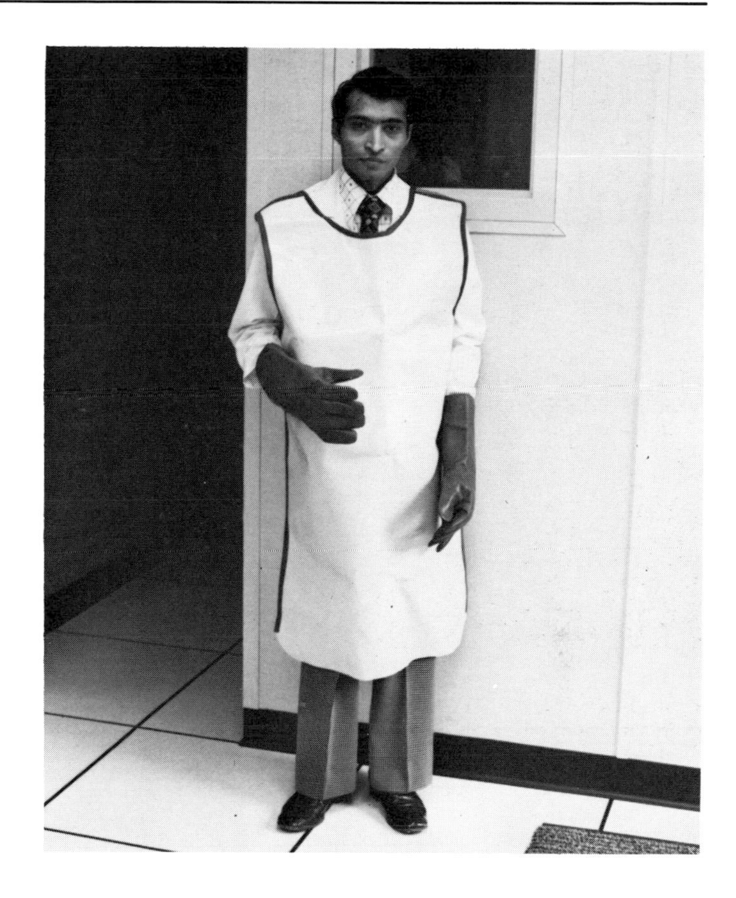

Figure 16–4. Operator protected with leaded gloves and body apron.

The Wheelchair Patient

A patient in a wheelchair usually cannot walk because of non-control or weakness of the legs. If the patient is totally unable to walk, the wheelchair can usually be brought close enough to the x-ray machine for radiography if obstructing equipment is moved away from the machine. Usually films can be exposed with the patient in the wheelchair; however, a short exposure time should be used to minimize image unsharpness due to increased patient movement. Note that the brakes of the wheelchair must be set to keep the chair from moving.

When the wheelchair cannot be brought to the x-ray machine, the immobile patient is transferred to the dental chair; two operators are needed, one behind the patient lifting under the patient's arms and the other in front of the patient lifting under the patient's knees. When lifting patients, the operator must be standing firmly on the floor and must not lean forward too much.

Wheelchair patients who can temporarily support their weight are transferred to the dental chair by placing the wheelchair beside

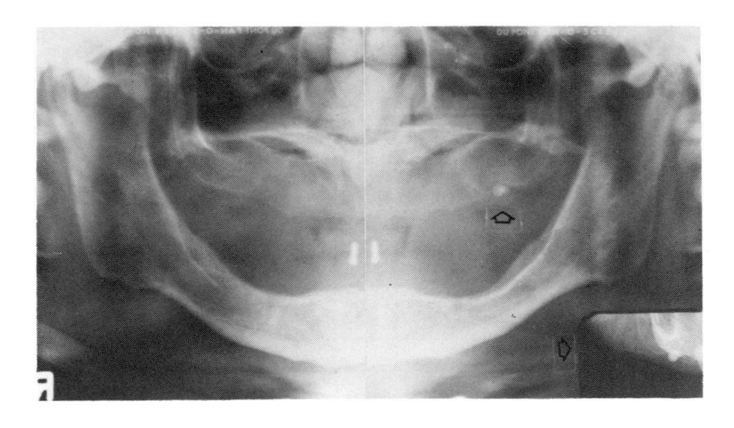

Figure 16–5. Radiographic survey of edentulous patient using panoramic radiograph and supplementary periapical view of unsharp image of small object (open arrows).

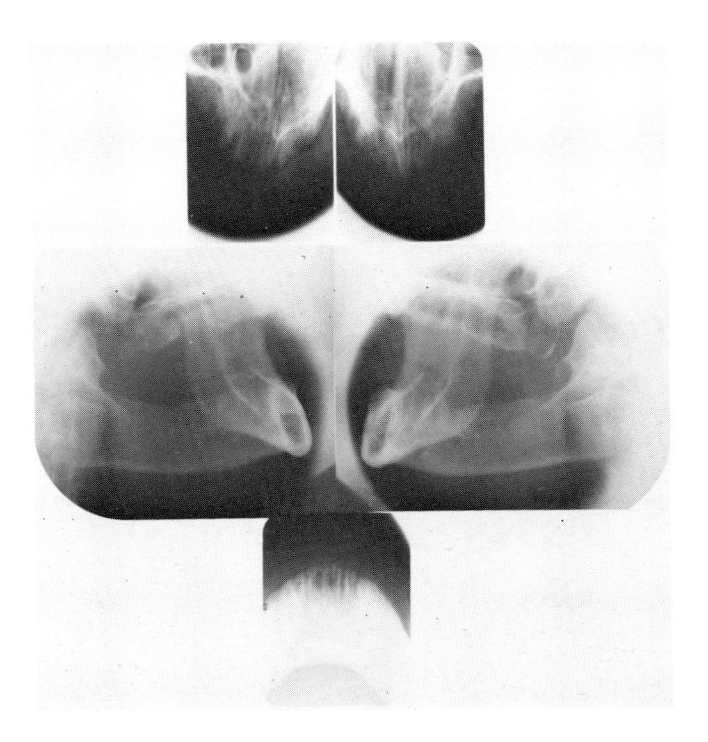

Figure 16–6. Radiographic survey of edentulous patient using two lateral jaw and three topographic occlusal radiographs.

the dental chair, setting the brakes of the wheelchair, elevating the dental chair to the wheelchair's height, moving the dental chair arm from between the chairs, and then having the patient move or slide sideways into the dental chair with the operator assisting while standing firmly in front of the patient. For panoramic radiography some machines have removable chairs to permit a wheelchair being substituted in the machine.

The Patient with Useless Hands

A patient may be unable to use his or her hands to support the film in the mouth. This can be due to a variety of conditions such as a broken arm, loss of fingers, or an uncontrollable hand. The assistance of a relative or other person to hold the film for the patient is sometimes needed. In most cases the operator can use a bite block type of film holder to keep the film in position. Most of these film holders require the patient only to bring the jaws together (Figure 16–3).

The Unconscious Patient

Dental radiographs are seldom made of an unconscious patient. The most common situation is the need for a radiograph during an operation when the patient is under general anesthesia. A bite block film holder is used; this requires only that the patient's jaws be closed upon the block. If the anesthetist must be close to the patient the anesthetist can hold the jaws together; in this instance the anesthetist should be provided with a leaded body apron and gloves and should keep both body and hands out of primary x-ray beam (Figure 16–4). If the anesthetist can move away from the patient, the patient's head can be positioned with wedge-shaped pillows and the jaws can be kept together by passing a soft rubber tube (of the type used with a Bunsen burner) under the mandible and tieing it above the patient's head. A quick exposure radiographic technic is used.

A portable dental x-ray machine mounted on wheels is sometimes used. Such a machine should have large wheels because small wheels tend to "trip over" tubing and other obstacles on the floor.

To keep radiography time at a minimum a portable small tank processing machine can

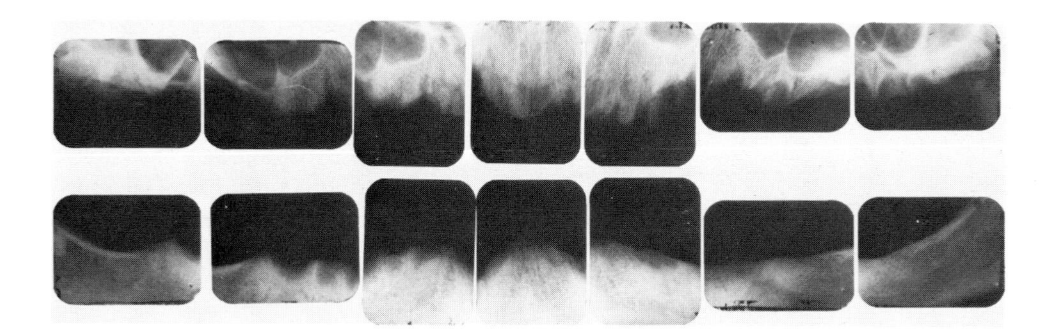

Figure 16–7. A 14-film intraoral edentulous survey.

be used in, or in an area close to, the operatory. Concentrated solution can be used to quick process the film.

THE EDENTULOUS PATIENT

Patients without teeth need to have their jaws examined to detect the presence of pathology or objects embedded in the jaws, to observe the quality of the bone, and to establish the position of the sinus, mental foramen, and incisive foramen relative to the crest of the alveolar ridge. A variety of radiographic surveys have been proposed for edentulous patients.

The Panoramic Survey

A panoramic radiograph is used by some dentists to survey the edentulous patient. This survey examines the entire jaws, but the radiograph does not provide sharp images of small objects. When the panoramic radiograph is used, it should be supplemented with intraoral periapical radiographs of any unclear suspicious objects seen in the panoramic radiograph (Figure 16–5).

Lateral Jaw and Occlusal Survey

Right and left lateral jaw radiographs plus anterior topographic occlusal radiographs of the mandible and maxilla have been used to survey the edentulous patient (Figure 16–6). As with the panoramic radiograph supplementary periapical projections may be needed to obtain sharper images of small objects seen in the lateral jaw radiographs.

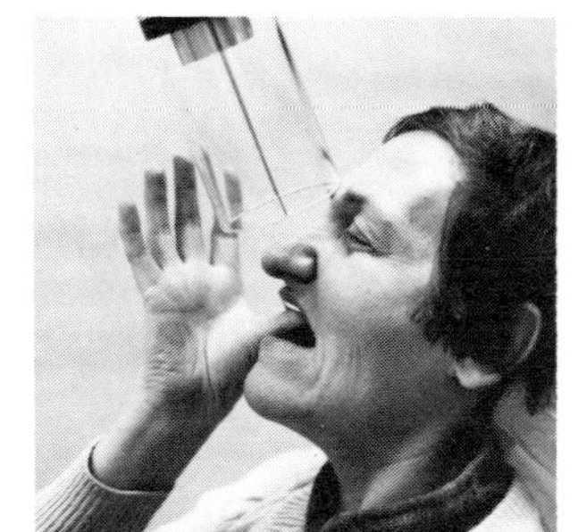

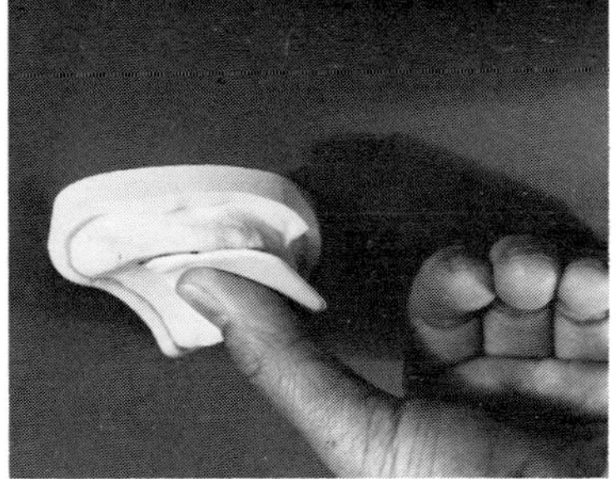

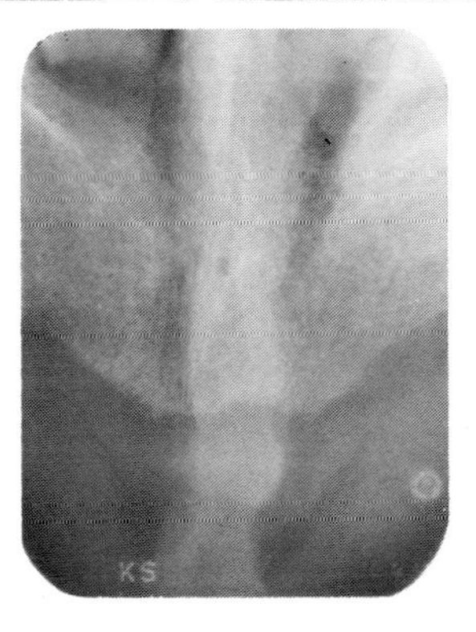

Figure 16–8. Film held by edentulous patient for maxillary anterior region and resultant radiograph.

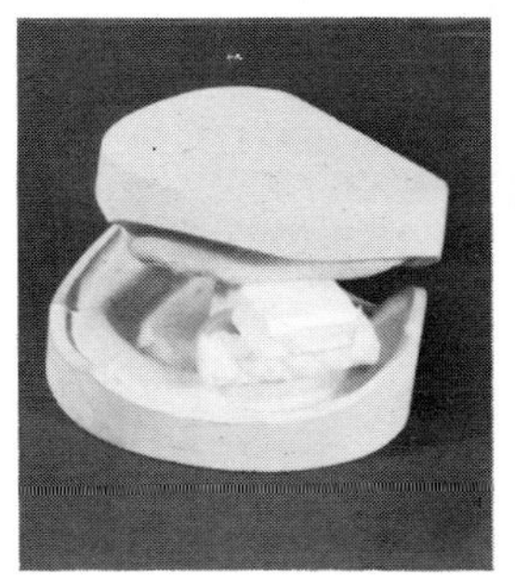

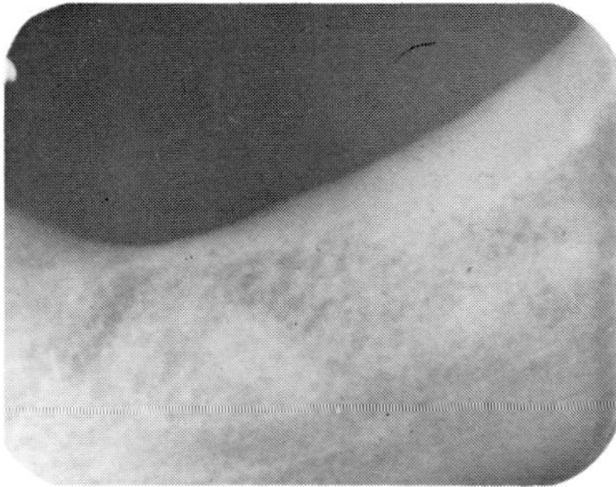

Figure 16–9. Film positioned for mandibular posterior area by using bite block; resultant radiograph.

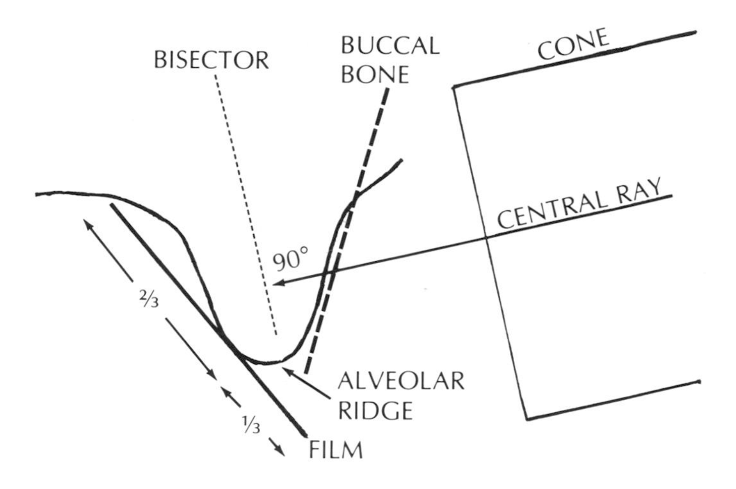

Figure 16–10. Radiography of edentulous area using buccal bone to form angle to be bisected and positioning of central ray perpendicular to bisector, or vertical edge of cone parallel to bisector.

The Intraoral Survey

A 14-film intraoral periapical survey will usually examine the tooth-bearing region of most edentulous patients (Figure 16–7). No bitewing radiographs are made because there are no interproximal areas to be examined. The survey provides the sharpest images available but does not survey all of the bone of the mandible and maxilla.

The intraoral technic generally used with the edentulous patient is the bisecting-the-angle technic. The film can be held by the patient's hand (Figure 16–8) or with a bite block (Figure 16–9). When the patient's hands are used, care must be taken to avoid excessive bending of the film against the palate or lingual surface of the mandible. Excessive bending of the film produces streaky distorted images. When a bite block is used, a cotton roll may be needed to replace the crowns of the missing teeth, support the bite block, and prevent patient discomfort from overclosure of the jaws with too much film extending into the floor of the mouth.

The film should be positioned with approximately one third of the vertical dimension protruding beyond the alveolar ridge; that is, the radiographic image should occupy two thirds of the film. Horizontal angulation positions the central ray perpendicular to the film in the horizontal plane. The vertical angulation is established, as in the bisecting-the-angle technic, using the buccal or labial bone instead of the long axes of the missing teeth to form one side of the angle

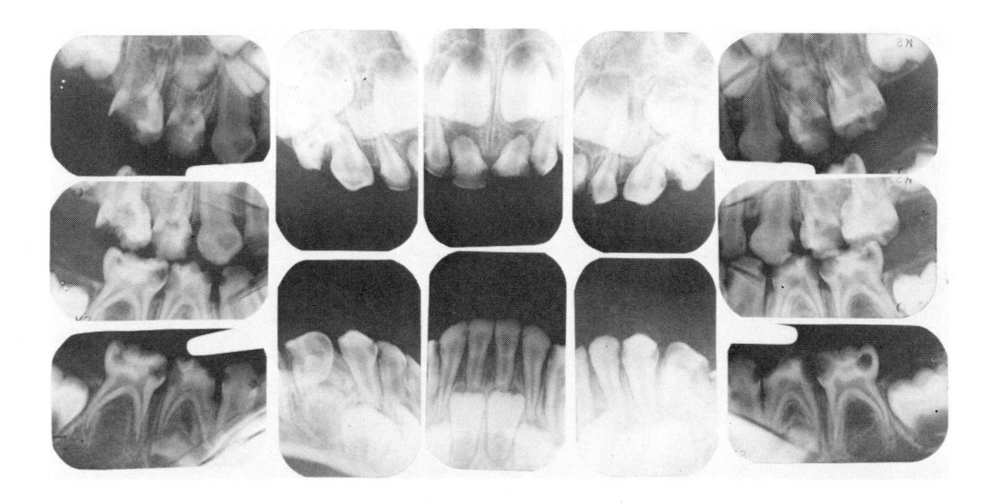

Figure 16–11. Intraoral survey of deciduous dentition using pedodontic 1.00 size film.

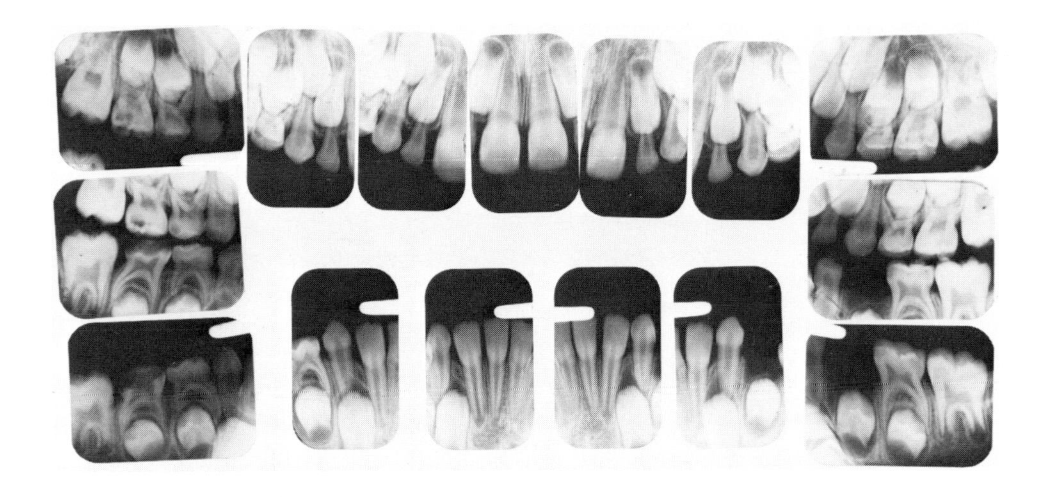

Figure 16–12. Complete mouth survey of child with mixed dentition using 1.1 and 1.2 size dental film.

(Figure 16–10). The central ray is positioned perpendicular (or the vertical edge of the cone parallel) to the bisector of the angle formed by the film and the outer surface of the alveolar ridge.

CHILDREN

Radiography of children is often difficult because of the small size of the oral cavity, lack of control of the tongue and other muscles, and the lack of cooperation. To be successful the radiographer must be able to control or adjust to these conditions whether they be great or small in the individual patient.

Film Size

Since the mouth is smaller in children, the smaller size (pedodontic) films are used. The ANSI 1.00 film (commonly called double zero and measuring 0.81 × 1.25 inches) is used in both the anterior and posterior teeth of children who have only deciduous or baby teeth. A complete mouth survey using this film is shown in Figure 16–11. If the dental office uses the slightly larger ANSI 1.1 film (0.94 × 1.56 inches) to radiograph the anterior teeth of adult patients, this film can usually be used instead of the 1.00 size film.

The child with a mixed dentition needs films that are large enough to record the permanent teeth. The adult size (ANSI 1.2) film

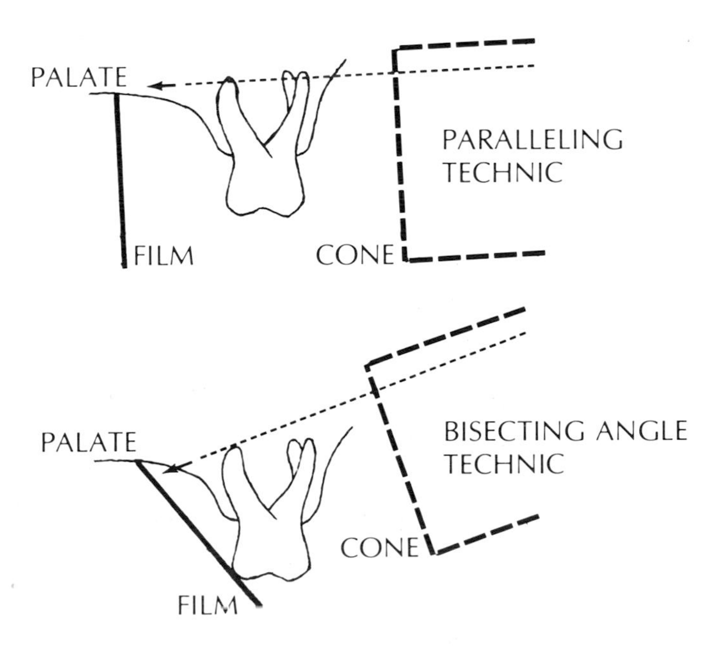

Figure 16–13. Difference in capability of paralleling and bisecting technics to project apices of permanent molar teeth in children with shallow palates.

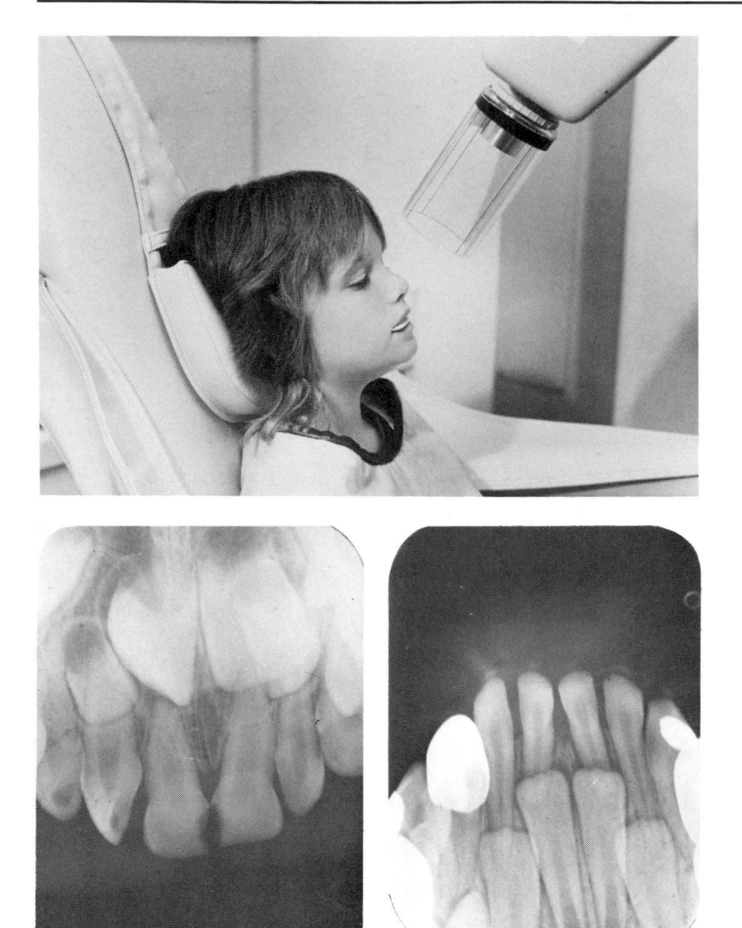

Figure 16–14. Child with No. 2 periapical film in occlusal plane and radiographs made with topographic occlusal technic for maxillary and mandibular incisors.

is commonly used. Because of the smaller size of the mouth the No. 1.1 size film is often useful in the anterior region (Figure 16–12). The commonly used adult periapical film should always be used in the posterior dental areas of children after the first permanent molar is fully developed; the length of this tooth requires the use of the larger periapical film.

Radiographic Technic

The bisecting-the-angle intraoral radiographic technic is used with children. The paralleling technic is not practical for two reasons. First, the apices of the permanent molar teeth tend to lie above the palate in the young maxilla and below the floor of the mouth in the undeveloped mandible; these positions prevent the image of the apices of these teeth to be projected into the oral cavity with the x-ray beam perpendicular to the long axes of the teeth (Figure 16–13). In adult patients the oral cavity is larger, but the teeth are the same size; the apices of the molars are lower in the maxilla and higher in the mandible, relative to the palate and floor of the mouth, respectively. The second reason for using the bisecting-the-angle technic is that it is desirable to examine the jaw area beyond the apices of deciduous teeth to observe the presence or absence of developing permanent teeth. The bisecting-angle technic

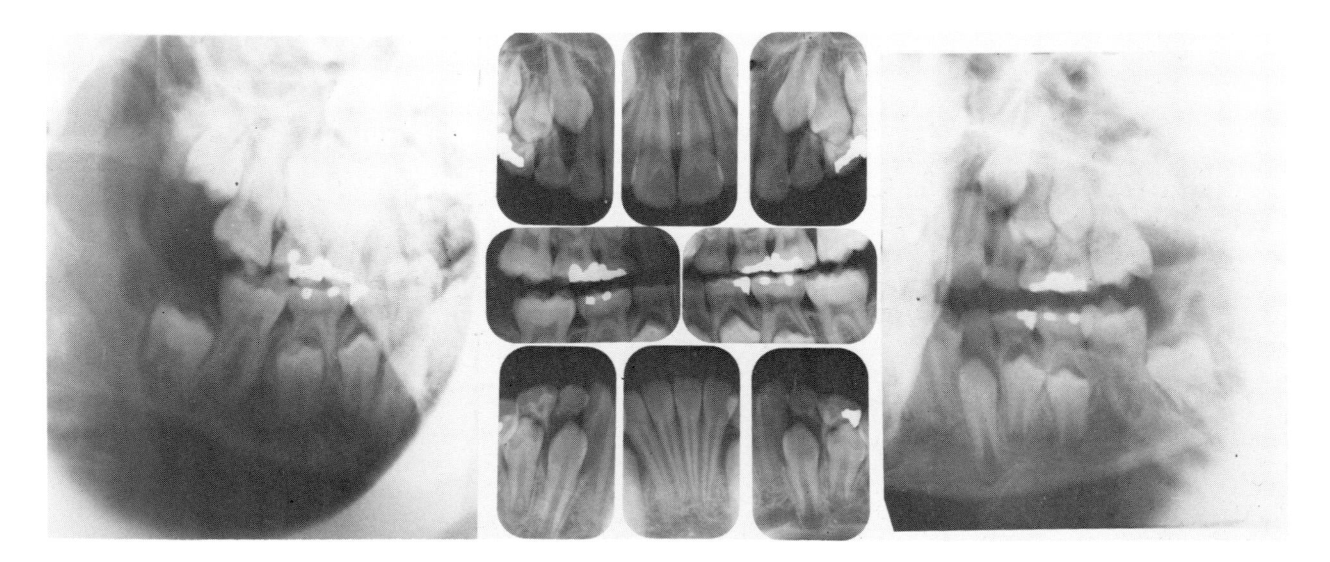

Figure 16–15. Radiographic survey of child using intraoral periapical views and extraoral lateral jaw projections.

can examine beyond the apices of the teeth without removing the images of the crowns of the teeth from the radiograph, that is, projecting the crown images beyond the occlusal border of the film.

When a child is cooperative but cannot hold the film in position, the bite block can be of great assistance, because this technic does not require the patient to use the hands.

With an apprehensive, uncooperative child it is sometimes possible to get the child to place the film in the mouth in the occlusal plane after the operator has demonstrated the procedure on himself or herself (Figure 16–14). After informing the child that he or she will not be touched, the operator positions the x-ray beam for a topographic occlusal radiograph without the cone or operator touching the patient. Useful radiographs of the anterior teeth can be obtained in this manner.

When the operator can obtain anterior and bitewing radiographs, but not posterior periapical projections, the posterior view can be obtained by extraoral technics using lateral jaw or panoramic radiography (Figure 16–15).

A small child may be cooperative but may have a mouth that is too small to comfortably hold a finger or bite block plus the film. In this case, the anterior teeth can be examined with the topographic occlusal technic using the adult periapical film (Figure 16–14). For

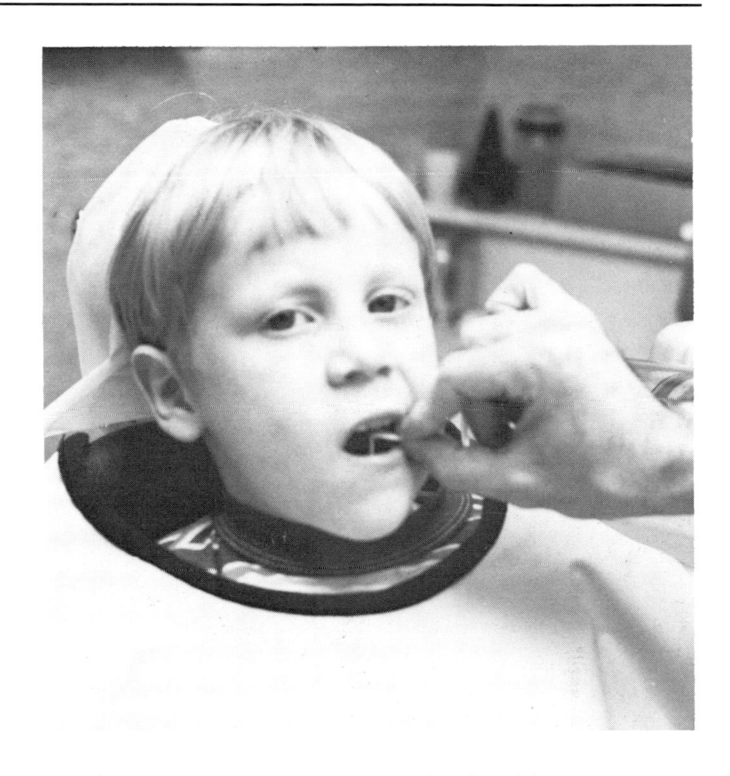

Figure 16–16. Number 1.1 film bent to make tab and the film positioned in small child's mouth.

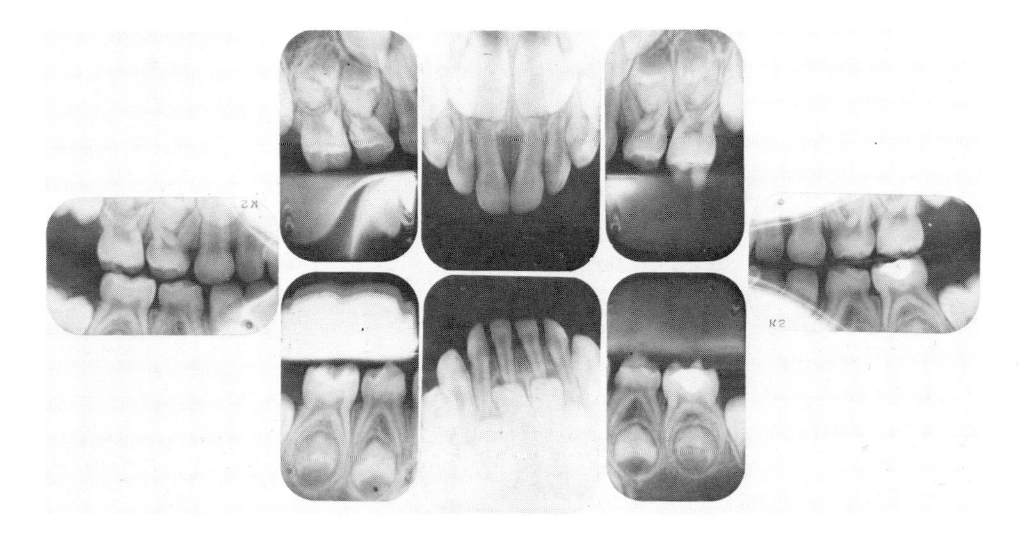

Figure 16–17. Radiographic survey of very small mouth using topographic occlusal and bent film technics with periapical films.

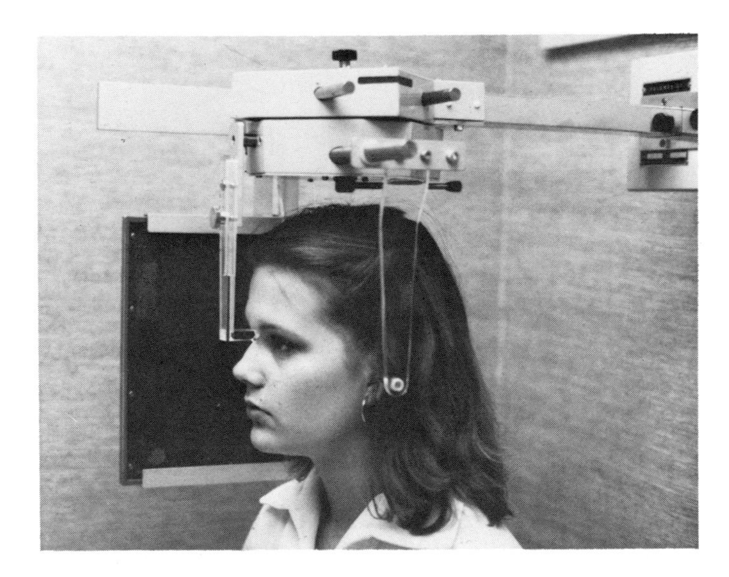

Figure 16–18. Patient's head positioned in cephalostat.

the posterior teeth, the No. 1.0 film or preferably the No. 1.1 film is used with the long dimension placed vertically; part of the film is bent to form a tab like a bitewing tab; the film is placed in the mouth with the patient closing the upper and lower teeth on the tab to hold it in place (Figure 16–16). In the maxilla and the mandible the tongue holds the useful part of the film in position when the patient closes the mouth. Only the film is in the patient's mouth. The operator cannot see the film with the patient's mouth closed and must be proficient in using extraoral anatomic landmarks to direct the x-ray beam. A complete radiographic survey of a small mouth is shown in Figure 16–17.

Restless or uncoordinated children often result in blurred radiographs due to movement by the patient. The intraoral radiographic technic in such cases should include the use of quick exposure procedures.

Occasionally a child will not permit film to be placed in position for periapical radiography. Many such children will cooperate for bitewing radiographs. Bitewing views plus a panoramic radiograph are often the best possible radiographic surveys with these children.

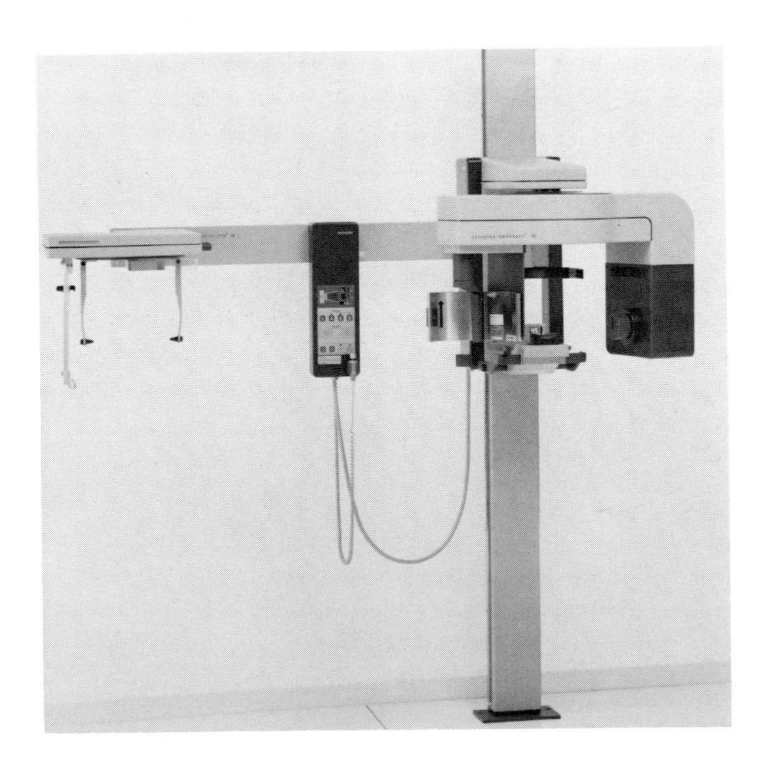

Figure 16–19. Orthoceph® x-ray unit used for cephalometric radiography.

THE ORTHODONTIC PATIENT

A patient under the care of an orthodontist is usually an older child or an adult. The general dental health of these patients is usually cared for by a general dentist or pedodontist who makes the standard diagnostic radiographic surveys. The orthodontist needs accurate skull measurements; when done radiographically, this procedure is called *cephalometric radiography.* Since orthodontic treatment can take many years to be completed, a scanning dental radiographic survey is useful to observe changes occurring due to treatment and growth of the patient and the development of any pathologic condition that might interfere with the treatment.

A scanning radiographic survey is commonly done with panoramic radiography. This radiograph examines the entire jaws from TM Joint to TM Joint; it is an extraoral technic and is easy and comfortable for the patient. A periapical intraoral survey is also used for this purpose and will give sharper radiographic images, but these radiographs will not survey the entire jaws and the technic is sometimes difficult to accomplish in a patient who has orthodontic appliances in the mouth.

The cephalometric radiograph commonly used is basically a lateral skull radiograph. The radiograph is made under rigidly standardized conditions. The patient's head is placed in a holder (cephalostat) to keep it motionless with the use of ear-rods (Figure 16–18). The x-ray tubehead is mechanically fixed for the central ray of the x-ray beam to superimpose the ear-rods upon each other. The central ray enters the right external auditory meatus of the patient and exits on the left side. The distance of the x-ray tube to the midsagittal plane of the patient's head is 5 feet. The dual need of a scanning radiograph and a cephalometric radiograph has resulted in the manufacture of combined panoramic and cephalometric units; an example is shown in Figure 16–19.

A lateral skull cephalometric radiograph is shown in Figure 16–20. The outlines of the anatomic parts of the skull are traced on semi-transparent paper placed over the illuminated radiograph. An orthodontic analysis of tooth-skull relationships is made with the identification of selected points on the tracing; planes formed by the joining of points, and angles formed by intersecting planes.

When a cephalometric radiograph is exposed to show the bone structures, the soft tissue images are too dense or dark. Since it is useful to see the soft tissue profile of the patient in the radiograph, x-ray exposure of the film in the profile soft tissue region is reduced. The best method is to remove some x rays from the beam before the beam reaches the patient; this is done by placing increased filtration in part of the beam in the machine's tubehead. However, this is somewhat difficult to do because of the great accuracy needed in positioning the additional filtration. Some radiographers use a wedge-shaped filter between the patient and the film to obtain less radiographic density of the soft tissue profile (Figure 16–21). The filter can be placed inside or outside the cassette.

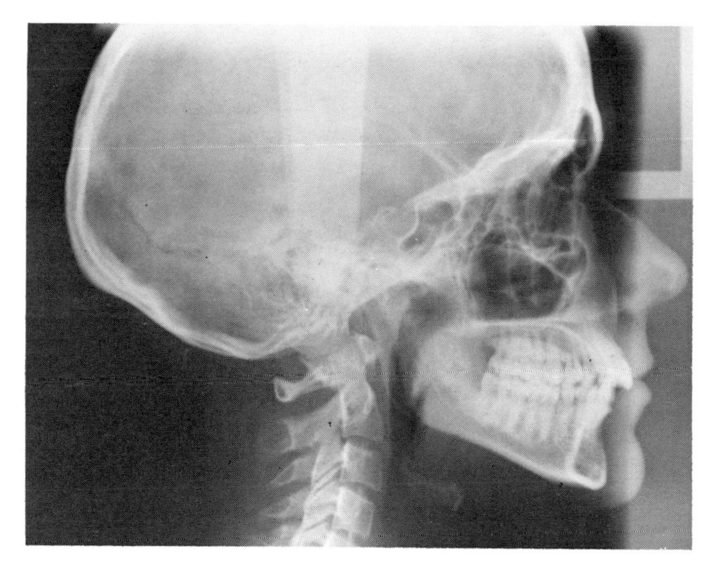

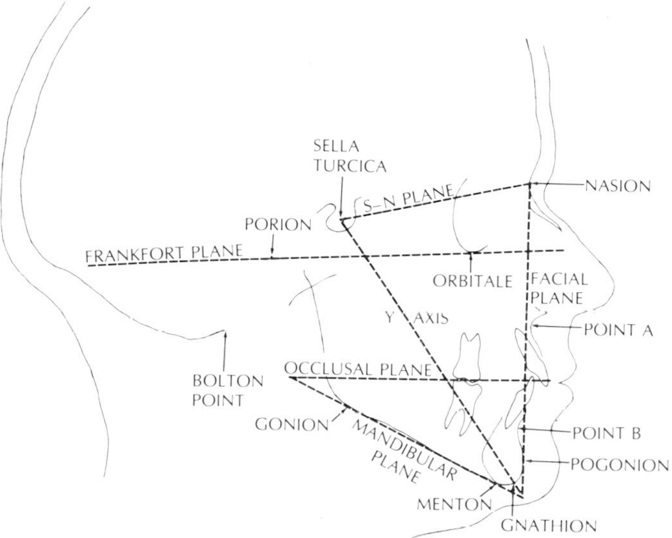

Figure 16–20. Cephalometric radiograph and tracing of the radiograph showing some orthodontic points, planes, and angles.

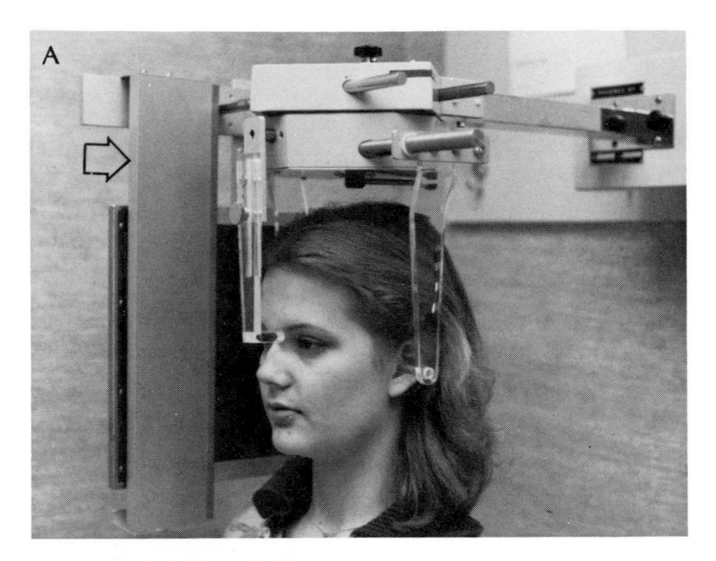

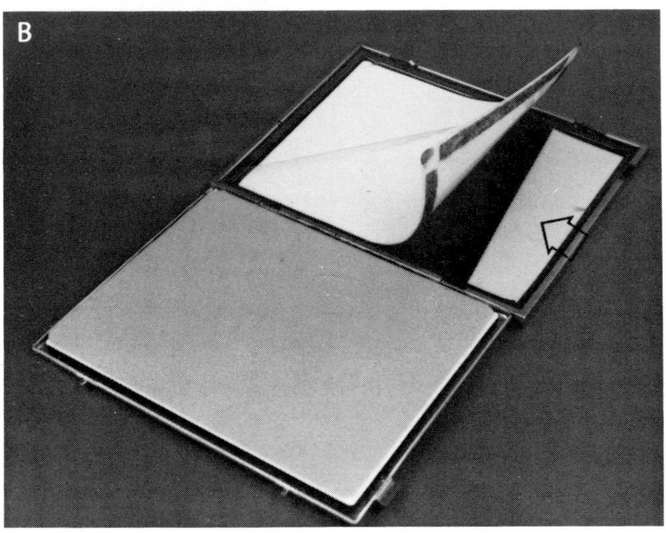

Figure 16–21. Wedge filters (arrows): A, removable filter in cephalostat; B, permanent filter in cassette. Radiograph showing reduced density in facial soft tissues is shown in Figure 16–20.

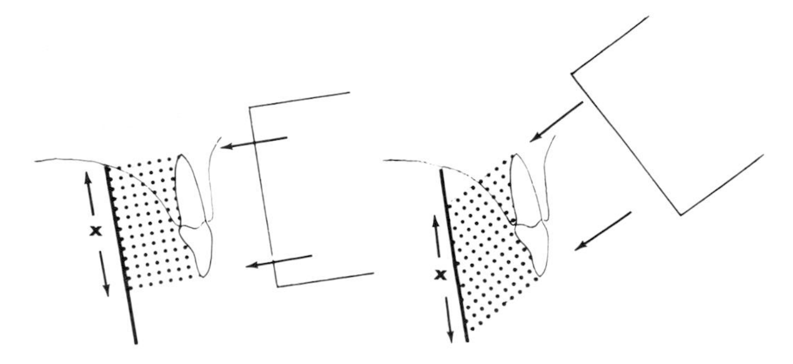

Figure 16–22. Diagram demonstrating why different vertical angulations do not change radiographic length of tooth when film is positioned parallel to long axis of tooth and long cone is used.

THE ENDODONTIC PATIENT

Visualization of the small root canal and root apex requires a radiograph that shows detail. Intraoral radiography is the technic of choice to provide the needed sharp images.

When the length of a tooth is being measured, the intraoral technic of choice is the paralleling technic. The reason is that changes in vertical angulation do not greatly affect the length of the root's shadow when the film is positioned parallel to the long axis of the tooth (Figure 16–22).

Modern root canal treatment requires the use of *working radiographs* to identify the position of endodontic instruments within the tooth. These radiographs must be made with instruments protruding from the crown of the tooth and with the tooth isolated by a rubber dam. Under such conditions the bisecting-the-angle technic is more practical. In addition, it is useful to use a film holder to position the film instead of the patient's hand, since the radiographic working area in the patient's mouth is reduced or restricted. The chosen film holder should not require the patient to bite upon it with the tooth being treated, since the tooth may have an instrument protruding from it. Two examples of film holders being stabilized by teeth other than the tooth being examined are shown in Figure 16–23.

A common problem in endodontic patients is the superimposition of buccal and palatal or lingual root apices (Figure 16–24). The root images can be separated on the radiograph by using a different horizontal angulation of the x-ray beam.

In some cases the root is thin or slender. The apex of such a root is sometimes difficult to distinguish from the surrounding bone in the radiograph. In such instances, maximum contrast between the root and bone is needed. Low kilovoltage and low radiographic fog can improve the contrast between tooth and bone. The kVp should be 60 or 65. The fog level can be greatly reduced by irradiating a smaller tissue volume of the patient, thus producing less secondary radiation; this reduction is achieved with the use of a smaller x-ray beam. Note that the area to be examined is the tooth apex, not the entire tooth; the operator does not need an x-ray

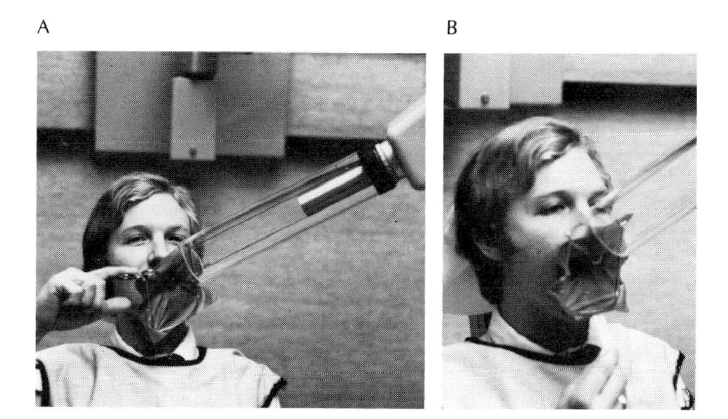

Figure 16–23. Endodontic working radiograph being made with (A) hemostat with bite block and (B) tongue blade with attached film. The examined tooth does not close on film or holder.

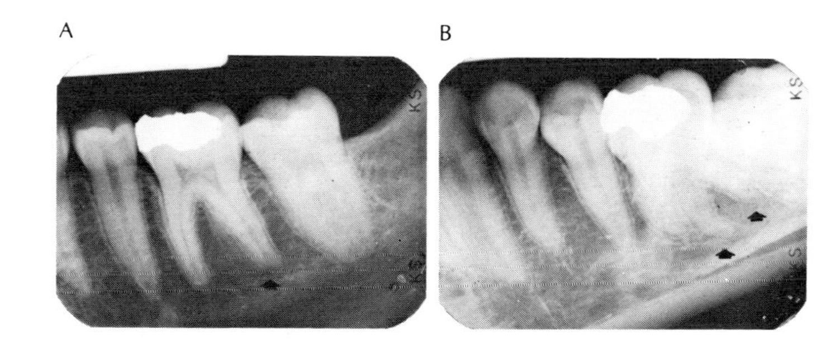

Figure 16–24. A, Superimposition of buccal and lingual apices of distal root apices of mandibular molar. B, Separated root apices showing two distinct distal roots obtained by changing horizontal angulation of x-ray beam.

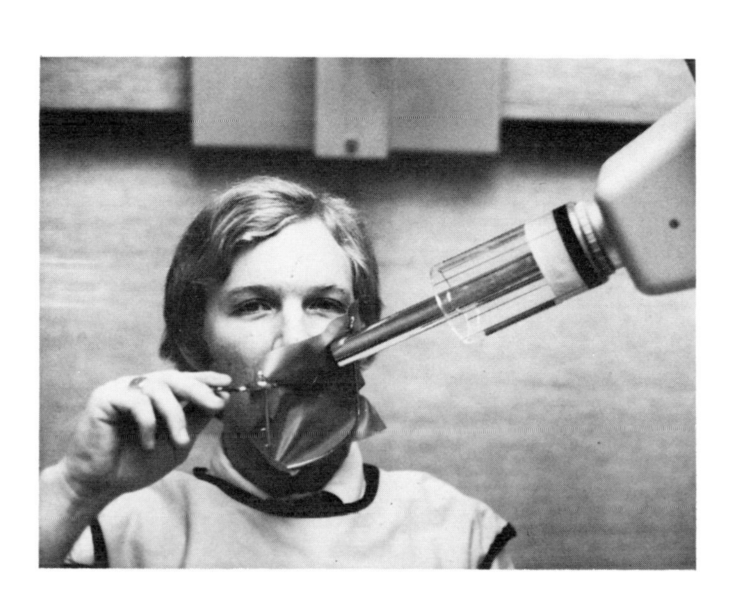

Figure 16–25. Small x-ray beam obtained by using brass cylinder collimator attached to base of cone.

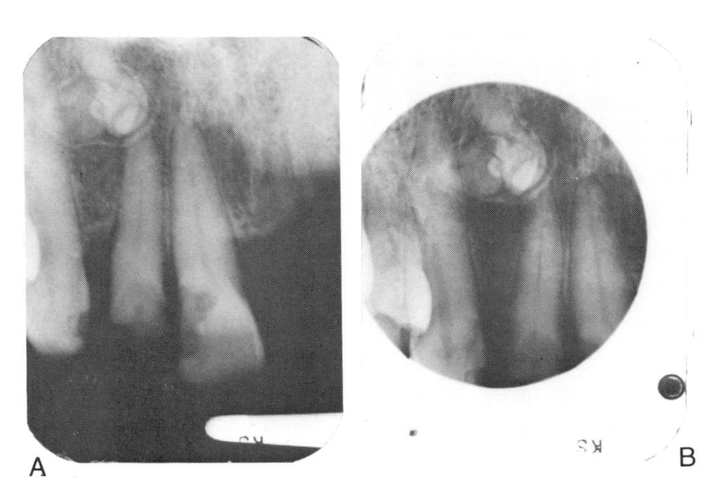

Figure 16–26. A, Radiograph of lateral incisor, made with standard $2\frac{3}{4}$-inch diameter x-ray beam, showing calcifying lesion in apical region. B, Radiograph of lateral incisor apex made with a one-inch x-ray beam showing area with more contrast due to less fog.

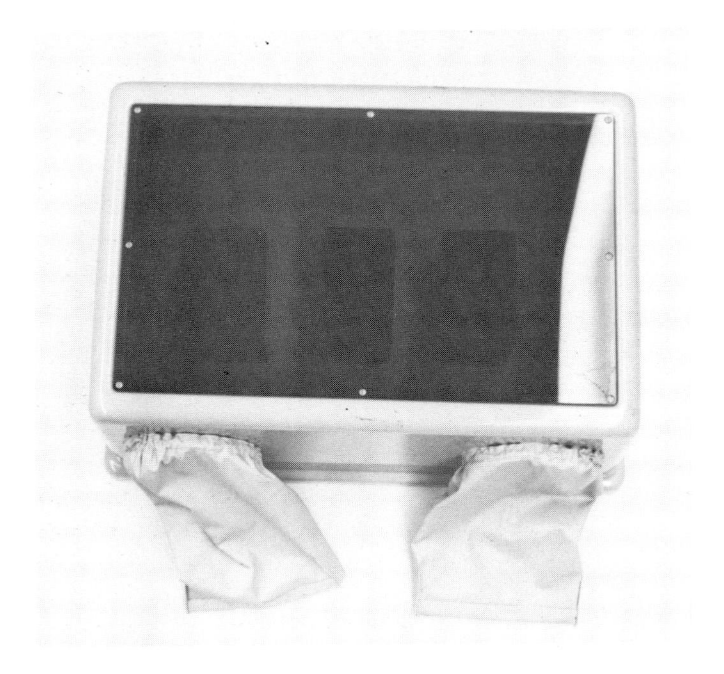

Figure 16–27. Daylight loader of Procomat® processor being used with small developer, water, and fixer tanks.

beam that is $2\frac{3}{4}$ inches in diameter. A 1-inch diameter x-ray beam is quite adequate. The small beam is obtained with a cylinder-shaped collimating cone (Figure 16–25). Radiographs of a root apex area made with a $2\frac{3}{4}$-inch beam and a 1-inch beam are shown in Figure 16–26.

Working radiographs made during endodontic therapy should be processed as quickly as possible to minimize the time the patient is uncomfortable with the rubber dam and saliva ejector in position. A manually operated small tank processor using concentrated solutions is useful in processing films within a minute (see automatic processing and quick processing, Chapter 2). Small solution containers can be used inside a daylight loader (used with some automatic processors) that is made light-tight (Figure 16–27). A small processor is capable of being operated in the x-ray room, and the needed radiographic information can be obtained quickly.

Chapter 17

Interpretation and Value of Radiographs

Dental radiography is an essential part of modern oral diagnosis. All radiographers should be able to recognize pathologic changes and be aware of the value of radiographs. Radiographs show pathologic lesions or foreign bodies that cannot be identified in any other way and assist in the localization of these objects. Radiographs are sometimes used to provide needed information during dental treatment; such is the case with the working radiographs made during endodontic treatment. Radiographs are also an important part of a patient's records.

Radiographs show the state of the calcified teeth and bone structures and are indispensable in evaluation of their growth and development. The radiographic images of normal structures are shown in Chapter 11 along with dental restorations and other materials. When abnormal or pathologic changes occur, the changes are often observable in radiographs and are referred to as radiographic signs.

Radiographic signs can be recognized by any person possessing knowledge of normal radiographic anatomy. However, the interpretation of the observed signs requires a good background of anatomy and oral pathology. Auxiliary personnel should be able to detect basic abnormal signs in dental radiographs; however, radiographs should be interpreted by a dentist who must plan patient treatment.

This chapter is not presented to completely teach x-ray interpretation. Radiographic interpretation requires a much greater presentation than is possible in a book of this size. This chapter presents basic dental x-ray interpretation and outlines the value of radiographs in dentistry. It shows common radiographic signs and some conditions with radiographic signs. The material also provides the reader with descriptive terminology commonly used in diagnostic radiology. For complete radiographic interpretation the material should be supplemented with a good oral pathology text.

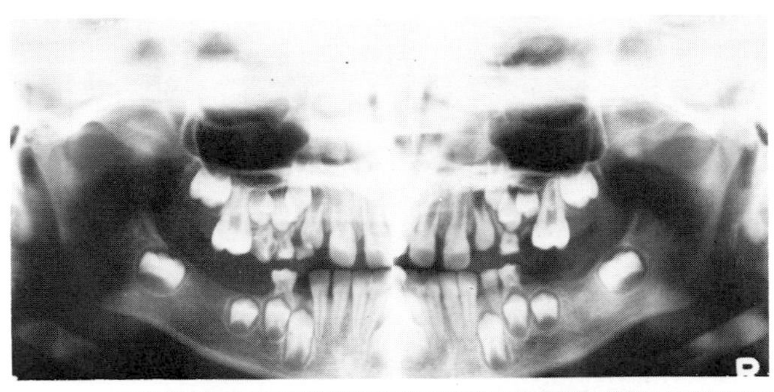

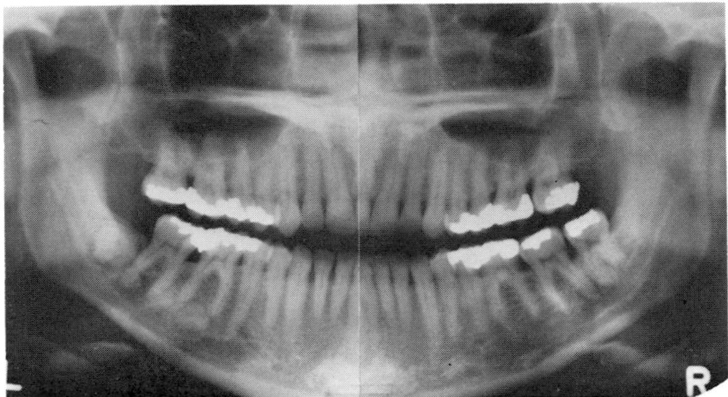

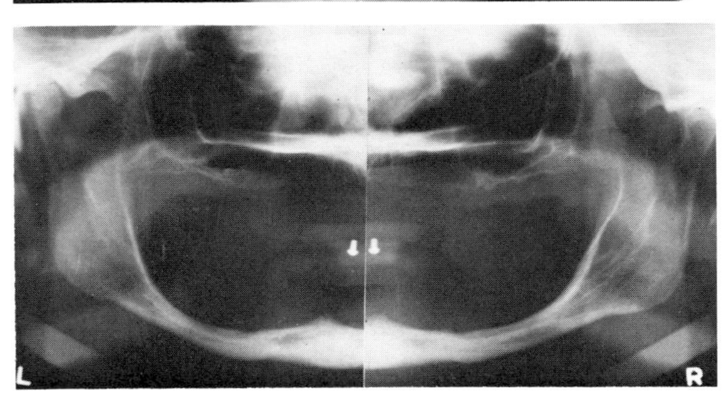

Figure 17–1. Panoramic radiographs of a child, an adult, and a geriatric patient.

RADIOGRAPHIC RECORDS

The value of radiographs as part of the patient's records cannot be overstated. The information contained in radiographs cannot be easily matched by written records and the x-ray record is usually more indisputable than a written statement in the event of a disagreement or lawsuit.

Radiographs show the condition of the patient at a particular time. Later radiographs compared with the x-ray records show the changes due to pathology or treament occurring in the patient with time. This information can be useful in caring for the total health of the patient.

Radiographs placed in a patient's records should be of good quality. They should be properly processed and mounted or stored in envelopes. They should also be properly identified and dated.

GROWTH AND DEVELOPMENT

The anatomy of patients of varying ages is important to both radiographer and diagnostician. Information of the size and number of teeth and their position in the jaws is useful in identifying if changes are taking place in the patient. Panoramic radiographs are used to give an overview of the basic changes that occur in the jaws with age (Figure 17–1). Examples of localized growth disturbances producing over or under development of an area are shown in Figure 17–2.

RADIOGRAPHIC SIGNS

Unusual or abnormal changes in the calcified structures of the patient can be observed as changes in the shape of bone and teeth, changes in size of these structures, changes in the number of teeth, changes in the position of the teeth, and changes in density due to pathologic conditions. When pathologic lesions are evident, they may appear as a radiolucency, a radiopacity, or a mixed radiopaque and radiolucent lesion. Changes in the soft tissues are not usually evident in radiographs; however, when radiopaque calcifications or foreign bodies are

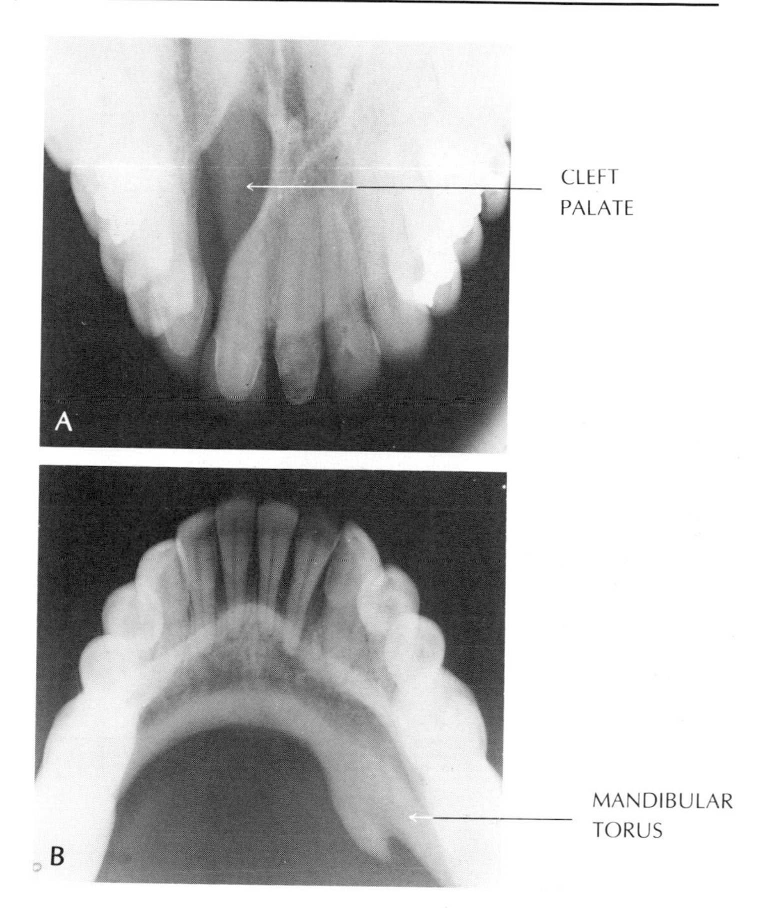

Figure 17–2. A, Local underdevelopment of bone in a case of cleft palate and B, local overdevelopment in a case of mandibular torus.

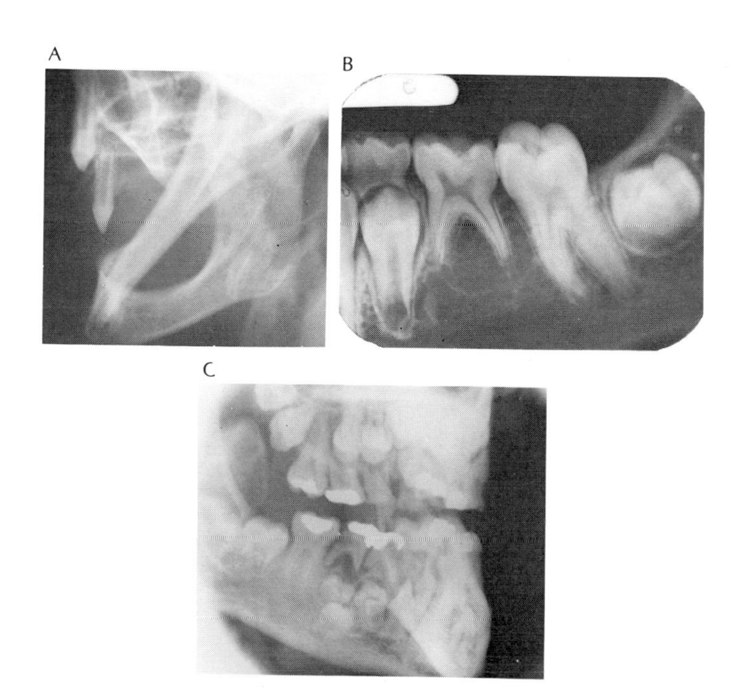

Figure 17–3. Some conditions affecting number of teeth seen in radiographs. A, Lateral jaw radiograph showing multiple missing teeth in patient with ectodermal dysplasia. B, Periapical radiograph showing retention of deciduous molar due to failure of development of permanent bicuspid. C, Lateral jaw radiograph showing multiple supernumerary teeth in patient with cleidocranial dysostosis.

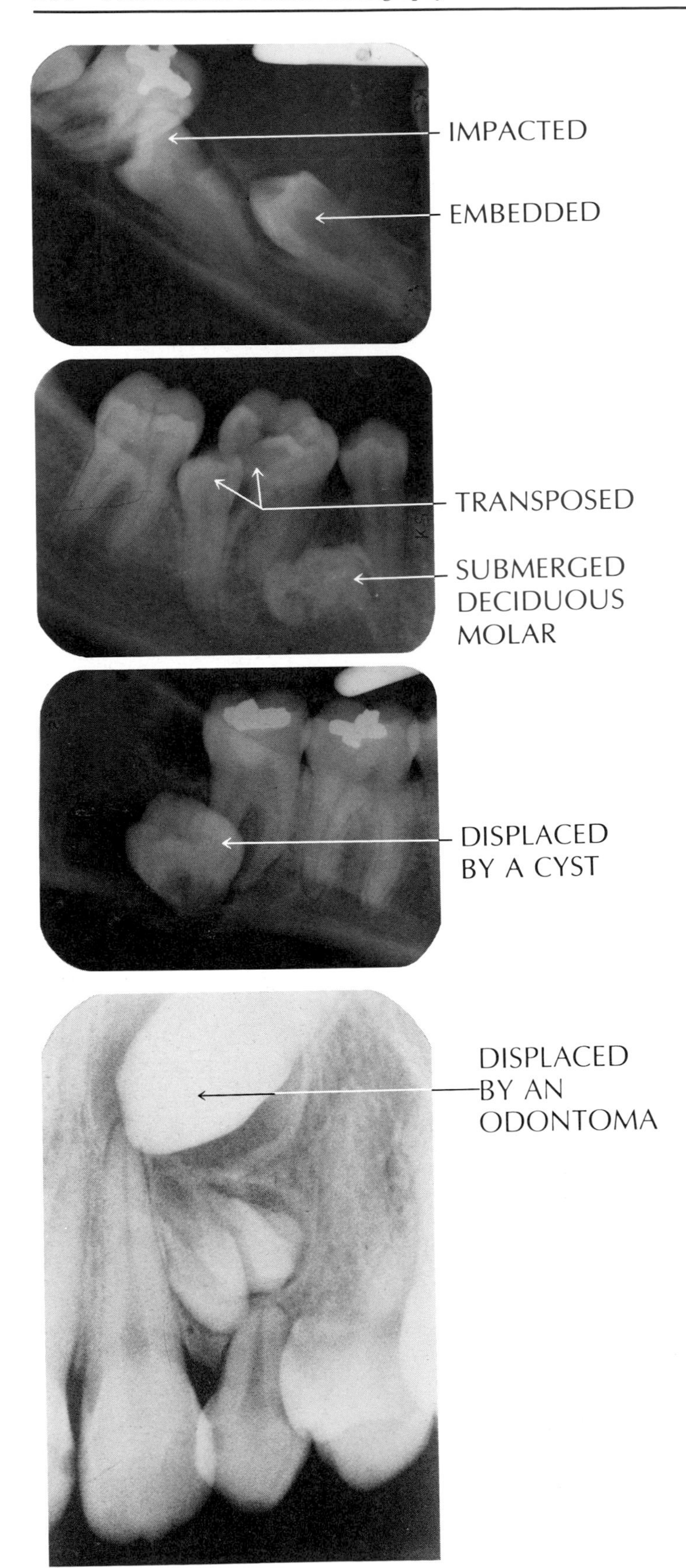

Figure 17–4. Examples of abnormally located teeth.

present in soft tissues, radiography is useful in diagnosis of the condition.

Alterations in Teeth

Number. Changes in teeth that are observed in radiographs can be seen as an alteration in the number of teeth. Absence of teeth (anodontia) or failure in development of some teeth (oligodontia) is seen in some developmental conditions (Figure 17–3A and B). The most common missing teeth are second bicuspids, third molars, and permanent lateral incisors. Extra or supernumerary teeth are not rare; they may be associated with a developmental disorder such as cleidocranial dysostosis (Figure 17–3C).

Location. Abnormal location of teeth can be seen as impacted teeth, embedded teeth, and translocated teeth. The relationship of these teeth to the sinus, nasal cavity, cortical bone plates, and vital structures such as the inferior alveolar canal is of great diagnostic importance (Figure 17–4). Radiographic localization procedures are often used when removal of abnormally located teeth is considered.

Shape. Alteration in the shape of teeth may be developmental in origin, e.g., dens in dente, dentinal dysplasia, taurodontism, dentinogenesis imperfecta, amelogenesis imperfecta, odontodysplasia, fusion, gemination. The alteration may be due to infections (e.g., hypoplasia) or to trauma (e.g., dilaceration). Examples of changes in the shapes of teeth are shown in Figure 17–5.

Structure. Loss of normal tooth structure is reflected in the radiographic images of teeth. The result is a radiolucent area in the radiograph where there is usually radiopaque tooth structure. Such is the case with caries, tooth resorption, and fractures (Figure 17–6). A major reason for making bite-wing radiographs is to observe the condition of the proximal surfaces of teeth. Studies have shown that small carious lesions on these surfaces are detected better with radiographs than by a clinical examination.

Calcification can occur on or inside a tooth. Calculus may form on the erupted portions of a tooth. The pulp can produce pulp stones or become totally calcified. The cementum may be stimulated to produce hypercementosis on the root surface. Examples

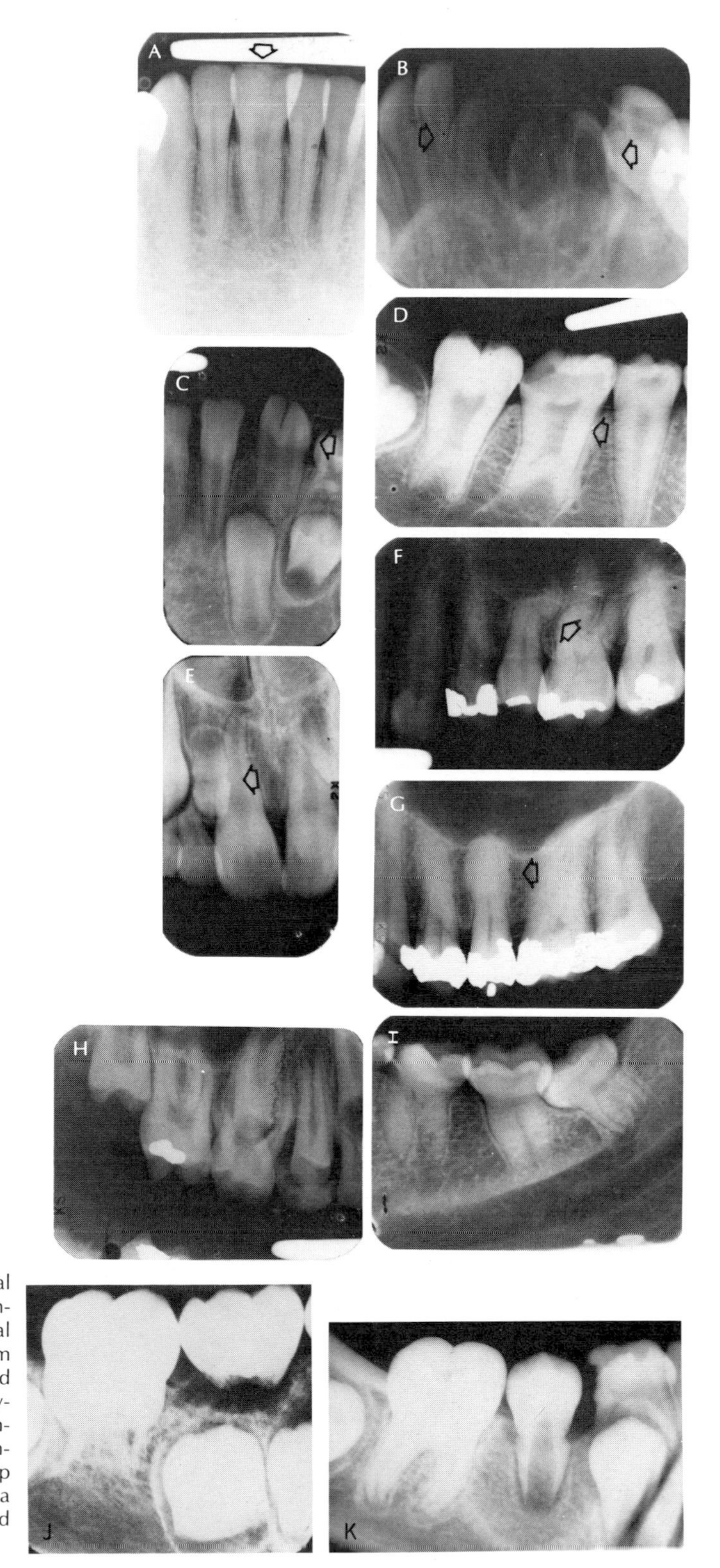

Figure 17–5. Examples of conditions showing teeth with abnormal shapes. A, Gemination of mandibular central incisor. B, Regional odontodysplasia showing typical "ghost teeth." C, Fusion of deciduous lateral incisor and cuspid with absence of permanent successor. D, Taurodontism showing teeth with large pulp chambers. E, Hypoplasia of unerupted lateral incisor. F, Dilaceration showing tooth with crooked root. G, Hypercementosis showing tooth with bulbous root. H, Amelogenesis imperfecta showing teeth with practically no enamel. I, Dentinogenesis imperfecta showing teeth with slender radiolucent roots and obliterated pulp chambers. J, Missing roots in dentinal dysplasia. K, Turner's hypoplasia or interrupted root development seen in a mandibular second bicuspid due to periapical infection in the preceding deciduous second molar.

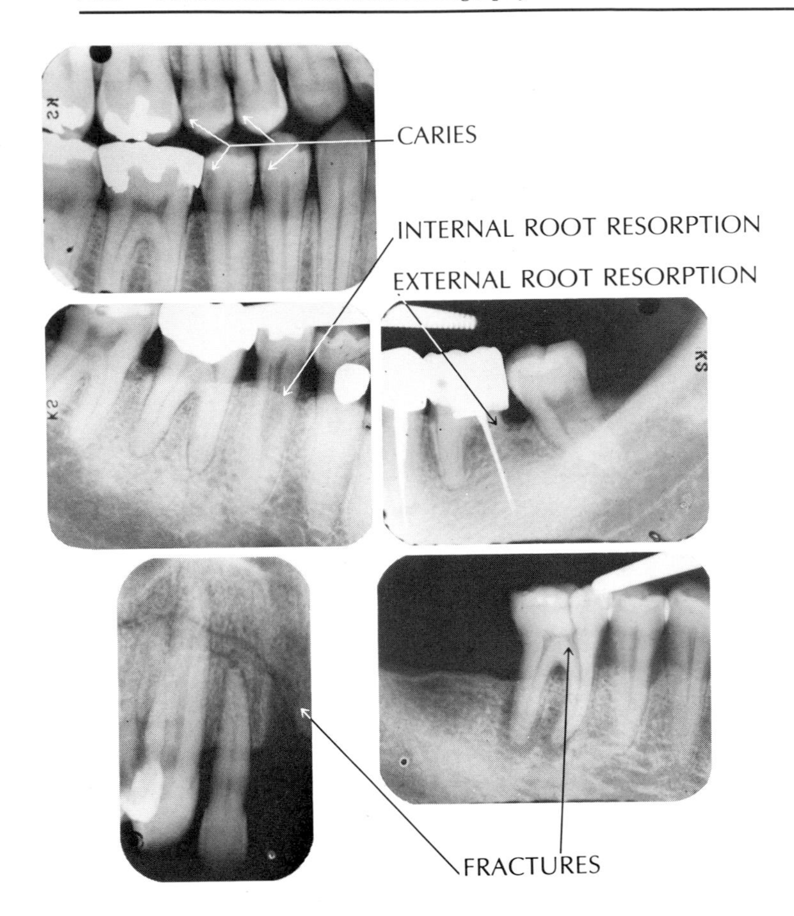

Figure 17–6. Some conditions producing radiolucent areas in teeth.

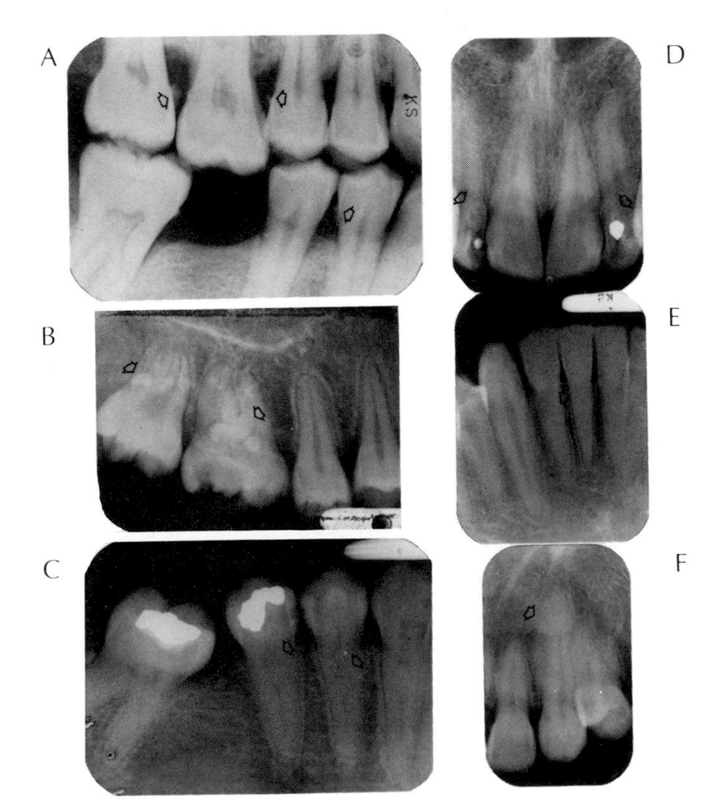

Figure 17–7. Examples of calcifications affecting teeth. A, Calculus. B, Enamel pearls. C, Pulp stones. D, Dens in dente. E, Calcified pulp. F, Hypercementosis.

of calcifications affecting teeth are shown in Figure 17–7.

Alteration of Periapical Tissues

The most common cause of changes in the periapical tissues is infection. The radiograph may show a widening of the periodontal space, destruction of the lamina dura, formation of a radiolucent area of bone destruction, or formation of a radiopaque area of bone resistance or sclerosis in the surrounding bone (Figure 17–8). The sclerotic or more radiopaque bone is commonly referred to as "condensing osteitis." Longstanding infections may produce resorption of the root apex.

Other common alterations of periapical tissues may be produced by a cyst, a cementoma, or trauma. Examples of such alterations are shown in Figure 17–9.

Alterations in the Periodontium

Periodontal changes visible in radiographs are seen in the alveolar bone. The height of the tooth-supporting bone is normally within 1.5 mm of the cementoenamel junction of a tooth. Disease processes or calculus and restorations with overhangs can produce bone loss. Early bone loss appears as a small triangular-shaped radiolucency adjacent to the neck of the affected tooth. Bone loss can progress and lower the height of the alveolar bone (horizontal bone loss) or produce an area of no bone trabeculae beside a tooth (vertical bone loss). Examples of bone loss seen in radiographs are shown in Figure 17–10A.

Bone loss can be radiographically measured in terms of the actual amount of loss of the height of the alveolar ridge. However, it is often more useful, for treatment evaluation, to measure bone loss as a percentage loss of the normal amount of bone. The normal bone is between the apex of the tooth and a point 1.5 mm below the cementoenamel junction of the tooth. The use of a graded transparent template placed over the radiograph can assist the operator in making this measurement (Figure 17–10B).

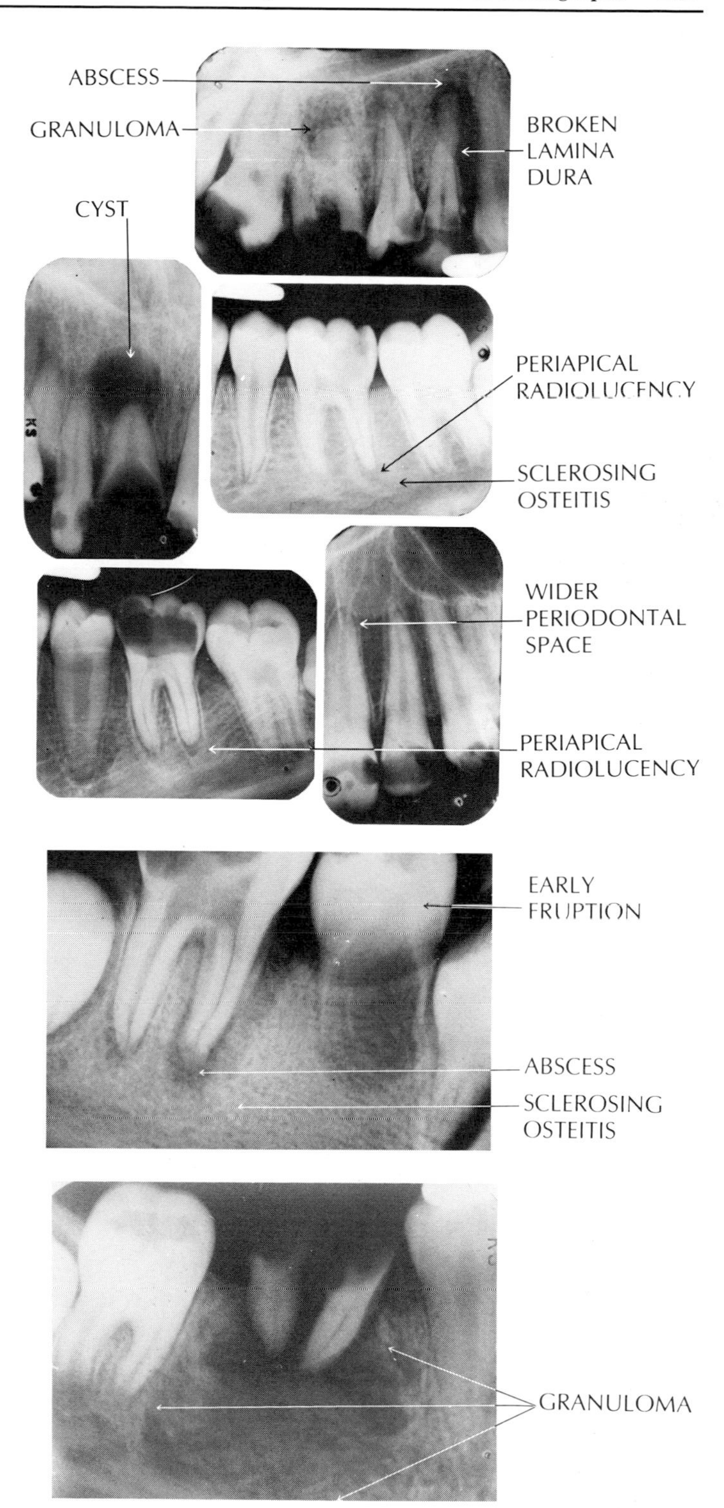

Figure 17–8. Periapical changes commonly seen with infection.

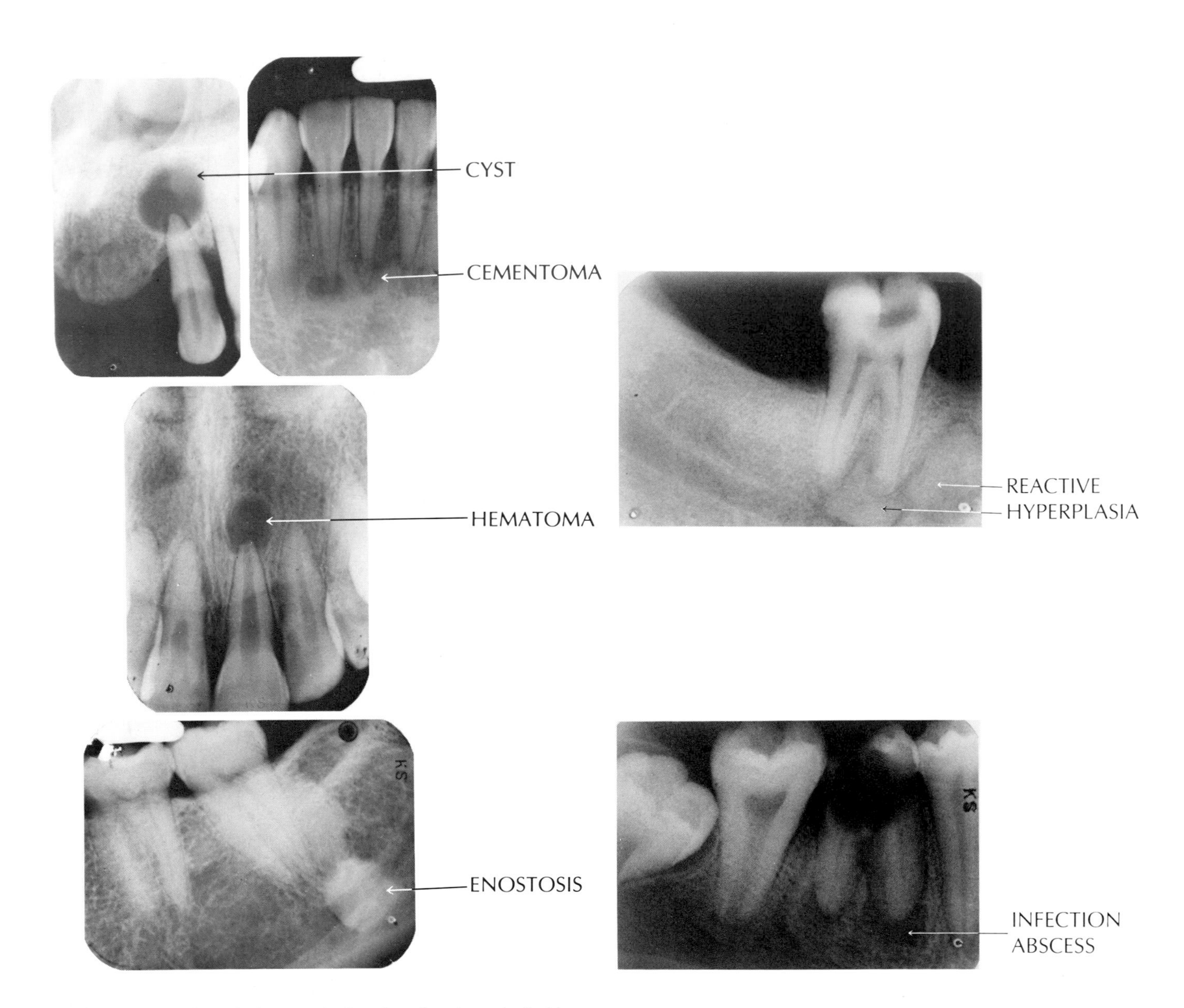

Figure 17–9. Some lesions producing alterations in periapical bone.

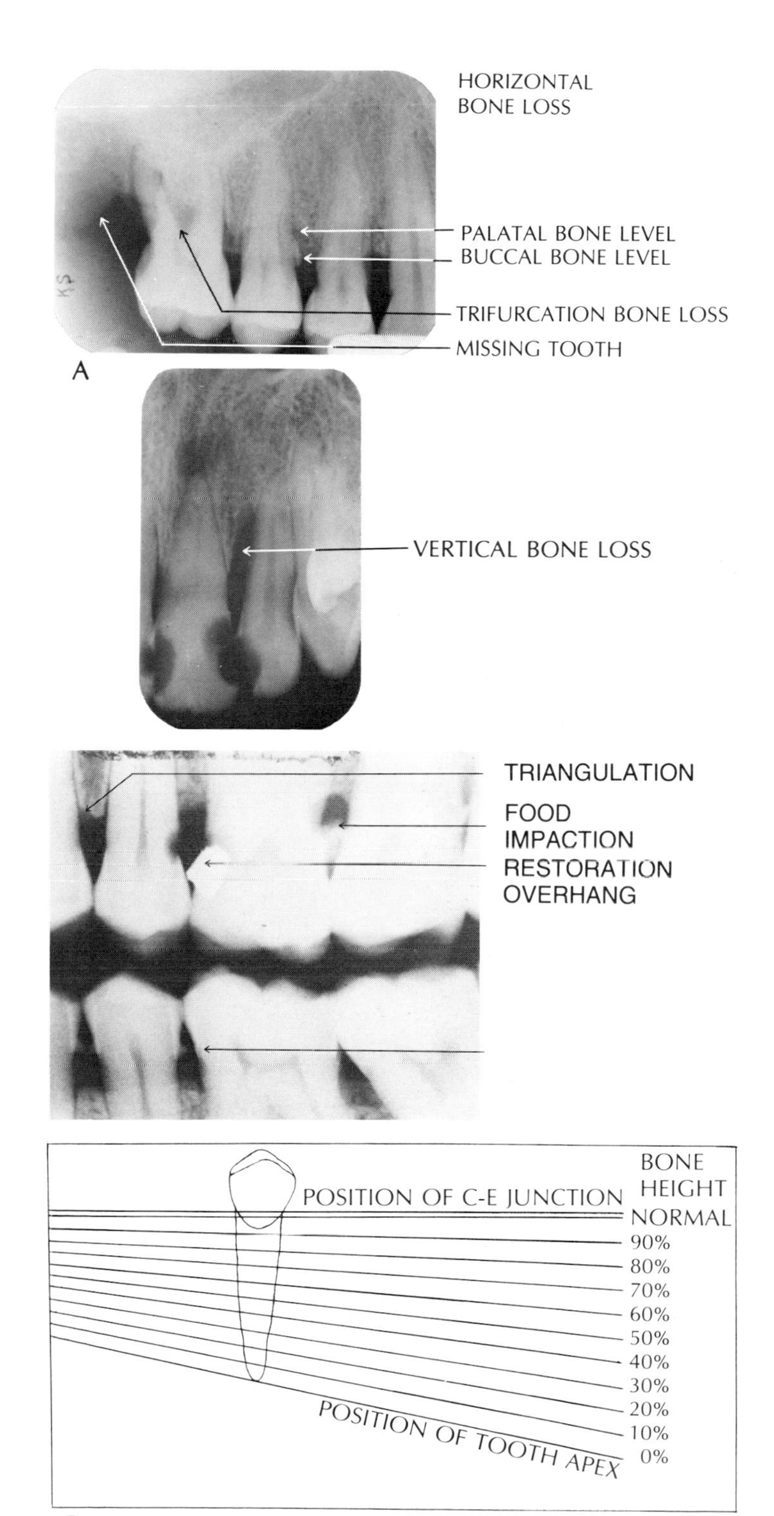

Figure 17–10. A, Examples of vertical and horizontal bone loss and some contributing factors to bone loss. B, Design of transparent template used in measuring percentage of bone loss.

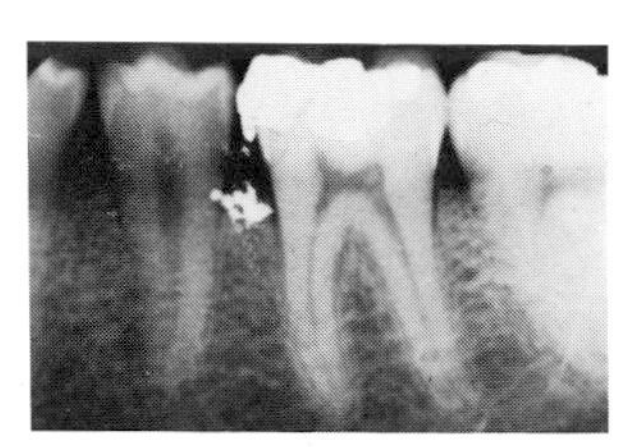

AMALGAM IN GINGIVA

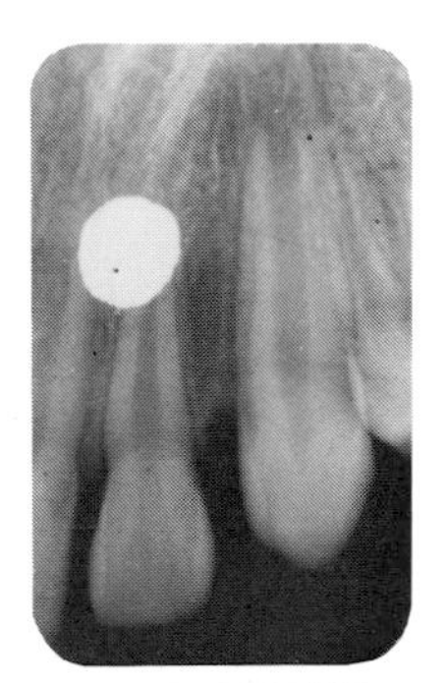

LEAD PELLET

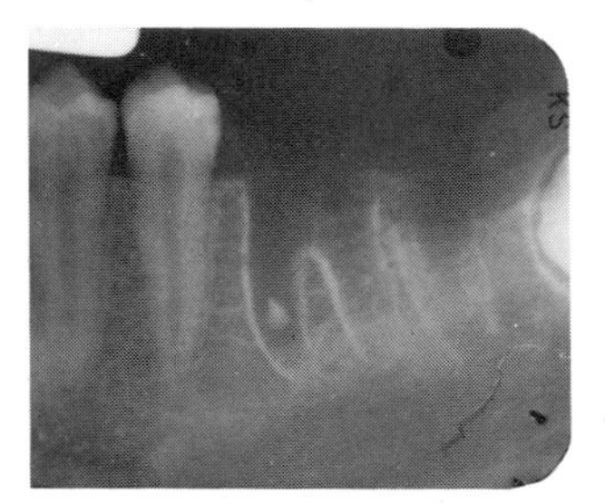

TOOTH CHIP IN SOCKET

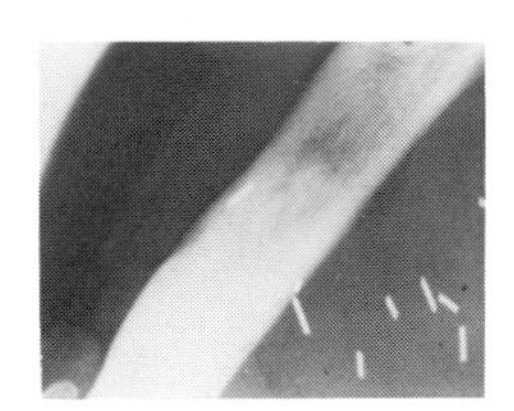

RADON CAPSULES IN TUMOR

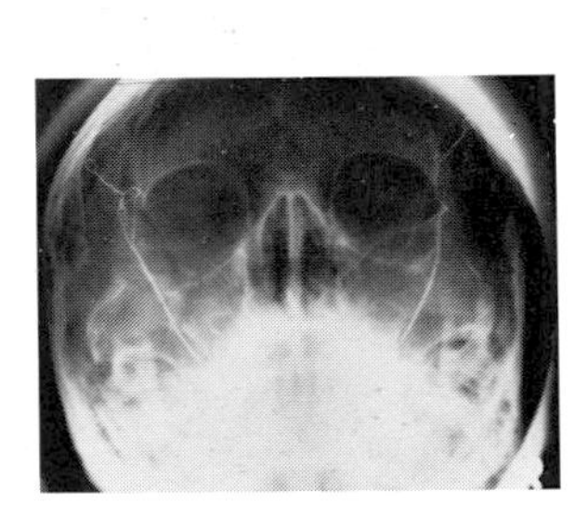

FRACTURE WIRES

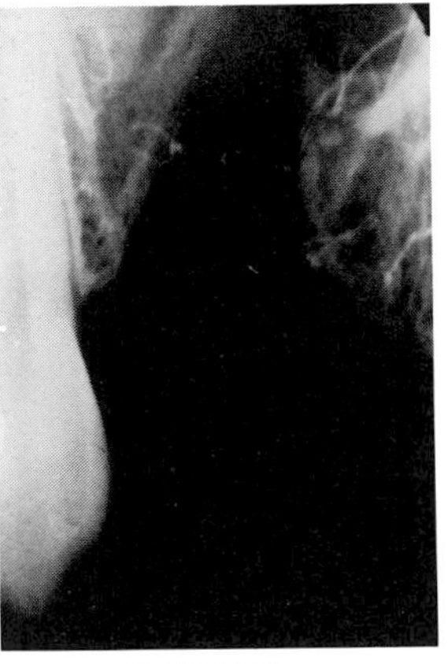

SUTURES

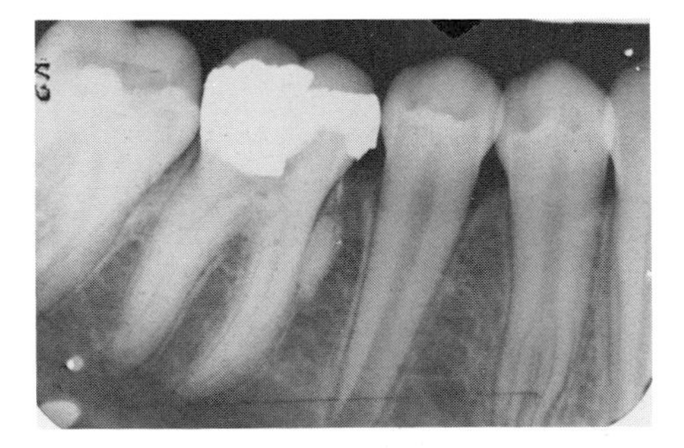

RETAINED DECIDUOUS ROOT

Figure 17–11. Foreign objects in oral tissues shown by dental radiographs.

Foreign Bodies

Radiography is the most important diagnostic tool available to the dentist in locating and identifying foreign objects within a patient's oral tissue. Localizing procedures have been described earlier in this book. One must remember that x rays are absorbed proportional to the atomic density of the object. Radiolucent foreign objects are not shown in radiographs unless they are positioned within a calcified or radiopaque anatomic structure. Examples of foreign objects found in dental radiographs are shown in Figure 17–11.

Alterations in Bone

Alteration of the normal radiographic image of the bone of the mandible and maxilla may appear as a change in the bone itself or as the presence of a lesion affecting the bone. Whole bones become more radiolucent as a result of calcium being removed (osteoporosis), or additional calcification can produce more radiopaque bone (Figure 17–12). It is difficult to assess the opacity of bone when only a small area of bone is seen, such as in a single intraoral radiograph. Whole bones may also be altered in shape. This may be due to abnormal development, fractures, or disease processes. Some conditions affecting the shape of the jaws are shown in Figure 17–13.

A bone may be altered to be radiolucent or radiopaque in different areas. Both radiopacities and radiolucencies are seen in the case of Paget's disease (Figure 17–14). In this example the radiopaque areas tend to have a "cotton-wool" appearance in the radiograph.

Lesions present in bone may show distinct patterns or forms of objects. Radiopaque lesions may show the formation of bone, e.g., tori and osteomas; they may show the shapes of teeth, e.g., odontomas, teratomas; or they may show indistinct calcified masses, e.g., cementomas, complex odontomas, and fibromas. Some examples of these radiographic signs are shown in Figure 17–15.

Bone can also be changed in the type of trabeculae. When very fine trabeculae are present, the bone is said to have a "ground glass" radiographic appearance (Figure 17–16). Normal trabeculae replaced by very

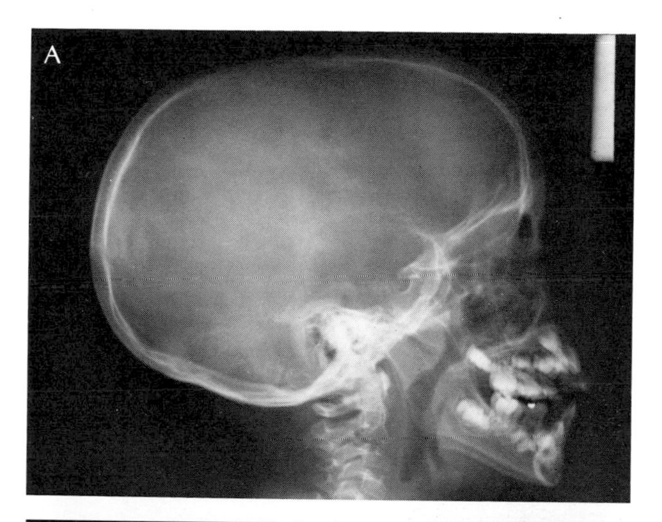

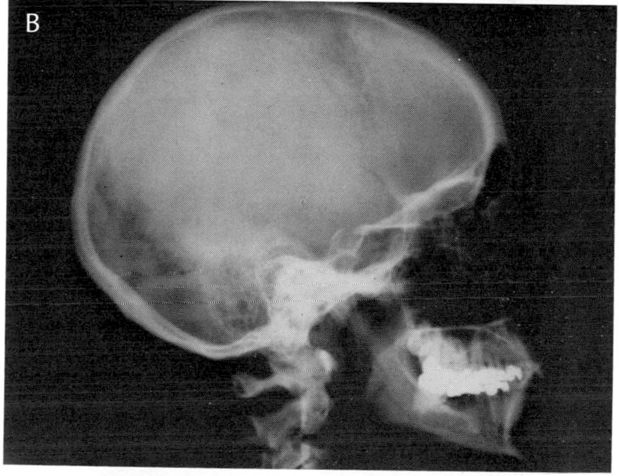

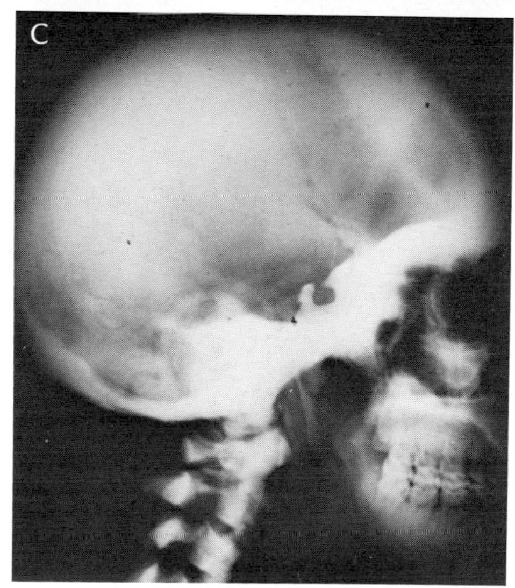

Figure 17–12. Lateral skull radiographs demonstrating alterations in bone density. A, Radiolucent skull in patient with sickle cell anemia. Note that soft tissues appear in radiograph. B, Normal density skull. C, Radiopaque skull of patient with osteopetrosis. Note that bone marrow spaces are obliterated.

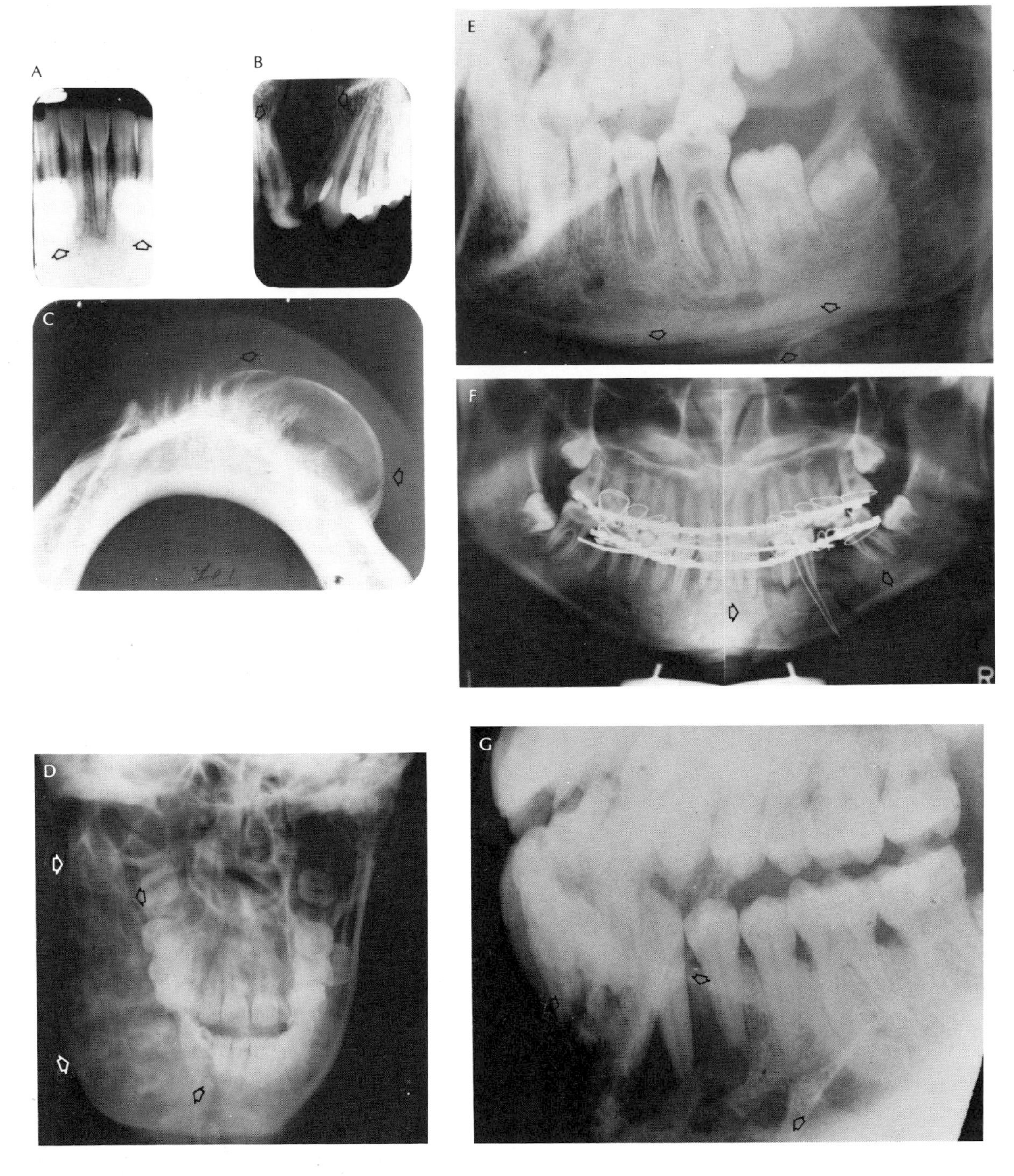

Figure 17–13. Some conditions affecting shape of bones. A, Periapical radiograph of mandibular incisors showing large lingual tori. B, Periapical radiograph of maxillary cuspid area showing cleft alveolar ridge and palate. C, Occlusal radiograph of mandible showing expansion of labial cortical bone by residual cyst. D, Posteroanterior radiograph of jaws showing enlargement of one side of mandible in patient with fibrous dysplasia. E, Lateral jaw radiograph of mandible demonstrating laminated calcifications on lower border of mandible in patient whose periostitis ossificans is associated with periapical tooth infection. F, Distortion of mandible seen in panoramic radiograph of patient with fracture. G, Lateral jaw radiograph demonstrating destruction of mandible in patient with cancer.

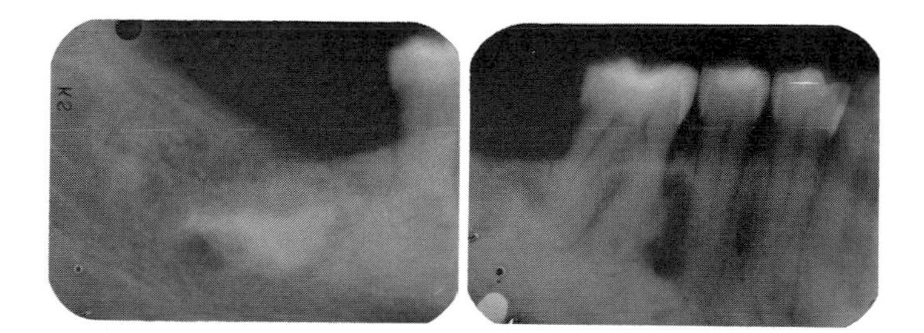

Figure 17–14. Radiograph of patient with Paget's disease showing radiolucent and radiopaque areas of bone having "cotton-wool" appearance.

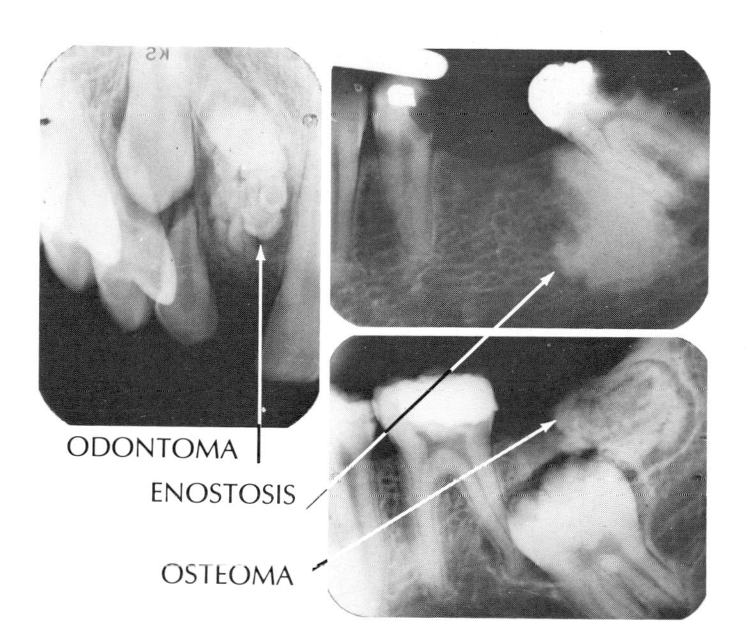

Figure 17–15. Radiographs demonstrating some calcifications within bone.

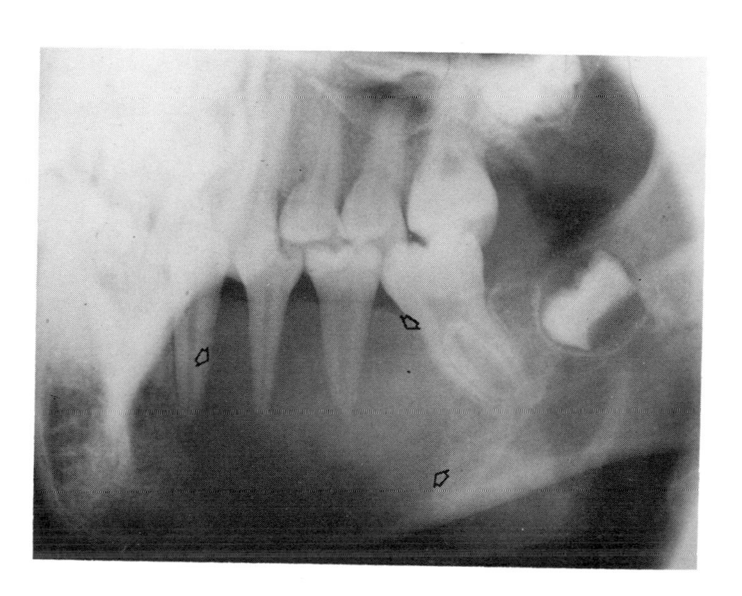

Figure 17–16. Radiograph of patient with fibrous dysplasia showing loss of lamina dura and bone with a "ground-glass" appearance (arrows) commonly associated with hyperparathyroidism, fibrous dysplasia, and rickets.

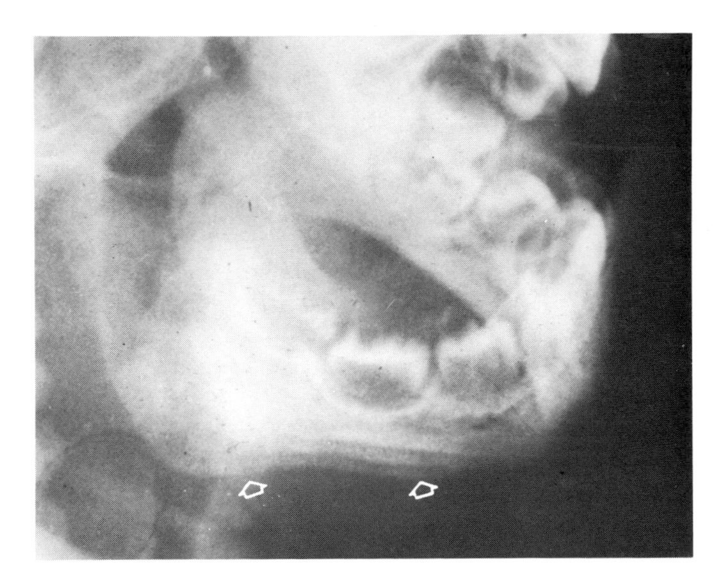

Figure 17–17. "Onion-peel" appearance (arrows) of bone cortex in patient with infantile cortical hyperostosis.

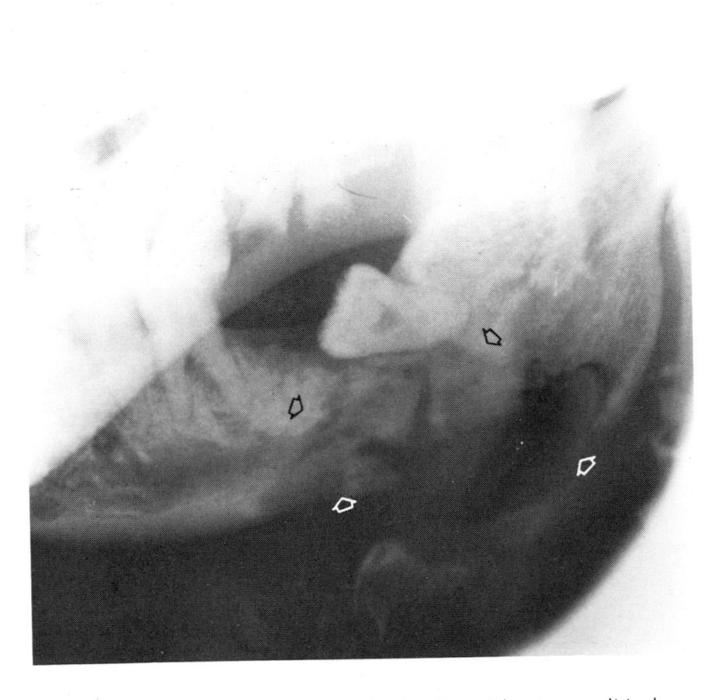

Figure 17–18. Lateral jaw radiograph of patient with osteomyelitis showing "worm-eaten" appearance of bone and destruction of part of cortical bone plate (arrows).

small trabeculae are often associated with hyperparathyroidism, rickets, anemias, and fibroosseous lesions, such as fibrous dysplasia, fibroma, and Paget's disease. In some cases the cortical plates of a bone may be affected. The patient's body may deposit layers of bone on the cortical plate, resulting in an "onion-peel" appearance radiographically (Figure 17–17). This radiographic sign is sometimes seen in patients with infantile cortical hyperostosis, periostitis ossificans, and Garré's osteomyelitis.

Radiolucent lesions in bone are produced by many different disease processes. Bone infections, or osteomyelitis, tend to show channels of purulent material in the bone producing a "worm-eaten" radiographic appearance (Figure 17–18). Infections tend to punch holes in the cortical plates of bone to establish a fistulous tract.

Whether a bone lesion is single or multiple is of great diagnostic importance. The use of panoramic radiographs and skull projections is mandatory whenever a lesion is detected in the dental area and the presence of other lesions is suspected.

A lesion may completely destroy the bone around a tooth. The radiographic image produced is sometimes called "floating teeth" (Figure 17–19). This condition may be due to extensive periodontal disease or one of the histiocytosis-X disease processes, such as eosinophilic granuloma. When eosinophilic granulomas occur in the cranium, they produce well-defined radiolucencies with sharp borders. These lesions are said to have a "punched-out" appearance (Figure 17–20).

Slowly expanding radiolucent lesions often have a "lamina-dura-like," thin layer of bone, resisting the expansion of the lesion at the periphery of the radiolucency. This radiographic sign is sometimes referred to as an "eggshell" bone layer and is most often associated with a cyst or slowly expanding benign soft tissue neoplasm (Figure 17–21).

Radiographic signs associated with aggressive lesions destroying bone tend to show only bone destruction. Malignant neoplasms such as carcinomas and sarcomas often cause this type of bone lesion. The borders of these lesions are usually indistinct, and when the cortical plate is involved, the lesion may produce a "notching" of the plate or may com-

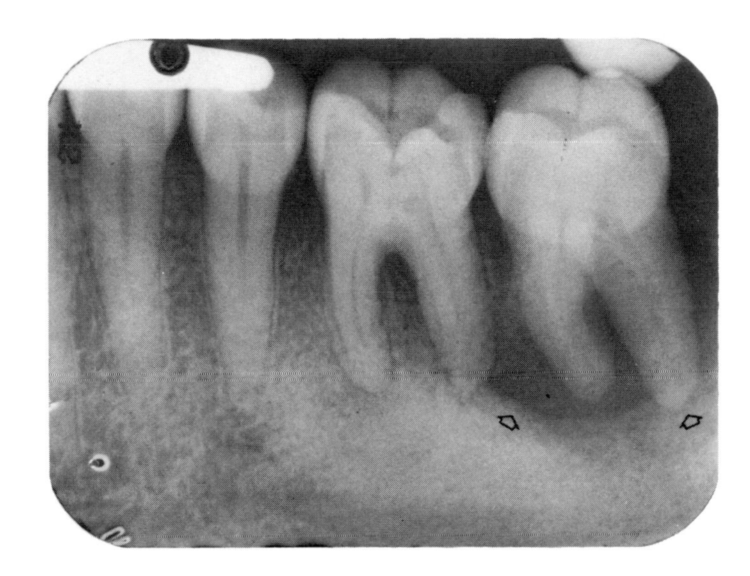

Figure 17–19. Radiographic picture of "floating tooth" due to extreme bone loss (arrows).

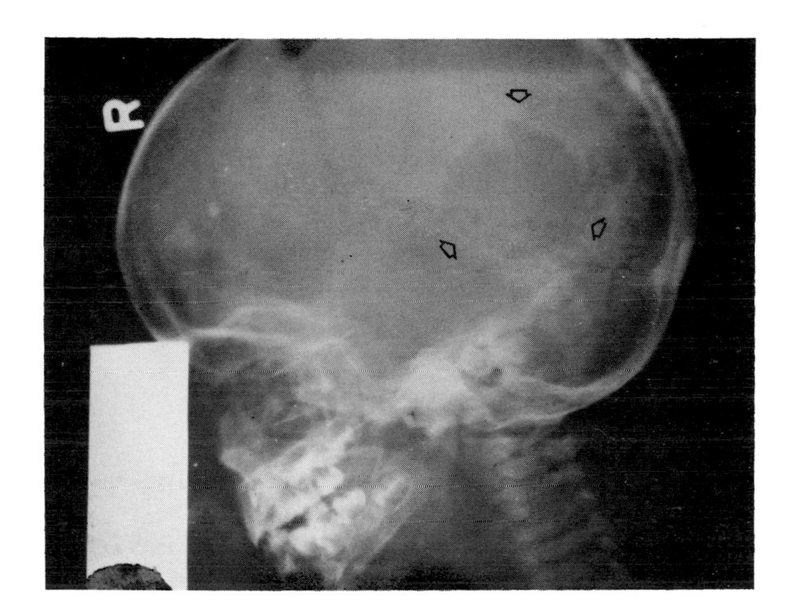

Figure 17–20. Skull radiograph of patient's cranium showing large lesion of eosinophilic granuloma that has "punched-out" appearance (arrows).

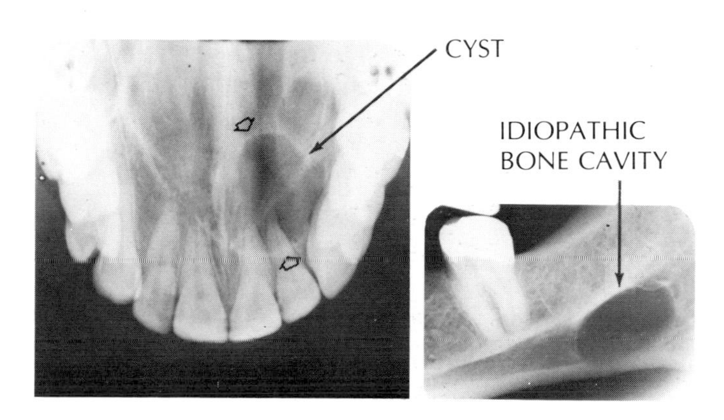

Figure 17–21. Occlusal radiograph demonstrating "lamina dura-like" or "eggshell" appearance of thin bone layer surrounding radiolucent cyst and periapical radiograph showing the "cyst-like" appearance of idiopathic bone cavity.

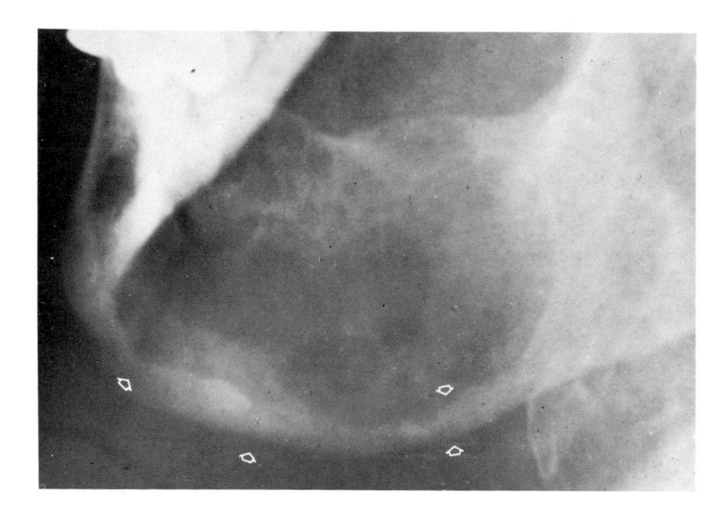

Figure 17–22. Bone destruction caused by an aggressive neoplasm with "thinning" and "notching" of cortical bone (arrows).

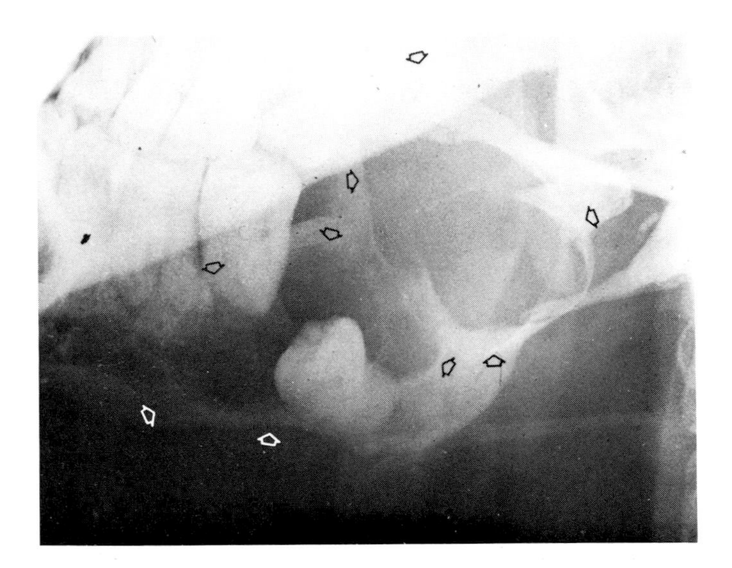

Figure 17–23. Cyst showing a multiloculated radiographic image. Lesion is divided by septa.

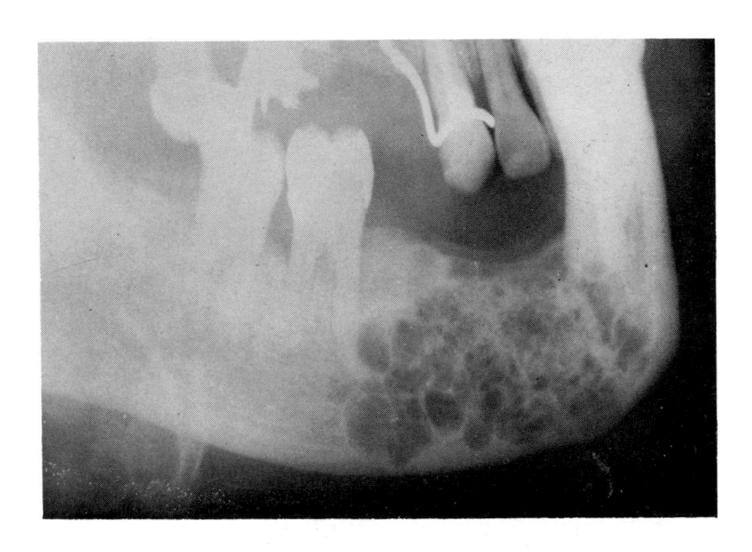

Figure 17–24. Radiograph of ameloblastoma showing a "soap-bubble" or "honeycomb" radiographic appearance. A soap bubble pattern may also appear with cherubism, hemangioma, or myxoma.

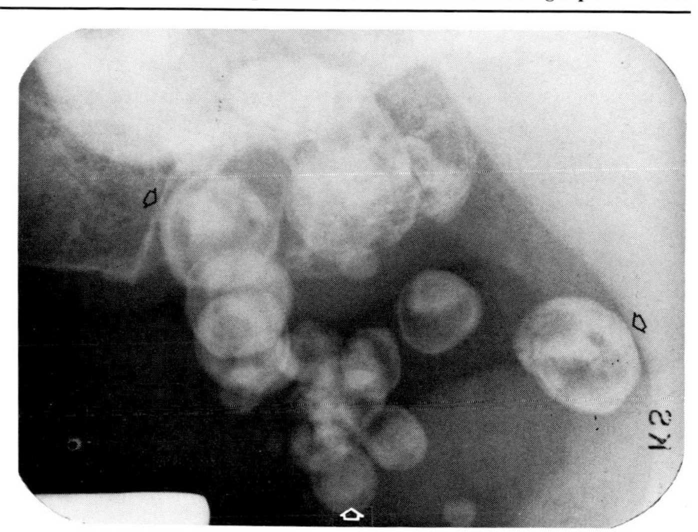

Figure 17–25. Periapical radiograph showing phleboliths appearing as laminated radiopacities within radiolucency of hemangioma.

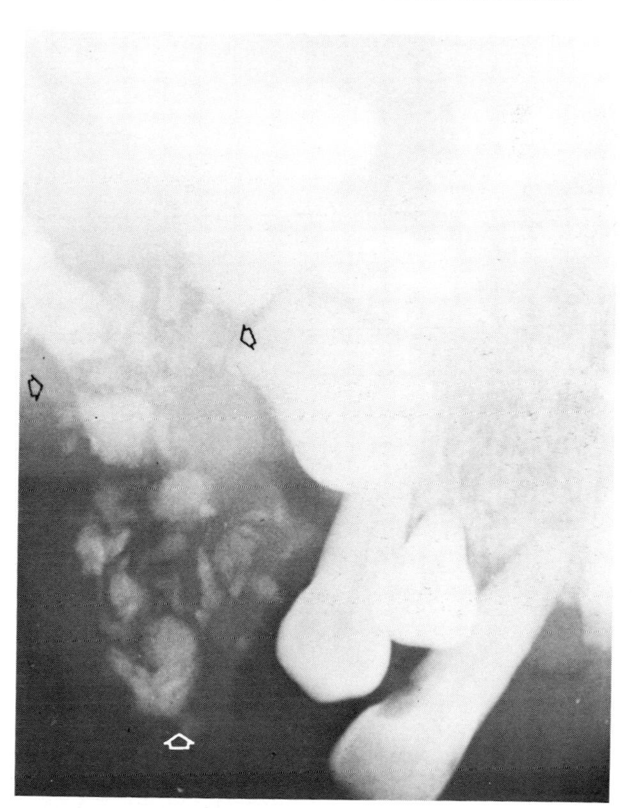

Figure 17–26. Occlusal radiograph showing indistinct amorphous calcifications within fibroma located between maxilla and cheek.

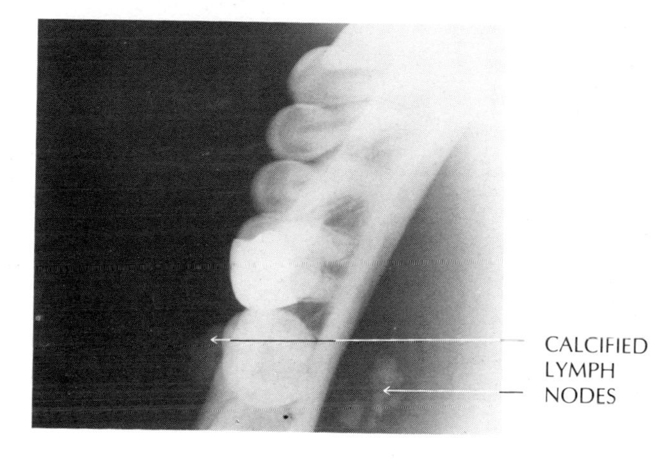

Figure 17–27. Occlusal cross section radiograph of the mandibular molar area showing buccal and lingual calcified lymph nodes.

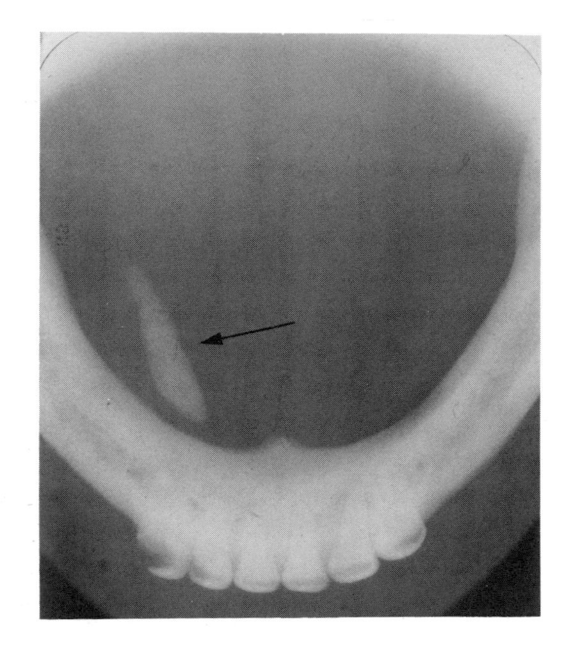

Figure 17–28. Occlusal cross section radiograph of the mandible showing an oblong calcified sialolith in Wharton's duct.

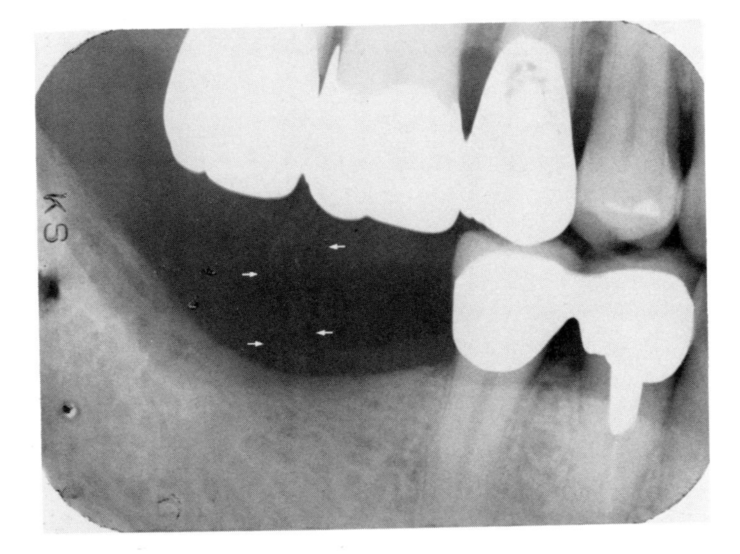

Figure 17–29. Bite-wing radiograph showing a slightly radiopaque worm-like calcification in the cheek of a patient with arteriosclerosis.

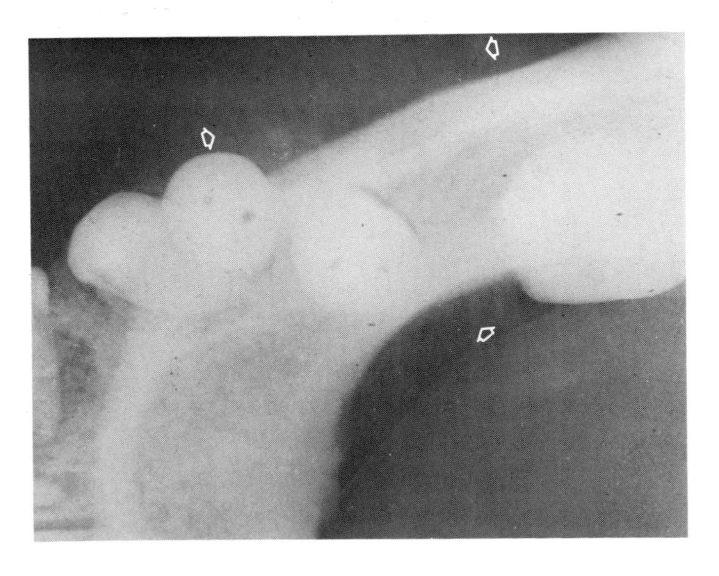

Figure 17–30. Radiograph showing "sun-ray" appearance associated with osteogenic sarcoma.

pletely destroy the cortical bone (Figure 17–22).

In some cases a radiolucent lesion may show distinct radiopaque calcifications within the radiolucency. When a well-defined radiolucency shows one or more bony septa dividing it, the lesion is said to have a multiloculated appearance (Figure 17–23).

A large number of septa can divide the lesion into many tiny compartments. This radiographic image has been referred to as a "honeycomb," "soap-bubble," or "polycystic" appearance by different writers (Figure 17–24).

A well-formed tooth attached to a well-defined radiolucency is seen in the case of a dentigerous cyst. Small teeth within a distinct radiolucency are seen in an odontoma. Small laminated radiopacities are sometimes the result of phleboliths within a radiolucent hemangioma (Figure 17–25). Indistinct amorphous radiopacities are sometimes the result of calcifications within a fibroma (Figure 17–26). Distinct localized calcifications within soft tissue are seen with calcified lymph nodes (Figure 17–27). Sialoliths appear round in the salivary glands and oval or oblong in the ducts of the glands (Figure 17–28). Slightly radiopaque worm-like calcifications in soft tissue may be shown by calcified blood vessels (Figure 17–29).

Bandlike calcifications radiating from the cortical plate of a bone are strongly suggestive of the presence of osteogenic sarcoma. The lesion is said to have a "sun-ray" appearance (Figure 17–30). Some disease processes, such as sickle cell anemia and thalassemia, may produce a widened diploe (Figure 17–31.) In the later stages of these disease processes there is destruction of the outer cortical plate of the cranium and the appearance of distinct hairlike calcifications radiating from the inner cortical plate. Such a condition produces a "hair-on-end" appearance in the radiograph (Figure 17–32).

Basic radiographic signs and the pathologic conditions usually associated with the signs are shown in Figure 17–33. The reader is reminded that the material in this chapter is presented to show the value of dental radiography in oral diagnosis and to acquaint the x-ray operator with radiographic diag-

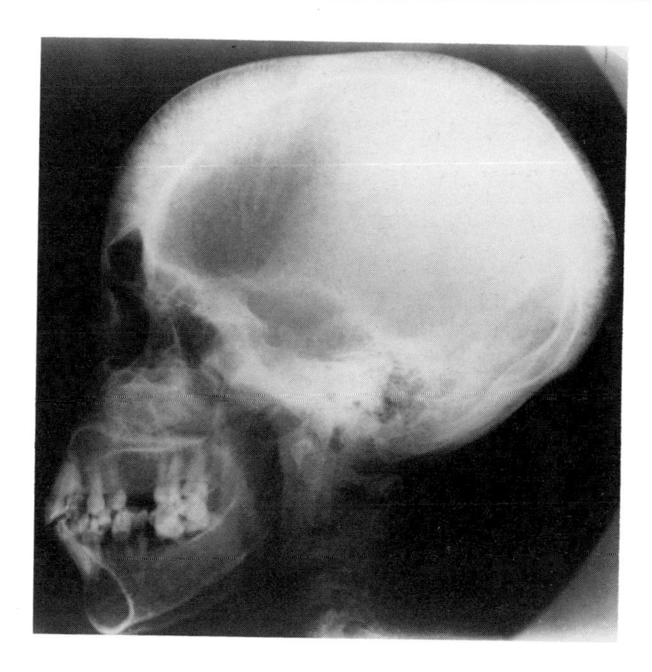

Figure 17–31. Wide diploe of the cranium and expanded mandible in a patient with thalassemia. A similar appearance is also seen with sickle cell anemia.

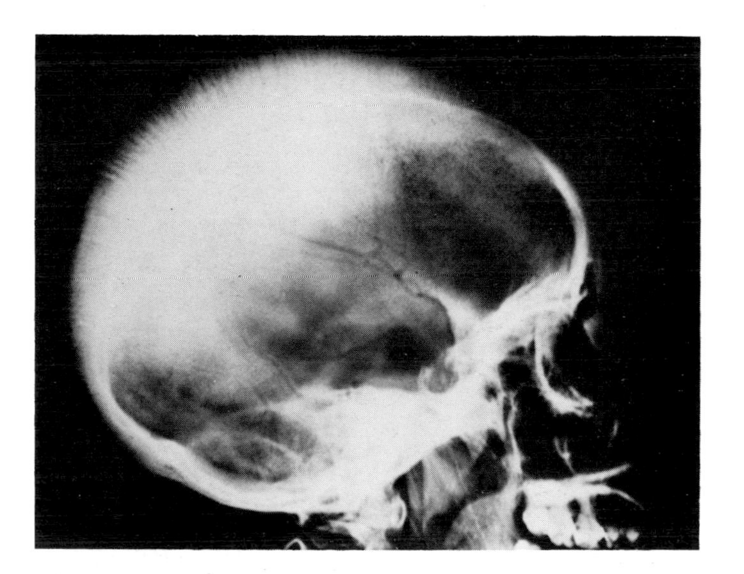

Figure 17–32. The "hair-on-end" radiographic appearance of cranium of patient with sickle cell anemia. A similar appearance is also seen with thalassemia.

nostic terms. This chapter is not intended to be a comprehensive diagnostic text. Readers involved with radiographic diagnosis should consult oral pathology texts and radiology texts written with the objective of teaching radiographic diagnosis.

RADIOLUCENT LESIONS

Single—well circumscribed
- Periapical granulomas
- Periapical scars
- Cysts
- Benign tumors
- Ameloblastoma
- Static bone cyst
- Traumatic cyst
- Non-calcified cementoma

Single—poorly circumscribed
- Abscess
- Cementoma
- Osteomyelitis
- Giant cell tumor
- Ameloblastoma
- Malignant tumors
- Bone marrow defect

Single Multilocular
- Ameloblastoma
- Dentigerous cyst
- Myxoma
- Hemangioma
- Giant cell tumor
- Aneurysmal bone cyst

Multiple
- Histiocytoses-X
- Hyperparathyroid brown tumors
- Metastatic tumors
- Multiple myeloma
- Multiple cementomas
- Multiple cysts
- Cherubism

RADIOPAQUE LESIONS

Abnormal and malpositioned teeth
Odontomas
Cementoma
Sclerosing osteitis
Garré osteomyelitis
Foreign bodies
Sialolith
Phlebolith
Rhinolith
Antrolith
Fibrous dysplasia
Tori
Bone sclerosis
Osteoma
Infantile cortical hyperostosis
Osteopetrosis

RADIOLUCENT AND RADIOPAQUE LESIONS

Cementoma
Odontomas
Odontogenic cysts
Calcifying odontogenic tumors
Ossifying fibroma
Osteoid osteoma
Sclerosing osteomyelitis
Paget's disease
Osteogenic sarcoma
Chondrosarcoma
Fibrous dysplasia
Osteoblastic metastases

LOSS OF LAMINA DURA

Hyperparathyroidism
Rickets
Fibrous dysplasia
Paget's disease
Multiple myeloma
Histiocytoses-X
Leukemia
Lymphomas
Osteoporosis
Osteomyelitis
Traumatic cyst

GROUND GLASS TRABECULAE

Hyperparathyroidism
Fibrous dysplasia
Rickets
Paget's disease

Figure 17–33. A list of pathologic conditions usually associated with basic radiographic signs.

Chapter 18

Patient Relations

The relationship between patient and dentist or office personnel is important at all times. Dental radiographic procedures are no exception to this rule. The dental radiographer, whether the dentist or an auxiliary, must not only be capable of technically making radiographs but must also be professional in appearance and attitude, be able to communicate with patients, and be capable of educating patients. In the area of the patient's education most radiography questions raised by patients can be handled by the auxiliary. However, questions relating to diagnosis and treatment are best handled by the dentist. There should be an understanding in the dental office of the types of questions that are to be answered only by the dentist. This division of functions should be kept in mind when reading the section on patient education in this chapter.

APPEARANCE AND ATTITUDE

A professional appearance should always be maintained in the presence of a patient. A clean uniform and a well-groomed appearance are important. Eating or chewing gum should not be done in a patient care situation, and attention must be given to personal hygiene such as washing one's hands before working in a patient's mouth.

The attitude of the radiographer must contain the qualities of empathy, honesty, and patience. Empathy can be defined as "the intellectual understanding of something in another person that is alien to one's self." It is most needed by the operator when the patient is a child or has a handicap such as being unable to see, hear, or speak. The operator should always exhibit a friendly attitude in facial expression and in speaking. Both politeness and firmness are often required in difficult radiographic situations; however, the procedure must be carried out with diplomacy, especially when the patient is in pain or the operator is dealing with the parent of a young child. The operator must be clinically proficient and carry out the work in an efficient manner if the patient's confidence is to be achieved. Failure to do this can result in a tense, uncooperative patient.

Honesty is the best policy. Radiography can cause the patient some discomfort in many situations, such as when tori are present, when the floor of the mouth in uncontrollably tense, or when the mouth is very small. Radiography rarely causes great pain to the patient. The patient should be informed of possible discomfort and cooperation and assistance requested. With a young patient a few tears are better than telling the child that the procedure will not be uncomfortable and then proceeding to hurt the patient. The patient's cooperation for any future dental work cannot be obtained when radiography is not done in an honest manner.

Apprehensive patients should be assessed regarding their degree of apprehension which can vary from mere concern to fear or phobia. The operator must obtain information about the characteristics and intensity of the patient's fear and set up a definite program to systematically desensitize and control the patient's fear. These patients should not be looked upon as time-wasters; they can become most enthusiastic patients when cured of irrational fears.

Patience is needed. Whenever a difficult or uncooperative patient is encountered, the operator must be ever mindful of his or her own mood. A reservoir of patience or "submissive waiting" must be present in the operator. Inability to obtain the desired radiographic results quickly should not produce an impatient attitude or loss of control in the operator. Exhibiting such behavior can only result in a more uncooperative patient. When patience is exhausted, it is best to stop radiography for a time and step out of the operatory in order to "recharge one's patience." It is often surprising how easily the difficulty is overcome when such a break is taken by both the patient and the operator.

COMMUNICATION

The patient and the operator must communicate during radiography. Communication can be accomplished by words, by signs, or by touching the patient. In any event, the information that the operator wishes the patient to know should be in a form or at a level that the patient can understand. For example, a young child may understand that "pictures of the teeth are being made by a camera," while being unable to comprehend "radiographs are being made with an x-ray machine."

The operator must be aware of the available medium of communication with some patients. Blind patients cannot see a smile; the operator's friendliness must be communicated through a gentle touch and a warm tone of voice. Likewise a deaf patient cannot hear warmth in an operator's voice; the operator must smile and be facing the patient at the same time so that the patient can see the operator's face. Consideration of a patient's needs can avoid many communication problems.

A picture is worth a thousand words; this old proverb indicates that pictures are more efficient than words. In a busy dental office it is often necessary to explain technics and answer the patient's questions in the short time available. The use of a "show and tell" method of communication is often useful in radiography. To help explain a radiograph, show a radiograph; to explain a technic, show the film and demonstrate film and machine placement. The operator may feel capable of quickly telling a patient what the patient wants to know, but often the quick explanation is not adequate. Showing while telling provides the patient with much more information and thus uses much less time.

In communication there is a transmitter and a receiver: in other words, it takes two to communicate. Radiography need not be carried out in an impersonal manner, and a normal conversational atmosphere is beneficial in relaxing the patient. However, during radiography the operator should not talk all the time. This implies periods of listening on the part of the operator. During these listening periods the operator should pay attention to the patient. If the operator must perform some task while the patient is talking, an occasional comment or question can indicate that the operator is still listening to the patient.

PATIENT EDUCATION

Many patients have questions about dental radiography. Some questions can be an-

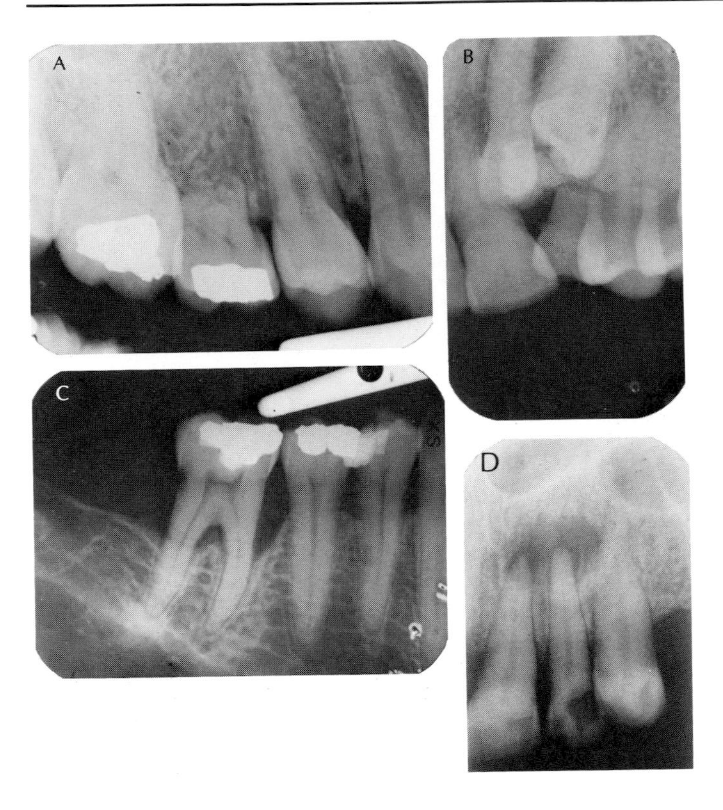

Figure 18–1. Examples of radiographs that are useful in patient education. A, Missing second bicuspid discovered at an early age resulting in the careful retention of deciduous second molar. B, Undetected development of small odontoma that prevented eruption of cuspid and lateral incisor and resulted in malocclusion. C, Great loss of supporting bone around molar. D, Asymptomatic radiolucency around the apices of the central and lateral incisors.

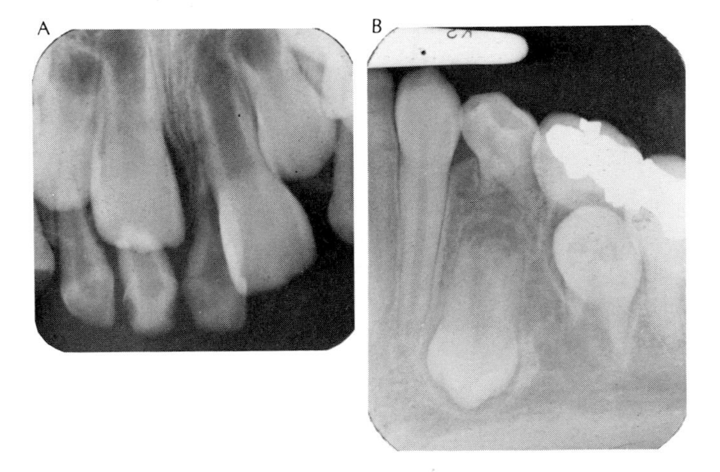

Figure 18–2. Radiographs of children: A, Abnormal resorption of palatal surface of deciduous tooth root with malpositioning of permanent successor requiring early removal of deciduous tooth to prevent possible malocclusion; B, Development of mandibular first bicuspid in inverted position.

swered by auxiliary personnel, whereas others are best handled by the dentist. This section will discuss some of the common questions asked by patients. Questions to be answered only by dentists should be established by the dentist and understood by office personnel.

Why do you need x rays?

An analysis of this question is very important. Why radiographs are needed in dentistry should be understood by all office personnel. Chapter 17 presents information on this subject. One must always remember that radiographs are made "when the benefits to the patient outweigh the possible potential hazards of x-ray exposure." In other words, *radiographs are not made for the dentist but for the benefit of the patient.* Answering this question must always emphasize this fact.

The operator must educate the patient regarding the value of radiographs. The use of an old or duplicate set of radiographs is helpful in demonstrating conditions that can be detected only in radiographs. The conditions shown to a patient should always be easy for the patient to identify and should always be easy for the operator to indicate that the type of information seen is beneficial to the care of the patient's health. Examples are radiographs of extra or missing teeth detected early when space maintenance can be anticipated, followed by radiographs of similar conditions seen later when malocclusion has occurred, due to loss of the deciduous teeth and nonreplacement of the absent permanent tooth, and when the condition was not diagnosed early from radiographs (Figure 18–1). Other easily demonstrated and understood conditions can be interproximal carious lesions, periapical radiolucencies, periodontal bone loss, and possibly a cyst or odontoma.

Why don't you examine me without x rays?

Many dental conditions produce no clinical signs or symptoms and are usually discovered only with diagnostic radiographs. When clinically undetectable conditions are present, early discovery through radiographs can cause less discomfort and cost. The x rays may show a problem that may not be discovered before it is too late to be treated.

Why do you need to x ray the baby teeth when they will soon be lost?

Radiographs show not only the condition of the deciduous teeth but also the developing permanent teeth. The retention of baby teeth until the proper time for shedding them is important to the future dental health of a child. Demonstration radiographs can show conditions such as the tipping of permanent teeth due to early loss of a deciduous tooth, a missing permanent tooth requiring extra care to protect and retain the deciduous tooth, and abnormal resorption of the deciduous tooth root with associated malpositioning of the permanent tooth requiring extraction of the deciduous tooth (Figure 18–2). Early identification and treatment of these problems can often avoid expensive orthodontic correction at a later date.

Why do you need to x ray when you are going to remove the tooth?

The simplest way for the patient to understand the need for radiographs in extraction cases is for the operator to show how the shape of a tooth's roots can influence the method of tooth extraction. Radiographs of teeth with multiple straight and curved roots clearly demonstrate when a tooth may be extracted whole and when each root must be removed independently (Figure 18–3). It is not difficult for the patient to understand that the same type and direction of force used in extracting the tooth with straight roots can easily break the tooth with curved roots. The benefit of radiography to the patient is obvious.

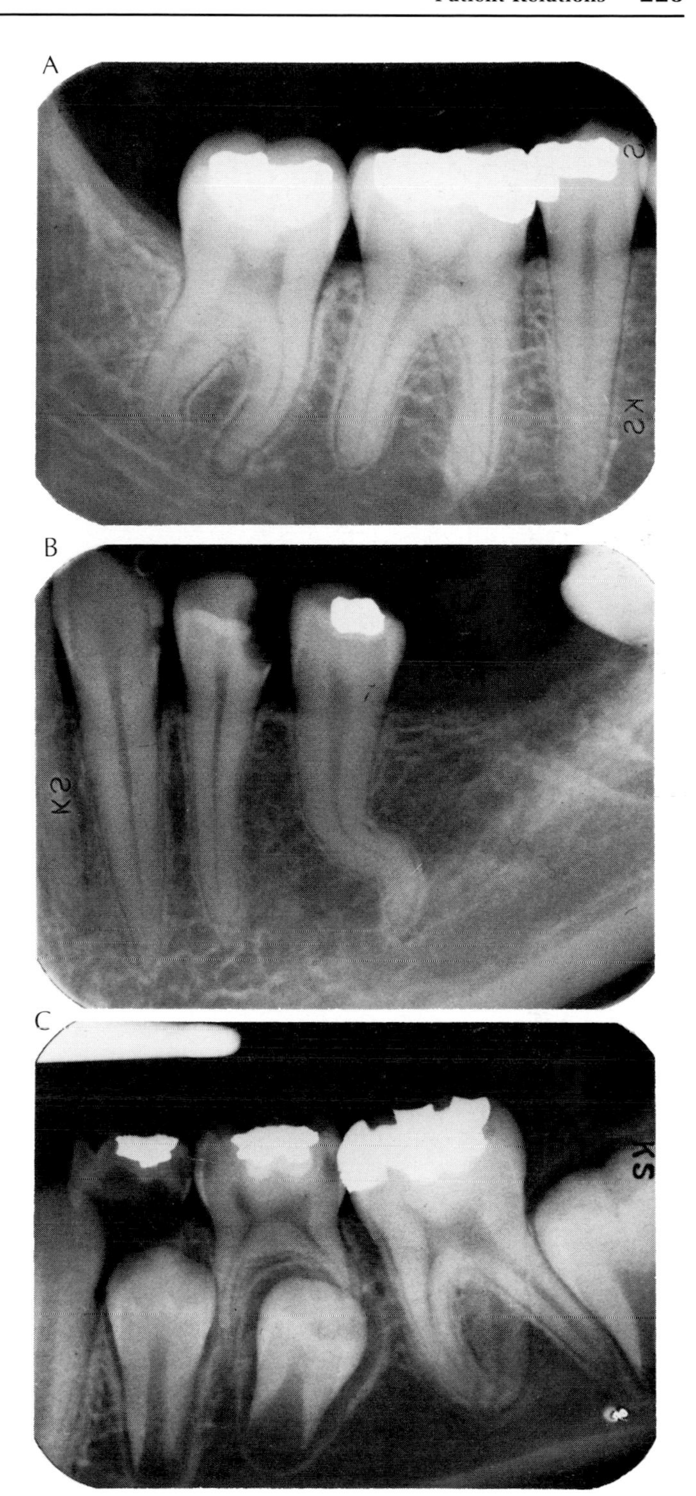

Figure 18–3. Radiographs showing root shapes. A and B, Straight roots permit simple tooth extraction and curved roots require separate removal of each root during tooth extraction or separate removal of parts of twisted root. C, Mandibular molar with three roots instead of two usually seen.

How often do you make x rays?

Everyone's dental condition is different. X rays are made only when the teeth are examined and the dentist determines that x rays are needed. There is no set time limit between x-ray examinations.

Are these x rays safe? Or, I think I am pregnant, will these x rays harm my baby?

It is not unusual for a patient to ask this type of question because many articles have been written in magazines and newspapers and many reports have been made on radio and television about the dangers of x rays. Patients are often confused about the hazards of dental x rays because of conflicting comments made by dentists and others regarding the potential biologic effects of x rays. These differences occur because there is not enough evidence to make firm conclusions about the effects of small doses of x rays.

Knowing that the benefits dental patients receive from radiographs can outweigh the possible hazard from the small doses of x rays used does not permit the operator to say that dental x rays are safe. No amount of x rays can be considered to be absolutely safe. The patient probably knows this, since most writers agree on this point. The operator should avoid making statements such as "These x rays are safe" or "Dental x rays do not harm you."

Patients asking questions about radiation safety need reassurance that radiographs of their teeth will be made in an approved manner. The operator must know the guidelines to be followed during radiography (Chapter 12). The statements of official agencies and national professional organizations can assist in calming the fears of the patient. An official of the American Dental Association has stated that "the ADA knows of not one instance of death or any serious injury resulting from a dental radiographic examination." In states where dental office radiation surveys are required, the operator can inform the patient that radiography is being carried out in an installation that is officially approved by the state.

If fast film is being used, the operator may state that the radiographs will be made with less than ⅕ the amount of x rays commonly used 20 years ago.

Pregnant patients or patients concerned about the genetic effects of dental x-rays can be informed that data collected and published by the U.S. Department of Health and Human Services indicate that when all medical x-ray films or technics are compared, there is no detectable contribution to x-ray exposure of the embryo, ovaries, or testes from skull radiography, even when the entire skull is exposed to four times the amount of x rays used in making a periapical radiograph (if the office is using fast dental films).

A discussion of relative hazards (comparing with other radiation hazards) is often useful in calming a patient's fear of the genetic effects of dental x rays. When the office uses fast films, the dental literature indicates that the genetic exposure from a complete set of intraoral radiographs is no greater than the background radiation exposure we receive from our environment each day. It is also similar to the increased radiation exposure we receive from outer space when we travel for a few hours in a jet plane, high above the clouds.

A lead apron can remove 95% of the gonadal exposure. The use of this device can further reassure the apprehensive, radiation-safety-conscious patient.

Are these big panoramic x rays more dangerous?

Panoramic radiographs expose the patient to much less radiation than a complete set of intraoral radiographs. Panoramic films use cassettes with screens and need much less radiation than periapical films to be exposed. Some writers estimate that a panoramic radiograph uses as little as one tenth the amount of radiation needed to expose a complete set of intraoral radiographs.

Why do you leave the room when you x ray my teeth?

The patient is necessarily exposed to x rays on occasional office visits and receives diagnostic benefits from the radiographs. The operator is repeatedly exposed to x rays every day and receives no diagnostic benefits from the radiographs that are made. Patients can be told that even though the scatter radiation received by the operator while standing away from the patient is small, it is entirely unnecessary to be receiving even these small amounts of x rays, and it is good radiation hygiene practice to avoid repeated doses of x rays even when the doses are small.

How do you measure x rays?

The radiation reaching each exposed square centimeter of the skin is measured in roentgen units. A roentgen is a small amount of energy (one electrostatic unit) deposited in a cubic centimeter of air. A similar small amount of energy deposited in a gram of tissue is called a RAD. The total amount of energy a person receives during the making of a radiograph is measured by adding the rads received by each exposed gram of tissue or multiplying the number of grams of tissue by the average rads. The result is expressed in terms of gram-rads.

How much radiation will I get from these x rays?

When a periapical radiograph is made, the x rays expose a small skin area. A federal government survey has shown that the average exposure is 330 milliroentgens. This is only a fraction of a roentgen and only a small part of the head receives this radiation. It takes hundreds of roentgens to cause the skin to become temporarily red and thousands of roentgens to cause visible permanent damage. When radiographs are made of other areas of the mouth the radiation exposure is not increased by adding the individual exposures since other skin areas are being exposed. They are only added when the same skin area is exposed again. Similarly an individual gram of tissue receives much less than the total rad dose. The amount of x-ray energy (measured in gram-rads) is added for individual radiographs but the energy is spread out over a larger amount of tissue when radiographs are made of different areas.

How often will I need x rays?

There is no fixed time interval to have x rays made. The dentist orders x rays according to the diagnostic needs of each patient. X rays are ordered when the anticipated information from radiographs outweighs any presumed risk of a harmful effect to the patient. Each patient's case is different and is evaluated separately.

Why do you use a lead apron?

Protection of the gonadal area from x rays is of special concern since any harmful effects are passed on to future generations. When dental radiographs are made the radiation reaching the gonads is from scattered x rays. The dose is small and is similar to what we are exposed to every day outside or in our homes. The risk of harm is obviously small and may be non-existent. In most states a lead apron is recommended but not required. It is used to give additional protection to these special tissues and make even this small gonadal exposure unnecessary.

Chapter 19

Infection Control

Radiographic examinations are often the first procedures conducted in the dental office. Knowledge of transmissible pathogenic organisms may or may not be known at this time. Infection control procedures should be examined and a written policy of precautions established for dental radiography to reduce the risk to the operator and other patients in the office. The Center for Disease Control and the American Dental Association have published recommended guidelines for infection control for all aspects of dentistry.* These guidelines are being established as the "standard of care" in dentistry and therefore carry both legal and ethical significance.

A dental radiographer is obligated to caring for other people. In becoming health care professionals, persons commit themselves to care for sick patients regardless of their disease. While the risks cannot be ignored, radiographers should not avoid treating a patient solely because the patient is infected.

MICROORGANISMS AND INFECTION

Microbiology is the study of microscopic forms of life. Three basic types of microscopic life exist; they are bacteria, virus, and fungi. Microorganisms multiply rapidly to form large colonies which may be seen without the aid of a microscope (Figure 19–1). Many varieties of microorganisms co-existing together make up the normal flora or microbiologic spectra of humans. The term pathogen is given to a microorganism which is known to cause disease. Some microorganisms are harmful and cause diseases in man (Figure 19–2). Vaccines have been developed for protection against some of these diseases.

An understanding of the terminology related to infection control is important.

*CDC, Current Trends: Recommended Infection-Control Practices for Dentistry. M.M.W.R., *35*:237–242, 1986. ADA Council on Dental Therapeutics: Guidelines for infection control in the dental office and the commercial laboratory. J.A.D.A., *110*:969–972, 1985.

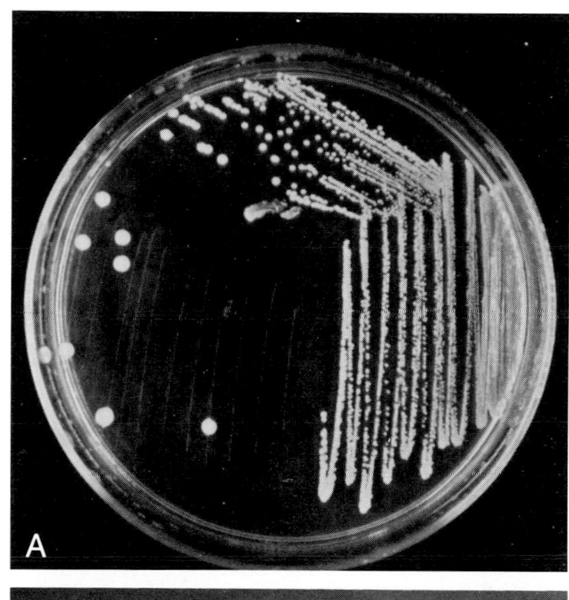

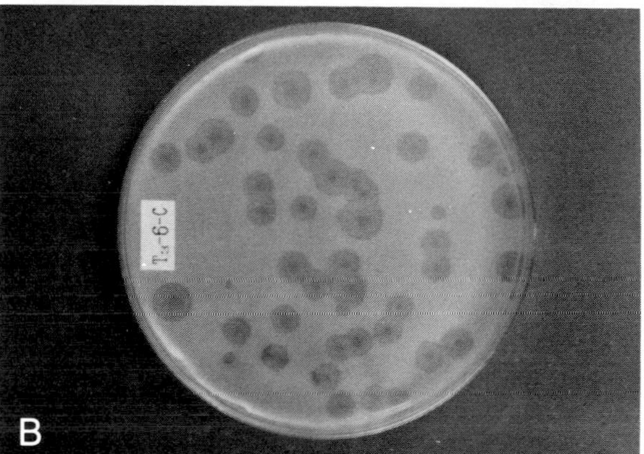

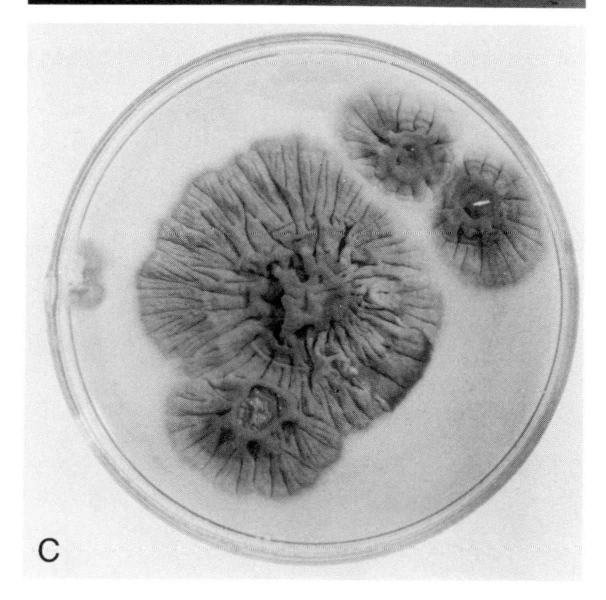

Figure 19–1. A, Bacterial colonies growing in a petri dish. B, Viral "plaques" or clear zones showing areas of virus activity. C, Fungal colonies growing in a petri dish.

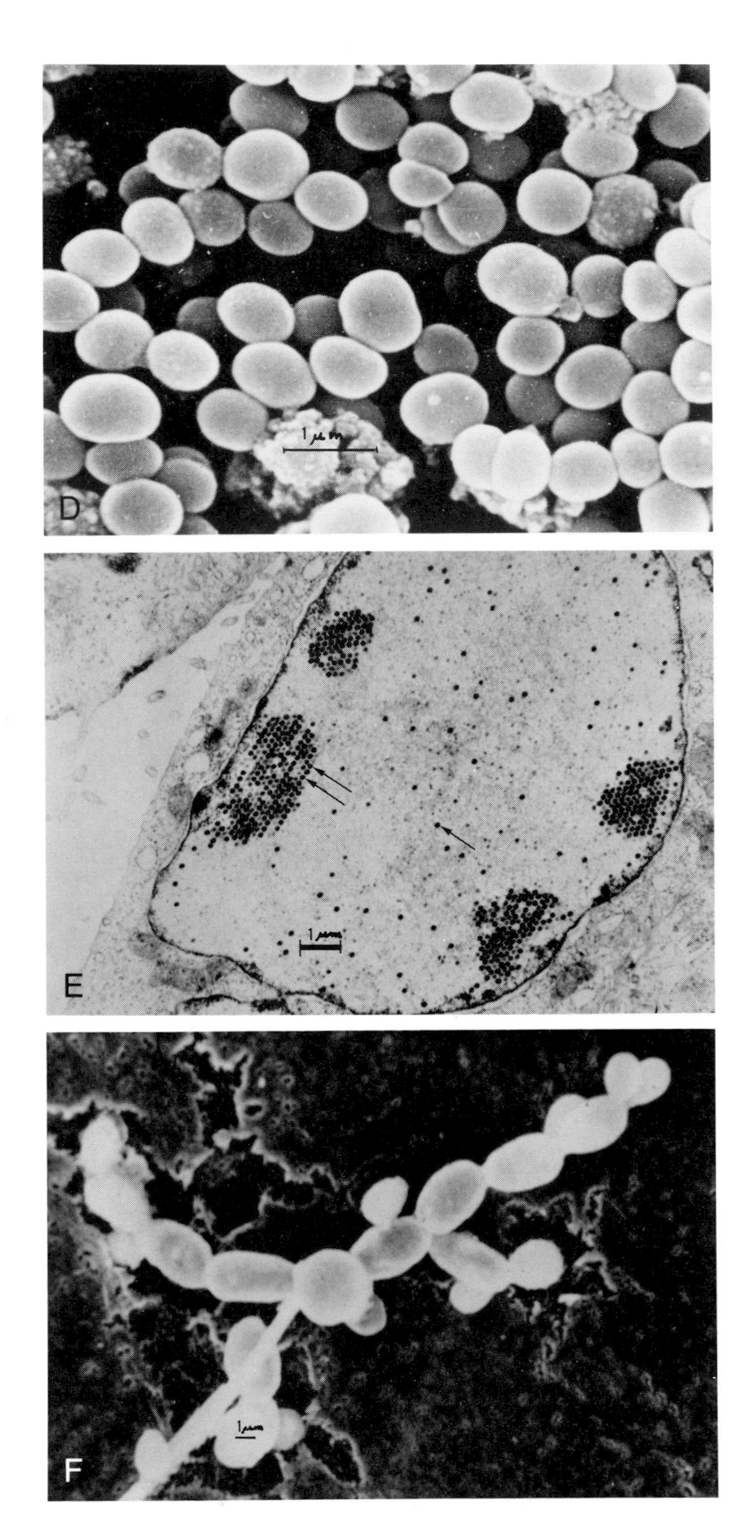

Figure 19–1 ***Continued.*** D, Scanning electron microscope photograph of bacteria. E, Virus particles seen within the nucleus of an epithelial cell. F, Scanning electron microscope photograph of the fungus Candida albicans. (Photographs courtesy of Koichi Nakashima, DDS, PhD)

Microorganism	Disease	Vaccine
Bacteria		
Streptococcus mutans	Dental caries	no
Bacteroides gingivalis	Periodontal disease	no
Streptococcus pneumoniae	Pneumonia	yes
Mycobacterium tuberculosis	Tuberculosis	no
Neisseria gonorrhoeae	Venereal gonorrhea	no
Staphylococcus aureus	Pus producing infections	no
Treponema pallidum	Syphilis	no
Virus		
Epstein-Barr	Infectious mononucleosis	no
Hepatitis A	Liver infection	no
Hepatitis B	Eventual liver carcinoma	yes
Herpes simplex	"Fever" blisters	no
Herpes simplex-2	Venereal herpes	no
Human immunodeficiency	AIDS	no
Rubeola—Rubella	Measles	yes
Mumps virus	Mumps	yes
Influenza	Flu—Common cold	yes
Fungus		
Candida albicans	Candidiasis—oral thrush	no
Tricophyton mentagrophytes	Athlete's foot	no
Microsporum audouini	Ringworm	no

Figure 19–2. Some microorganisms and the diseases they cause in man.

"Asepsis" means no sepsis or absence of pathogens in living tissues. The term is sometimes applied to the *prevention* of infection of tissues by pathogenic microorganisms. "Sterilization" is the total absence of all microbiologic life forms including spores. Because spores are often the most difficult form to destroy, they are used as a standard by which the completeness of a sterilization procedure is judged. Spore strips on instrument packaging before sterilization will change color when conditions of sterilization have been met (Figure 19–3). "Cold Sterilization" is a misused term which is usually applied to procedures resulting in disinfection, not sterilization. "Disinfection" refers to the absence of pathogenic microbiologic life forms, but not necessarily spores. Microorganisms not causing disease may still be present. Disinfecting agents are usually employed on instruments and surfaces, but are too toxic for living tissues. "Antiseptics" are agents used on human tissues and are bacteriostatic or bactericidal; they are most commonly used for handwashing procedures and wound cleansing. "Sanitation" describes the reduction of microorganisms to levels of concentration considered to be safe. Public health departments often inspect restaurants

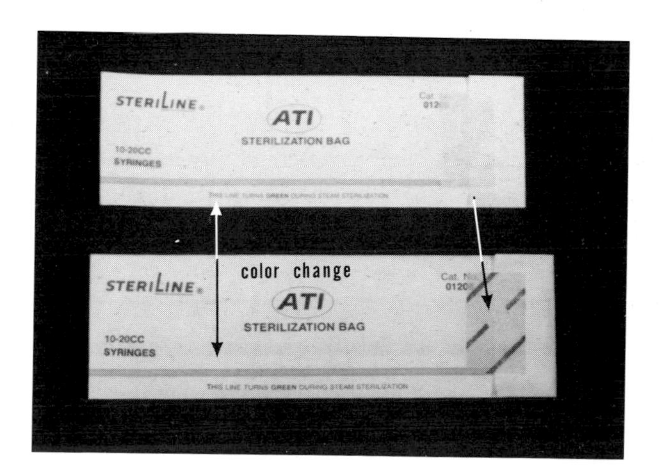

Figure 19–3. Instrument sterilization bags with spore strips and spore tape. Above: Before sterilization, spore strip along bottom of the bag is pink and spore tape sealing package is uniform tan. Below: After sterilization, spore strip has changed to green, and spore tape shows dark brown diagonal lines when conditions of sterilization have been met.

and food processing facilities for adequacy of sanitation.

To establish a relative degree of risk associated with transmission of infection, vectors, or transmission items or modes may be categorized as critical, semi-critical or noncritical. Critical items are those which penetrate soft tissue and bone and must be sterile. Semi-critical items are those which contact intact mucous membranes. It is desirable that these items be sterile, but high-level disinfection is usually acceptable. Noncritical items are those which contact the patient's intact skin but are not involved with treatment procedures. Examples are charts, the dental chair and other surfaces. For noncritical items, a cleansing wipe with disinfectant should achieve adequate sanitation.

MICROORGANISM CONTROL METHODS

Sterilization, disinfection, and preservation procedures are designed to eliminate, prevent, or frustrate the growth of microorganisms. Infection control is the prevention and reduction of disease-causing microorganisms to safe levels. The axiom that an ounce of prevention is worth a pound of cure holds true for infection control procedures. It is easier and less time-consuming to prevent microorganism contamination than to clean contaminated objects.

Many objects in the dental office are potential sources of infection or have the potential to transmit microorganisms to another location. These objects are called vectors and routes of transmission by such objects may be traced. Some vectors are: saliva, blood, nasal and respiratory secretions, dust, hands, hair, clothing, patient charts, films, x-ray machines, countertops, dental instruments, and the dental chair. Cross-contamination occurs when vectors transmit pathogenic organisms from one patient to another or to dental personnel. The potential for cross-contamination is greatly reduced if infection control procedures are established and carefully followed.

Barriers to infectious microorganisms may be employed to prevent contact and contamination with these organisms. Barrier techniques include gloves, masks, eye protection, and surface covers (Figure 19–4). If contamination has occurred, steps must be taken to

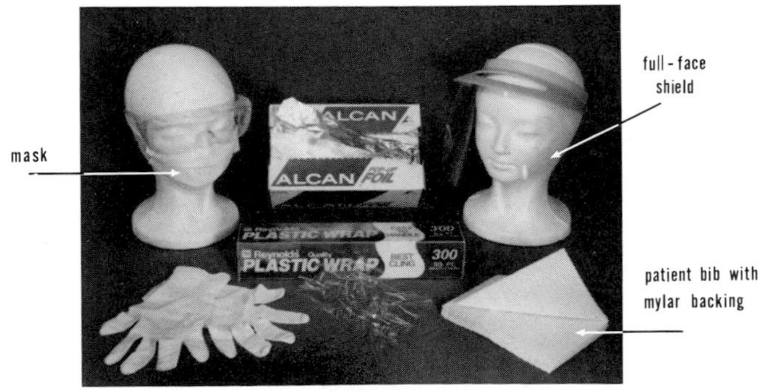

Figure 19–4. Some barriers useful for infection control in dental radiography.

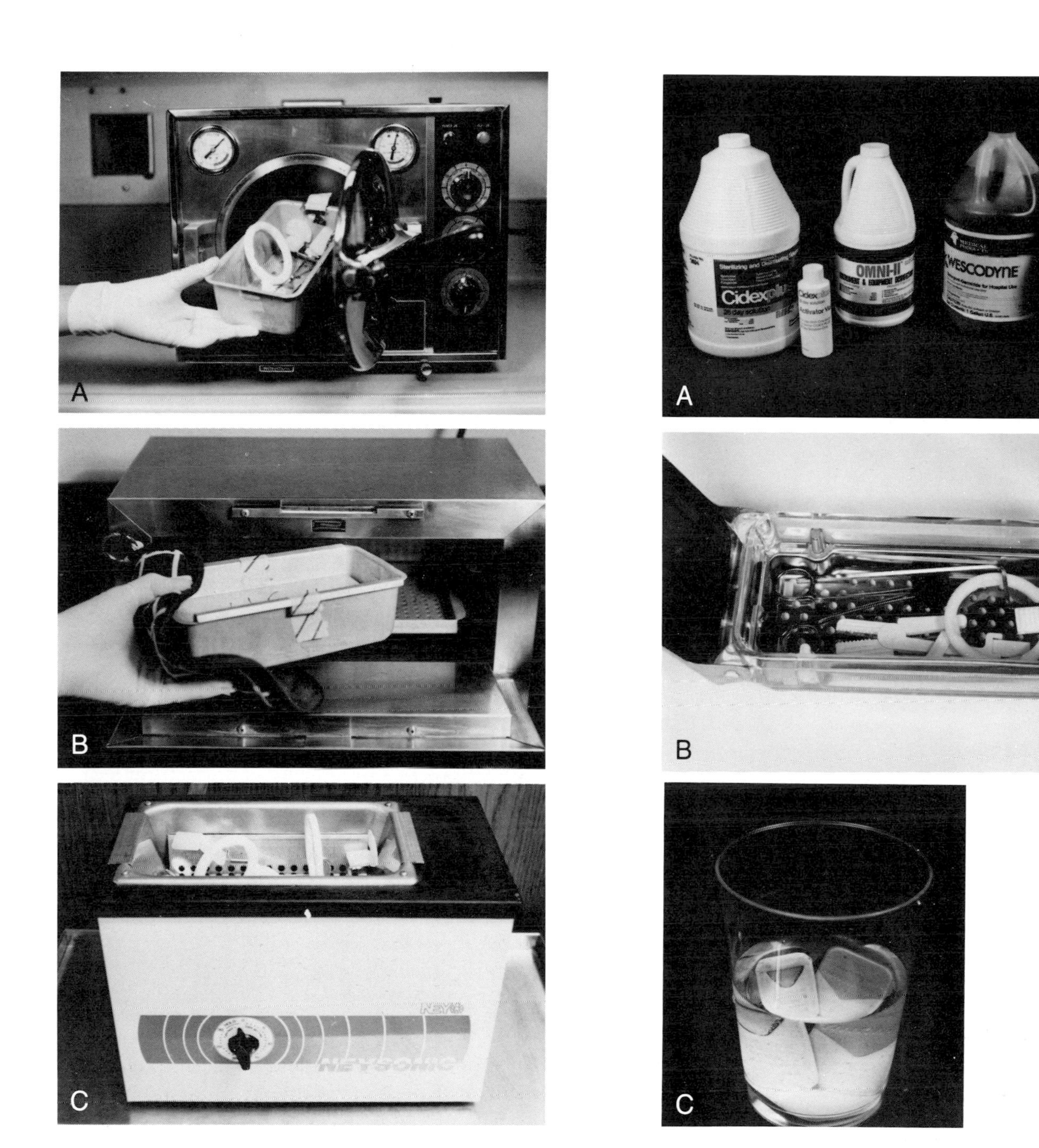

Figure 19–5. Some physical methods of sterilization. A, Steam autoclave. B, Dry heat oven. C, Ultrasonic bath for instrument preparation.

Figure 19–6. Some chemical methods of disinfection/sterilization. A, Assorted chemical agents. B, Glass soaking tray filled with chemical agent and radiographic film holders. C, X-ray film immersed in disinfecting solution.

Item	*Management*
Patient	Review medical history
Working surfaces	
Counter tops	Barrier protect or disinfect
Dental chair	
Instruments	
Films	Barrier, disinfect/sterilize, or careful handling
Film-holders	Sterilization preferred or disinfect
Cotton rolls	Dispose with other contaminated waste
Operator's hands	Wash before and after procedure, use exam gloves
X-ray tubehead	Barriers or disinfect
X-ray control panel	Barrier preferred or disinfect
Darkroom	
Entrance	Enter with uncontaminated hands
Counter tops	Barrier or disinfect
Automatic processor	Feed only uncontaminated films with clean hands
Solutions	Maintain uncontaminated films
Paper waste	Dispose contaminated waste carefully

Figure 19–7. Items of infection control significance in dental radiography.

remove the infectious agent to prevent further transmission.

Methods by which sterilization and disinfection are achieved may be classified into physical and chemical methods. The most common physical methods of sterilization used in dentistry involve heat in the form of steam or dry heat. The steam autoclave uses moist heat under pressure and provides sterile conditions in less time than dry heat alone. Less common physical methods of microbial elimination include microwave and ultraviolet radiations. Ultrasonic vibration is often a preparatory step used in conjunction with physical sterilization methods to dislodge debris from instrument surfaces. Some equipment used for physical methods of sterilization is shown in Figure 19–5.

Many chemical disinfectants and sterilants are accepted for use by the American Dental Association.* In addition, ethylene oxide gas is used in some autoclaves for the purpose of sterilizing porous materials and materials that would otherwise melt or burn under normal steam autoclave conditions. The concentration, dilution, length of contact time, temperature, and freshness of any chemical agent are all factors in determining the effectiveness of the agent to inhibit growth or destroy microorganisms. Office personnel should be familiar with each chemical agent used for infection control and the manufacturer's directions for its use. Improper use of chemical agents gives a false sense of security that microorganisms are under control. Figure 19–6 shows some chemical agents and their application in dental radiology.

INFECTION CONTROL IN RADIOGRAPHY

Radiography presents some unique opportunities for cross-contamination and items of infection control significance must be identified and assessed (Figure 19–7). Every patient may be considered a potential source of pathogenic microorganisms until proven otherwise. The patient's complete medical history must be reviewed for past infectious disease, current symptoms and risk factors

*ADA Council on Dental Therapeutics: Guide to chemical agents for disinfection and/or sterilization. JADA, *116*:244, 1988.

associated with infectious disease. The overall risk of treating a particular patient must be identified and necessary precautions established before radiography. If a medical history is not available or is suspected of being inaccurate, the case should be treated as if the patient is in the high-risk category. Some authorities advocate treating all patients as high-risk.

Standard dental radiographic procedures do not require the use of any vectors in the critical category. That is, no instruments penetrate soft tissue or bone. Semi-critical vectors or instruments that come in contact with the intact mucous membrane of the oral cavity during dental radiography include x-ray films, film holding devices, cotton rolls, and the hands of the operator. Radiographic working surfaces are potential vectors for transmission of microorganisms. Working surfaces are non-critical items and include the patient's chart, dental chair, lead apron, cone (PID), tubehead, control panel, exposure switch, and counter top surfaces. These non-critical items may be considered semi-critical if they come in contact with saliva.

Levels of disinfection should be achieved for working surfaces or appropriate barrier protection provided. The patient's chart is best left untouched and out of reach during operator-patient contact. Chart entries can be made when radiography is completed and the operator's hands thoroughly washed. The dental chair may be disinfected with appropriate solutions giving particular care to those surfaces contacted by the patient's skin.

X-ray film and film holder manipulation within the mouth frequently stimulates salivary secretions. In some patients salivary flow is quite copious. Care must be taken when removing the exposed film from the mouth or saliva may be deposited on the patient's chin or the lead apron. The lead apron should be thoroughly disinfected after each use. As an added precaution, the patient may wear a mylar-backed bib over the lead apron during radiography; this is especially advised for young children who are particularly prone to drool. Salivary contamination can also occur on all parts of the x-ray machine and control panel which are handled during the normal course of positioning the tubehead and selecting exposure factors.

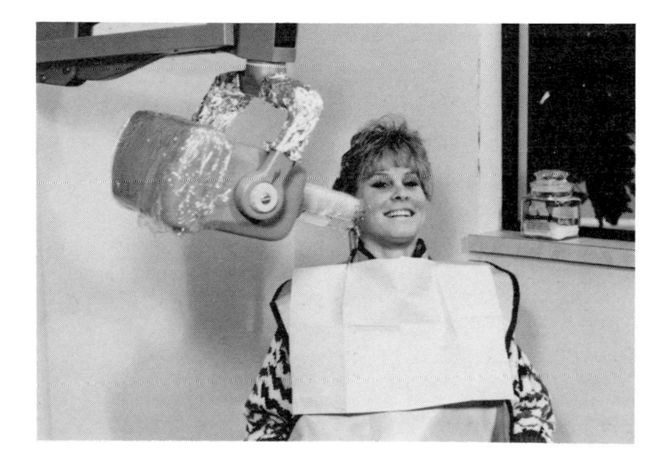

Figure 19–8. Radiographic operatory with barrier protection.

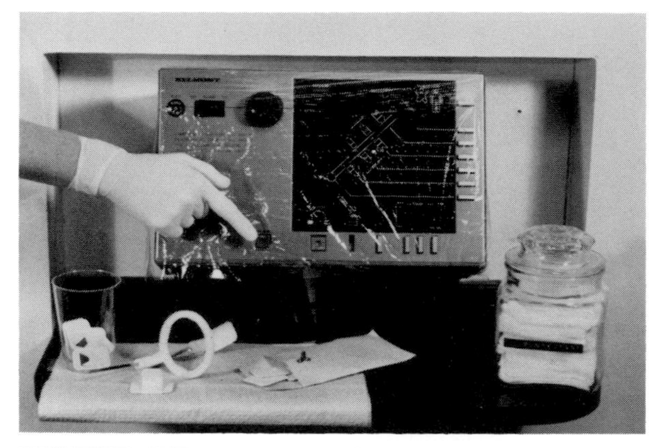

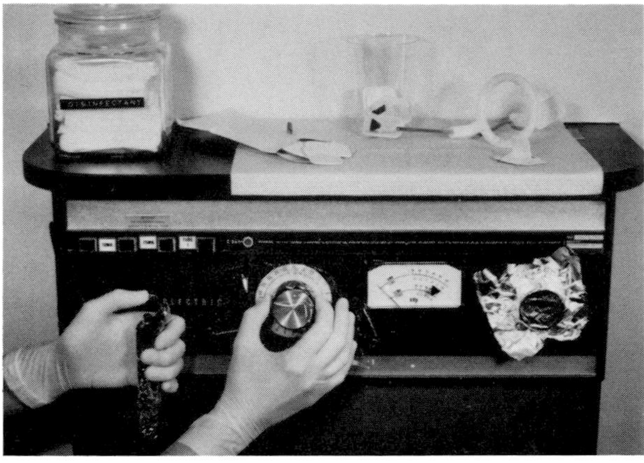

Figure 19–9. Barrier protection of x-ray machine control panel. Above: Push-button control panel with plastic wrap protection and working surface barrier with mylar-backed patient bib. Below: Conventional control panel with knurled knobs and exposure switch barriers.

The best way to reduce microorganism transfer is to touch as few surfaces and controls as is absolutely necessary. Those surfaces which must be handled may be covered with a barrier of clinging plastic-wrap prior to radiography or should be cleansed thoroughly with a disinfectant after radiography is completed. Figure 19–8 shows the use of plastic-wrap barrier protection for the cone, tubehead and yoke of the x-ray machine. The control panel and exposure switch may also be protected in the same fashion with minimum effort (Figure 19–9). A barrier is the preferred method for the machine control panel since electrical connections and irregular surfaces do not lend themselves to thorough saturation with liquid disinfectants. Counter tops and other surfaces where films, film-holding instruments, and supplies are laid should be covered with a mylar-backed patient bib or cleansed by wiping with a liquid disinfectant.

The hands of the operator are usually protected by washing with antimicrobial soap and barrier protection with latex or vinyl examination gloves. Once the gloves come into contact with the patient, care should be exercised not to touch the walls of the room (especially when exiting the room), the sill of the observation window, or the operator's own face. The operator's face is most important since the mucous membranes of the eyes, nose, and mouth can be ready receptors of cross-contaminating microorganisms.

Film, film holders, cotton rolls, and other supplies should be set out on the counter top or working surface prior to contact with the patient. If supplies dispensers or cabinet doors must be opened and closed with saliva-contaminated hands during the course of the procedure, then each surface touched should be disinfected. By planning in advance, radiography will be conducted more efficiently and the time consumed unnecessarily disinfecting surfaces will be saved.

Film holding devices may be routinely sterilized with other dental instruments in the autoclave or other physical method of sterilization. Some plastics, used for biteblocks, etc., will not withstand the high temperature required for sterilization. Disposable biteblocks of styrofoam are useful and are easily discarded with other contaminated waste after radiography.

Intraoral dental x-ray films, as vectors of transmission, present one of the greatest challenges for infection control in dental radiography. They must be handled both in the operatory and in the darkroom, and also transported from one area to the other. In addition, pathogens may be physically spread from the film packet, to the film, to the feed slots of automatic processors, or to the developing solutions. The developer and fixer have not been proven to act as sterilants as some people have assumed. There are four ways to prevent film packet transmission of microorganisms into and out of the darkroom. These are sterilization of exposed film packets, disinfection of exposed film packets, barrier protection of film packets, and controlled handling of film packets. Each method has limitations as well as advantages.

Sterilization or disinfection of an exposed film packet prior to darkroom handling is time consuming and difficult to accomplish without damage to the film emulsion and latent image. Ethylene oxide gas sterilization may be used if the diagnostician can wait 24 to 48 hours before film processing and has access to the expensive equipment. This procedure may be considered in large institutions for patients of known high-risk. Other physical forms of sterilization, such as autoclaving and dry heat, results in overall film blackening and renders the film undiagnostic.

Disinfection of intraoral film packets by chemical methods can be successfully employed if the film packet is tightly sealed and the time immersed in the solution is short. Exposed intraoral films may be dropped into a disposable paper cup of dilute (1:10) chlorine bleach. Ten minutes must elapse before the film is removed for processing. For a complete-mouth series, a procedure sequence is suggested. Expose one-half of the series, deposit the films in a cup with the bleach solution, expose the second half of the series, and deposit these films in a second cup of disinfectant. By the time the second half of the series is completed, all films in the first cup will have been immersed in the disinfectant for the necessary length of time and may now be developed. The second cup of films may then be developed, having been immersed for the necessary length of time during development of the first half of the

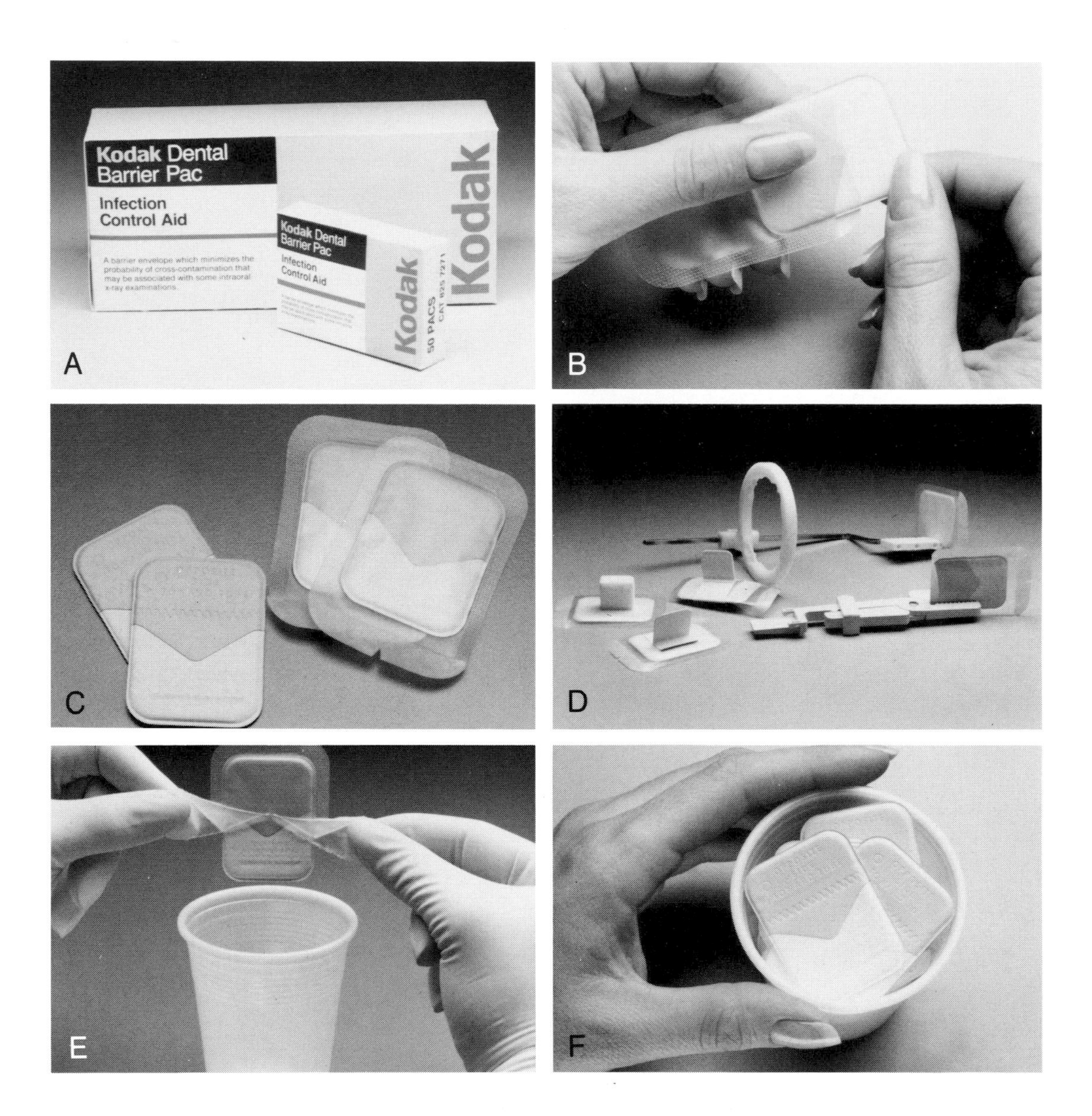

Figure 19–10. Commercial barrier envelope for dental film. A, Packaging of Kodak barrier envelope. B, Insertion of film into envelope. C, Protected and unprotected film. D, Bitewing and periapical applications of protected film. E, Film packet removal from envelope without contamination. F, Uncontaminated film ready for processing. (Photographs courtesy of Eastman Kodak Co., Rochester, New York)

film series. This procedure eliminates any objectionable delays in obtaining diagnostic radiographs and permits disinfection.

Barrier protection for film packets prior to placement in the mouth may be a suitable alternative to disinfecting or sterilizing contaminated film packets. One method is using a latex finger cot over a film packet which is then tied in a knot. After use, the barrier is removed by cutting the knot and removing the packet. A barrier envelope for film packets is commercially available (Figure 19–10). The film is inserted into the envelope and sealed by means of an adhesive strip. After intraoral use, the polypropylene envelope material is easily torn, allowing the film packet to drop untouched and uncontaminated into a clean receptacle. The film barrier technic may not be practical when large numbers of intraoral film need to be exposed. However, for single periapical exposures and bitewing series, the barrier technic appears to be a reasonable infection control system.

Careful handling is mandatory for contaminated film packets. Conscious effort is required to remember what may and may not be touched and which areas in the darkroom are and are not contaminated. Recommended procedures have been developed and instructions are to remove gloves or wash gloved hands before entering the darkroom or daylight loading box of automatic processors; place films onto a designated work surface covered with an impenetrable barrier or clean the work surface when film processing is complete with a disinfecting solution; open all film packets while being careful to touch only the wrapping materials and not the film itself; desposit film on a clean working surface; dispose all contaminated trash and used surface barriers (or disinfect); remove gloves and/or wash hands if a sink is available in the darkroom; feed the clean films with clean hands into the automatic processor or attach films to clips of manual processing racks.

Not every method is practical in every office. A variety of infection control methods useful for dental radiography have been presented so that the operator may determine what methods can work for their specific set of circumstances. A written office policy for infection control should be established. Policies, when followed, can reduce the risk of

Infection Control Checklist for Dental Radiography

I. Medical History Review
   [ ] Average risk?
   [ ] Potential high risk?
   [ ] Confirmed high risk? or unknown

II. Operatory Preparation
   [ ] Provide appropriate surfaces with barrier protection
   [ ] Set out all anticipated supplies
   [ ] Seat patient
   [ ] Wash hands thoroughly with an anti-microbial soap
   [ ] Use disposable latex or vinyl exam gloves

III. Procedural Precautions
   [ ] Handle only covered surfaces, film and patient during exposure procedures
   [ ] Place exposed films in paper cup or other disposable receptacle.

IV. Post Examination
   [ ] Wash hands prior to entering darkroom or daylight loader if sterilization, disinfection or barrier protection of film packets is not used.
   [ ] Observe "clean" handling techniques during processing.
   [ ] Dispose all contaminated barriers in examination room and/or disinfect.

Figure 19–11. Infection control checklist for dental radiography.

infection to the operator and patient. Initially it may be more time consuming to follow strict infection control protocols, but once new habits are developed, the cost of time will be insignificant. It does not take any more time to cover a control panel or working surface in advance than it does to wipe with disinfectant after radiography and the protection afforded by a barrier is more complete than attempts to properly disinfect crevices and knurled knobs found on control panels. Figure 19–11 is a checklist of important principles to incorporate into an infection control policy for dental radiography. Because no aerosol spray from a rotating bur or blood elements are encountered during normal radiographic practices these procedures are relatively easy to accomplish and provide good infection control.

Chapter 20

Quality Control in the Dental Office

In recent years standards of equipment performance for x-ray machines have been developed by federal agencies. The development of recommendations for a quality assurance program is presently under study. Radiation safety is the responsibility of the dentist or owner of the x-ray equipment. A written ionizing radiation policy should be developed for any x-ray installation. In large clinics the policy should include guidelines for ordering or prescribing radiographs. Dental offices should monitor radiographic procedures to document that x-radiation is being used properly. This implies that the x-ray machine, darkroom, and operator efficiencies should be periodically tested for quality assurance. Quality assurance can be defined as a series of tests performed to determine whether x-ray machines, processing procedures and film exposure technics are functioning properly. When a quality assurance program is established, it is necessary to maintain adequate records. Charts or logs must be kept to indicate the tests and the dates they are carried out and the results of the tests. These records can help in determining if corrective action is needed to maintain high quality radiography. Much testing equipment has been developed for medical radiography; however, low cost equipment suitable for individual dental offices is not yet available. In the absence of legally required tests, this chapter presents simple and inexpensive tests that can identify some dental radiography problems and can be carried out in the dental office.

THE TEST OBJECT

Most tests of a dental radiographic installation require exposing and processing dental films. A phantom object instead of a patient is used in these tests. While phantoms made from teeth, bone, and a variety of soft tissue substitutes can be used, it is preferable to use an object that provides sharply delineated areas and equally graded exposure lev-

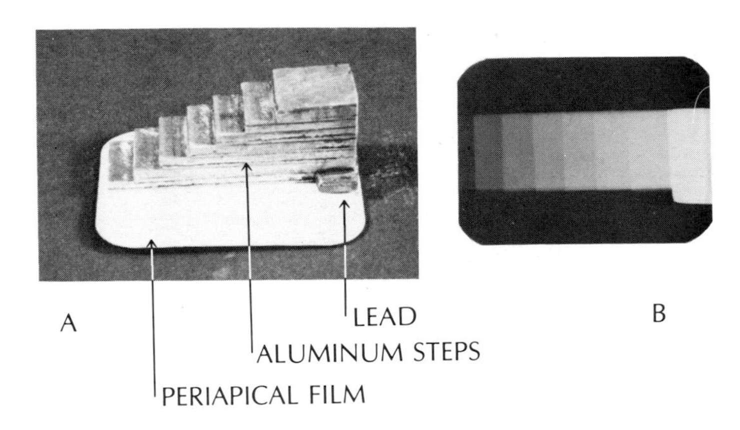

Figure 20–1. A, Aluminum step wedge of seven steps, made by gluing together 2-mm thick steps and piece of 2-mm thick lead placed upon intraoral periapical film. B, Radiograph of step wedge. Any exposure of area under lead is due to film fog.

els in the film. Such an object is the step wedge. A step wedge consists of uniformly different thicknesses of an x-ray absorbing material, usually aluminum. One-millimeter thick aluminum, such as is found in some pie pans, can be used to make a small wedge of 7 steps that are 2 mm, 4 mm, 6 mm, 8 mm, 10 mm, 12 mm, and 14 mm thick. These thicknesses produce similar amounts of x-ray absorption to the teeth and bones of the jaws. When the wedge is radiographed, the different steps absorb different amounts of x rays from the beam and thus different film densities appear in the radiograph (Figure 20–1). It is beneficial to have a small part of the wedge constructed of a minimum of 1 mm thick lead. The lead should be placed in contact with the film and thus cast its shadow on the film to produce an unexposed area in the radiograph; this area permits the operator to view the fog that is inherent in the film. Changes in radiographic density and contrast are much more easily seen in a step wedge image than in the images of teeth and bone.

DARKROOM QUALITY CONTROL

The application of quality assurance tests to film processing can greatly assist the dentist in obtaining consistently high quality radiographs, low patient exposure levels, and low operating costs.

Correct functioning of a darkroom depends upon proper light tightness of the room, proper safe lighting, proper strength of the processing solutions, and proper processing procedures being used by the operator. Testing of the darkroom should be done independently of x-ray machine testing, since the production of a processed film with poor density or contrast may be due to a machine malfunction and not to film processing failure.

Darkroom Light Safety

Film light-safe conditions can be checked with the "coin test." With all lights off in the darkroom, unwrap a dental film and place it on the workbench. Place a small coin (penny or dime) on top of the film (Figure 20–2A). Leave the film in position for 5 minutes or as long as you might have an unwrapped film in the darkroom during film processing. Re-

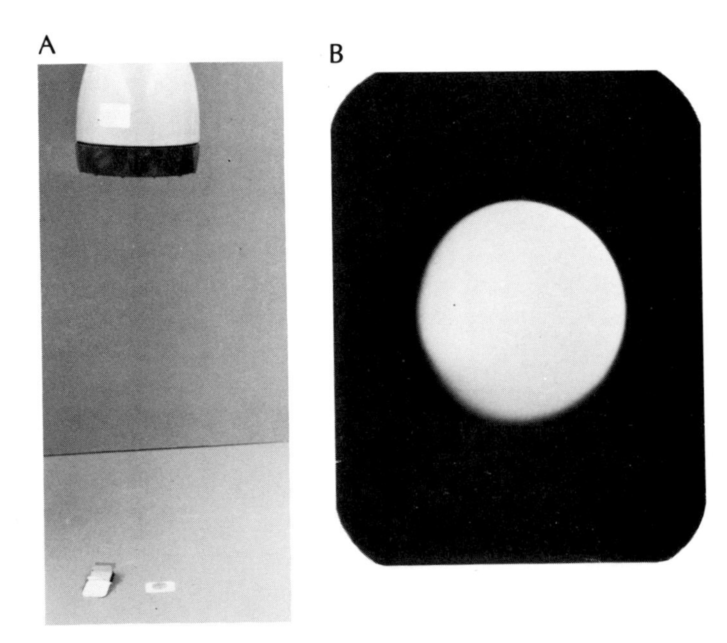

Figure 20–2. A, Coin on top of unwrapped dental film positioned beneath safelight on workbench in darkroom. B, Processed film showing exposure of film outside of coin area.

move the coin and process the film. A perfectly clear film indicates that no light has reached the film to cast a shadow of the coin onto the film. A fogged light density film showing a clear area under the coin indicates that light is reaching the film from some source other than the darkroom lights (Figure 20–2B). Note that fluorescent lights often have an invisible afterglow. With the light off, look around the room for light leaks in the darkroom. Seal all light leaks and repeat the test.

Note: If darkroom safety is tested with the safelight turned on and the outline of the coin is seen on the film, the exact source of light (safelight or outside light or both) cannot be determined.

The safety of the safelight must be tested only when light tightness of the darkroom is established. With only the safelight turned on in the darkroom, unwrap a dental film and a screen film (if used in the office) and place them on the workbench directly under the safelight. Place a small coin on each film. Leave the films in this position for 5 minutes or as long as you might have an unwrapped film in the darkroom during film processing. Remove the coin and process the films. Perfectly clear films indicate that no light has reached the films. The safelight is thus correct for both films. A fogged, light density film with a clear area under the coin indicates that the particular film is receiving unsafe light from the safelight.

Note: Many safelights used for periapical dental films are unsafe for screen and some non-screen films. Examine the safelight to see if the correct filter is being used, if the filter is cracked, if the correct wattage bulb is being used, and if the safelight is positioned at a safe distance from the work area.

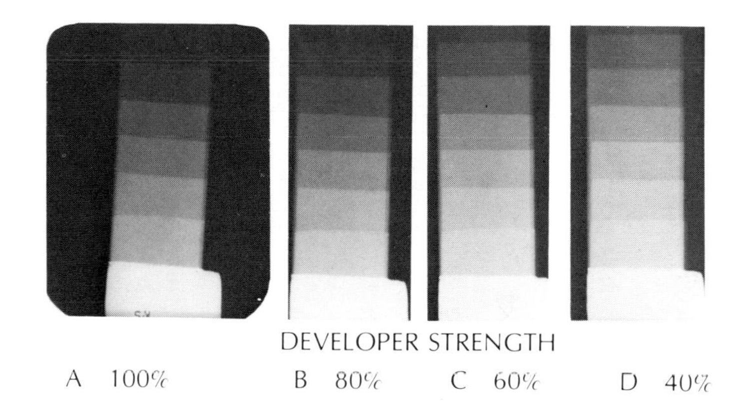

Figure 20–3. Four radiographs of step wedges that were exposed at same time and processed at different times. A, Radiograph processed when the processing chemicals were changed and complete development of image was obtained. B, Radiograph processed 2 weeks later when developer solution was weaker by 20%. An increase of 20% developing time is needed to obtain full development of latent image. C, Radiograph processed 4 weeks later when the developer is 60% of original strength. Full development requires 40% increase in developing time. D, Radiograph processed in developer of 40% strength showing obvious underdevelopment of latent image.

Developer Solution Strength

If a developer solution loses its strength the time-temperature recommendation of the manufacturer will no longer be accurate. A rough evaluation of developer solution strength can be made by matching the densities of radiographs made of similar sized patients at different times; this technic is described in Chapter 2. The same basic system, using a standard step wedge, can more accurately identify the weakening of a devel-

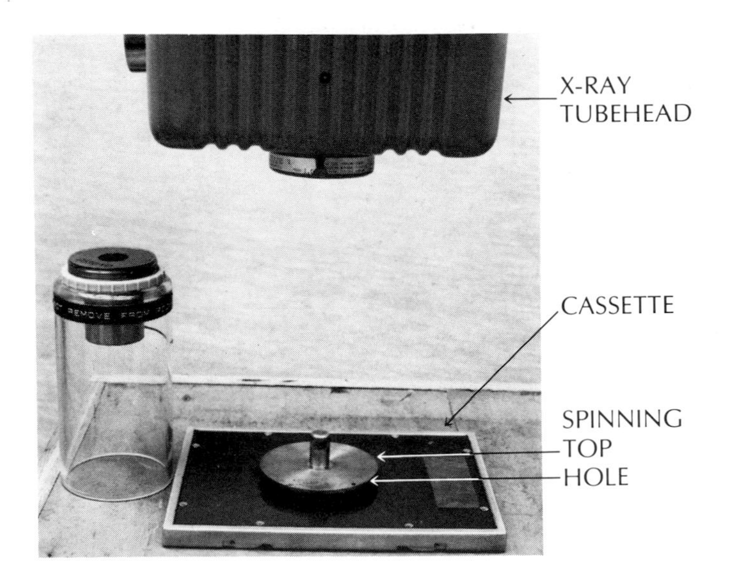

Figure 20–4. Commercially available brass spinning top being radiographed with cone removed from tubehead and screen film in cassette. Top is exposed when it is spinning at approximately one revolution per second.

oper solution. When the processing solutions are freshly mixed, seven periapical films are exposed using a step-wedge object and the same exposure factors of mA, kVp, distance, and time. One film is processed and stored. The other films are stored in a cool, dry area of the office. Each week a film is processed and compared to the first radiograph. A lessening of the densities of the step-wedge image in a later processed radiograph indicates a weakening of the developer solution (Figure 20–3). The earliest visible density loss is seen when the developer is weakened about 20%; a 40% loss in strength is clearly visible. It is recommended that processing solutions be changed before a 40% loss occurs. In an office with a heavy workload solutions may have to be changed every 2 weeks, whereas in low volume radiography practices the developer solution may still be 80% strong after a month. Processing solutions should be changed at least every 6 weeks, since they deteriorate with time and the cost of the solutions is not great relative to the income generated from dental radiography.

The test can be used in hand processing with tanks and nonreplenishing automatic processing machines. A record of when the solutions were tested should be kept posted next to the processing tanks or processing machine. The record should also indicate when the tanks or machines were cleaned.

Fixer Solution Strength

The depletion of fixer chemicals is usually automatically evident during routine film processing. This is seen as a lengthening of the time it takes to make a radiograph transparent in the unexposed areas. With full strength fixer solution a radiograph should clear within 2 minutes without film agitation. Overly long clearing time, for example, 4 minutes, indicates a weak fixing solution and the necessity of changing the solution.

To periodically test the fixer solution for quality control documentation, the operator can use a measurement of the time the solution takes to make an unexposed and undeveloped film transparent. The film is placed in the fixer solution immediately after unwrapping. This test does not need safelight conditions and can be done in a white light illuminated darkroom.

X-RAY MACHINE PERFORMANCE

Standards for machine performance have been established and must be met when an x-ray machine is installed in a dental office. The machine manufacturer's representative evaluates machine performance with special electrical and electronic testing devices. Special training is needed to operate and analyze the results of these tests. Complex methods of testing equipment are not practical for the average dental office. However, there are simple and inexpensive tests that dental personnel can use to detect some machine defects or malfunctions. Evidence of a possible malfunction can alert the dentist to the need of a thorough machine evaluation. Periodic testing of the performance of the x-ray machine is necessary in conducting a quality assurance program. The tests described in this chapter require exposing and processing films; thus, film processing needs to be standardized and proper darkroom conditions must be established before the tests can be used.

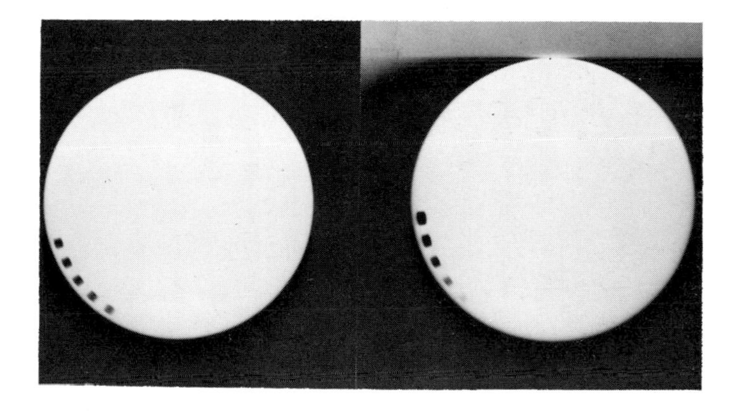

Figure 20–5. Radiographs of spinning top made with exposure time of five impulses or 1/12 second. Left radiograph was made on machine with an accurate timer and shows five images of hole in top that have equal film density. Right radiograph was made with machine whose timer also produced five impulses of radiation, but x-ray pulses were not of equal intensity and produced images of hole of different film density.

Timer Accuracy

Most trained operators can measure the approximate time of a one-second exposure. Major time differences between the timer being set at one second, or above, and the machine being activated for the set time can usually be detected by the operator. Errors in times below one second (or up to 60 impulses) cannot be easily detected or measured without a test.

A "spinning top" is used for measuring the number of x-ray pulses the machine produces. A spinning top consists of a rotating radiopaque disk with a hole or notch at the periphery of the disk. The top is exposed while spinning on a film (Figure 20–4). The top is spun by the operator and the exposure is made when the top slows and is rotating about one revolution per second. Because a sensitive film is needed, a screen film in a cassette is used. Each radiation impulse produced by the x-ray machine makes an image of the hole or notch; the hole is located at a different position for each pulse of x rays and

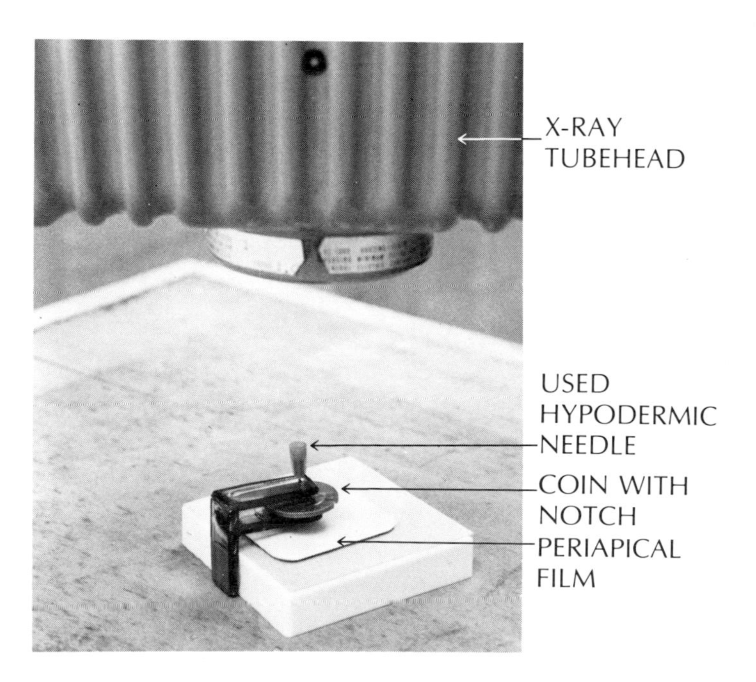

Figure 20–6. Small spinning top made of easily available materials being radiographed with short tube-film distance using speed D periapical film.

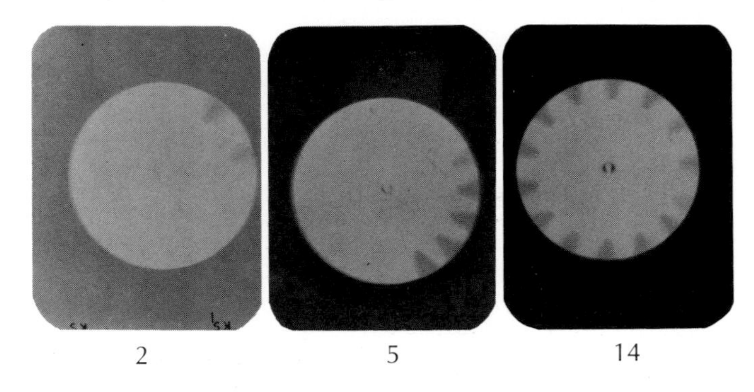

Figure 20–7. Radiographs made with spinning top shown in Figure 20–6 using exposure times of 2, 5, and 15 impulses. Machine's timer was accurate for 2- and 5-impulse exposure times, but showed a one less impulse error at 15-impulse setting.

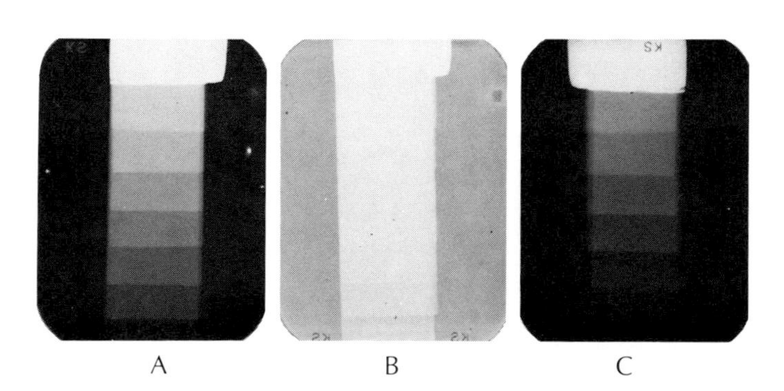

Figure 20–8. A, Reference radiograph of step wedge made when x-ray machine and processing facilities are functioning normally. B, Low density radiograph produced by drop in voltage in electric line used by x-ray machine. C, Increased density radiograph produced by removal of filters in beam of older model x-ray machine.

thus the processed radiograph shows the number of impulses (Figure 20–5). Timer accuracy can be easily checked by this method. Relatively inexpensive spinning tops can be obtained from medical radiology supply stores or can be made from a disk cut from a sheet of heavy metal, a threaded bolt with a sharpened point, and a small block of wood with a depression in it for stabilizing the base.

When a screen-film is not available, an ultra speed dental film can be used, but the film must be positioned close to the radiation source and a small spinning top used. The construction of such a top from materials found in a dental office is shown in Figure 20–6. The disk is made of heavy metal and is the size of a quarter or 25-cent coin. The middle part of a disposable injection needle is used to spin the disk by drilling a hole in the center of the disk, with a burr the size of the needle, and later attaching the needle to the disk with epoxy or super glue. A V-shaped notch is cut in the periphery of the disk. The "spinning top" is suspended over the film by thin plastic arms cut from small disposable plastic spoons or forks and assembled with epoxy glue. The plastic frame is glued to a small box filled with stone or plaster. The film is exposed with the top spinning slowly, the cone is removed from the x-ray machine, and the x-ray tubehead is placed close to the device. Films exposed to 2 pulses or $^{1}/_{30}$ second, 5 impulses or $^{1}/_{20}$ second, and 15 impulses or $^{1}/_{4}$ second are shown in Figure 20–7.

Radiation Output

When a spinning top and screen film are available, the radiation output of a machine can be measured in terms of the number of impulses it produces for any given time. In addition, variations in the amount of x rays produced with each pulse can be detected as differences in the densities of the images of the hole in the spinning top (Figure 20–5).

Radiation production can also be checked with a penetrometer or step wedge. A reference radiograph is made when the machine and darkroom facilities are known to be functioning properly. The wedge and film are placed at the end of the cone and the kVp, mA, and exposure time are set to be the same as when the maxillary posterior area is radiographed. The processed radiograph should clearly show all the steps of the wedge; it is stored and kept as a reference. When the machine output is being tested at a later date, the wedge is again radiographed, using the identical radiographic factors as those for the reference radiograph. The new radiograph will closely match the reference radiograph if the machine output is the same. Less radiation output can easily be identified as an overall loss of density. Increased x-ray output can be seen as an increase in overall density (Figure 20–8). Note that the effectiveness of this test depends upon using the same radiographic factors for the reference and test radiographs; this includes the darkroom and film processing conditions.

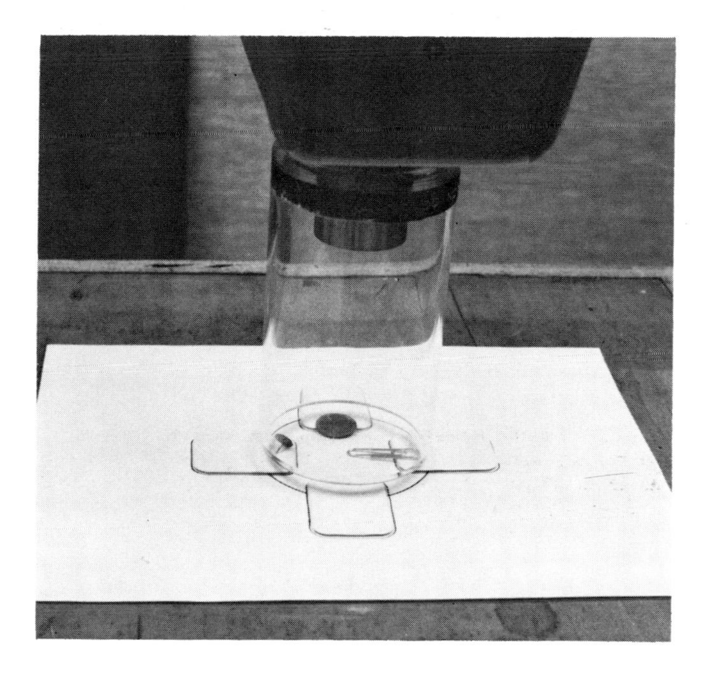

Figure 20–9. Four periapical films being exposed at end of open-end cone. Positions of films and cone end are traced on sheet of paper. Coin, thumbtack and metal paper clip are used to cast identifying images on individual films.

Collimation and Beam Alignment

The position and size of the x-ray beam is measured and compared to the size and position of the open end of the cone or position indicating device. Four dental films are placed on a sheet of paper, in the shape of a cross, with the edge of the cone crossing the middle of the films (Figure 20–9). The outlines of the cone-end and films are marked on the paper. Radiopaque objects, such as paper clips, coins, pins, or nails, are placed on the films inside the x-ray beam. The films are exposed with one-half the exposure time used for an anterior radiograph. The radiographs are processed and relocated in their original positions on the paper, using the images of the different radiopaque objects. The exposed areas of the films identify the edge of the x-ray beam in the cone. Incorrect alignment of the x-ray beam in the cone or incorrect width of the x-ray beam at the end of the cone is easily detected (Figure 20–10).

Direct observation of the beam's position can be made on a fluorescent screen if the room is made dark (Figure 20–11). Lines drawn on the screen can show if the beam is properly collimated and positioned. This system is useful when the operator can make the observation from behind a shield.

Focal Spot Condition

The condition of the focal spot of the x-ray tube, where the x-rays are produced, can be

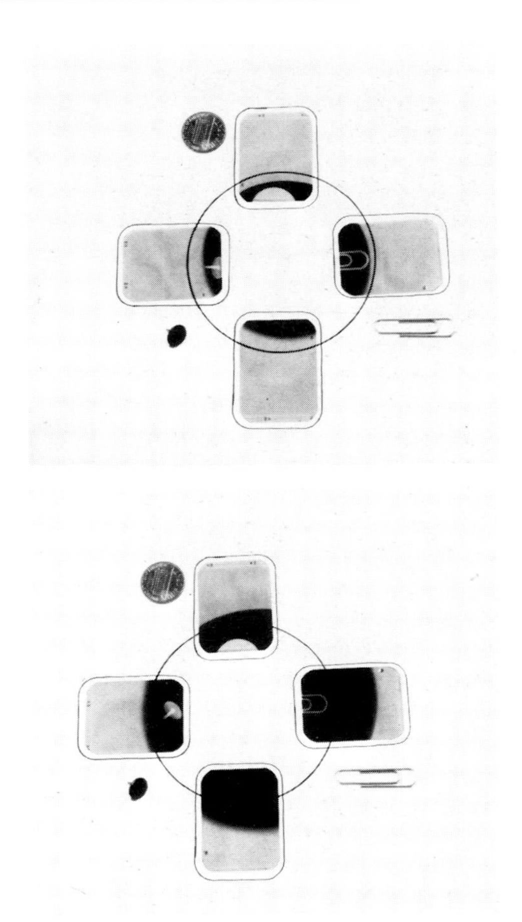

Figure 20–10. Reassembled beam alignment radiographs made on two different x-ray machines. Top, Correct alignment of x-ray beam. Primary radiation is located in center of cone and collimated within edge of cone. Bottom, X-ray beam that is greater than 2¾ inches in diameter at end of cone and is not centered in cone.

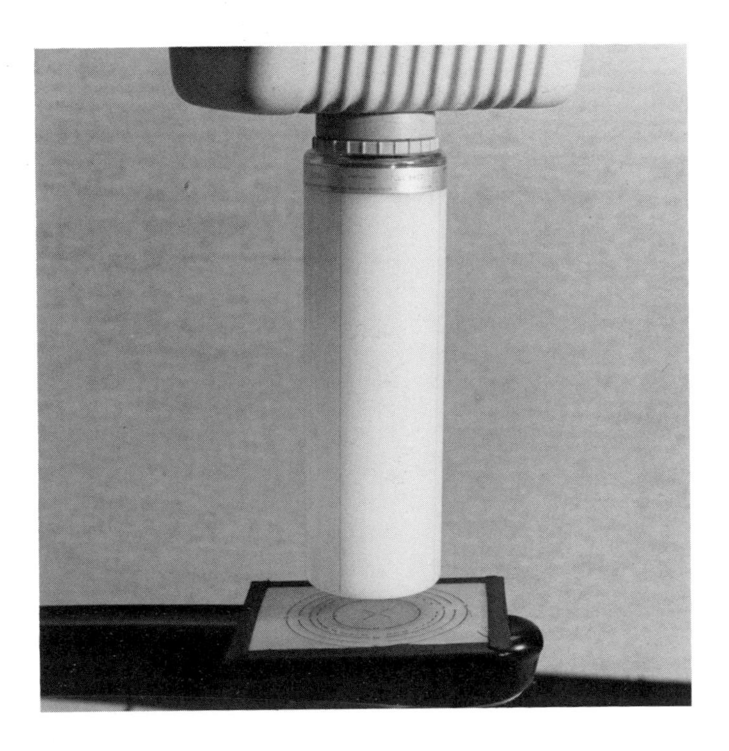

Figure 20–11. Fluorescent screen positioned close to the end of an x-ray machine cone. Various diameter circles on the surface of the screen are used to quickly observe the size and position of the x-ray beam when the beam is activated and cause the screen to fluoresce or glow in a darkened room.

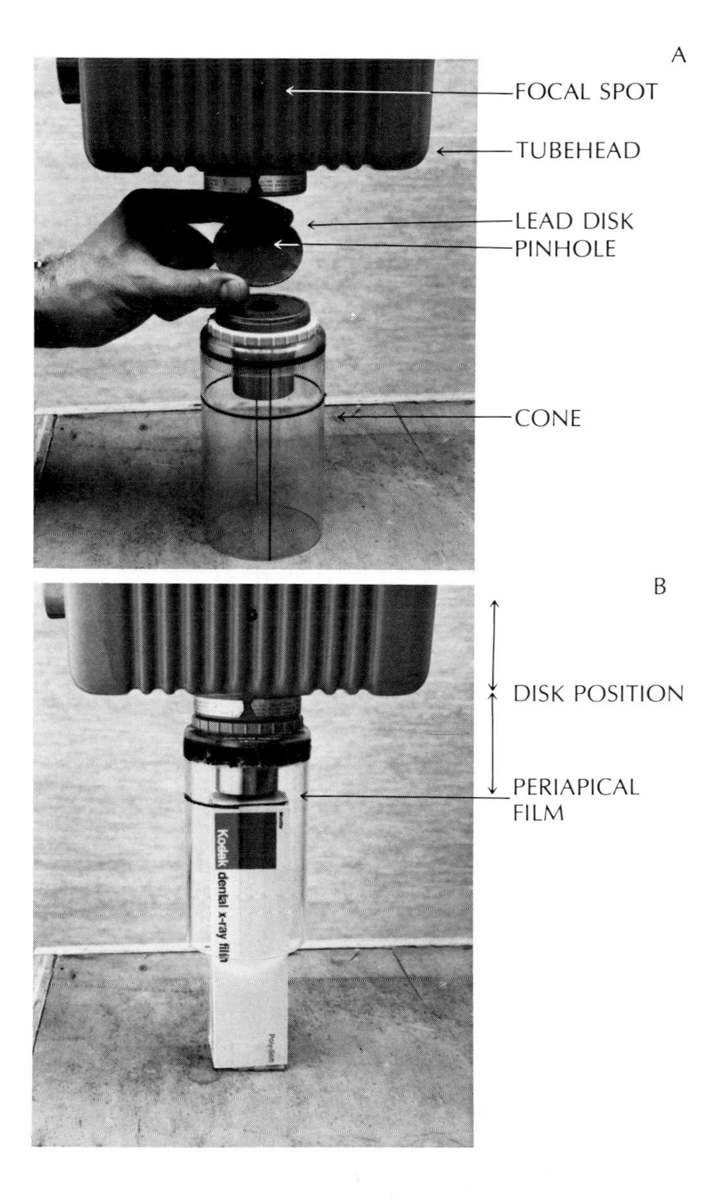

Figure 20–12. A, Lead disk with pinhole in center. Disk is placed between cone and machine tubehead. B, Speed D periapical film placed on top of empty film box in open-end cone at position that is same distance from pinhole as x-ray source. Note that x-ray source position is marked on the tubehead.

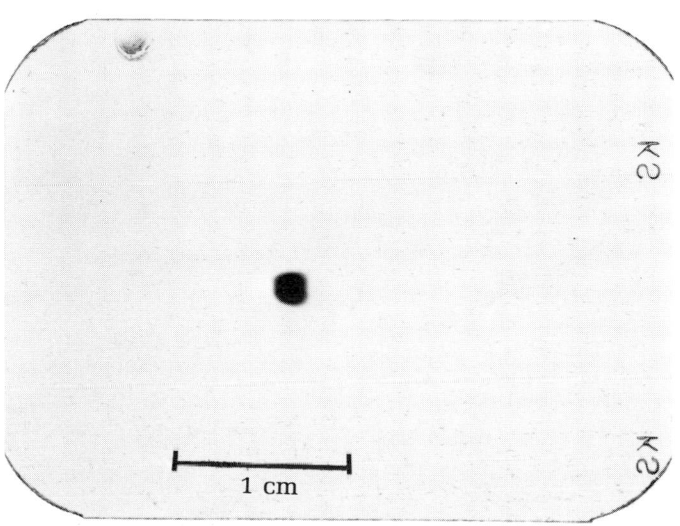

Figure 20–13. Radiograph of 1- × 1-mm focal spot x-ray source made with pinhole ½ mm in diameter.

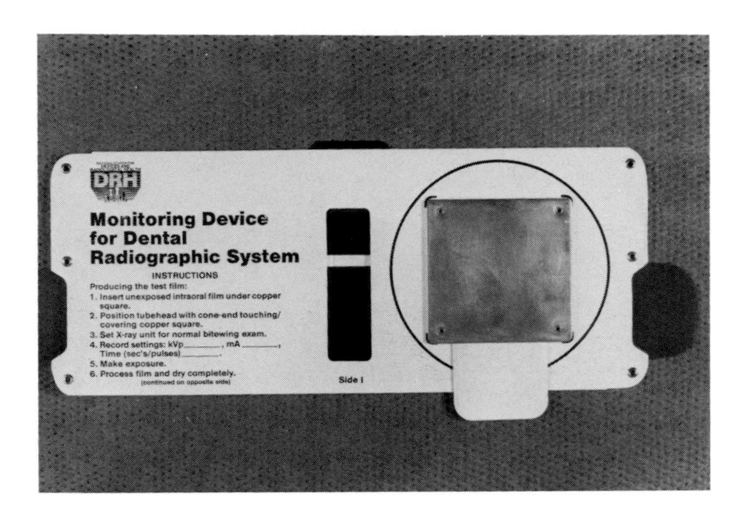

Figure 20–14. The DRH monitoring device.

checked by making a picture of the spot using the pinhole camera technic. A piece of lead approximately 1 mm in thickness is placed over the collimator opening in the base of the cone; a small hole no larger than ½ mm in diameter is made in the center of the lead. A dental film is placed on a small box in the middle of the cone at the same distance from the lead hole as the focal spot (marked on the tubehead) of the x-ray machine (Figure 20–12). When speed D film, 65 kVp, and 10 mA are used, an exposure time of approximately 5 impulses is usually needed to produce a clear image of the focal spot in the processed film. The dimensions of the image of the focal spot will be larger than the size specified by the machine's manufacturer due to the large size of the hole used; however, the dimensions should be close to the manufacturer's specifications plus the diameter of the hole. The image of a dental x-ray tube's focal spot is usually 1 mm by 1 mm. A focal spot image made in the described manner is shown in Figure 20–13.

THE DRH MONITORING DEVICE

The National Center for Devices and Radiological Health has developed a dental monitoring device (Figure 20–14). A sheet of copper is used as an object. Periapical films are periodically exposed under the copper with the end of the cone on the device and with normal bite-wing exposure factors. The processed film is matched for density to a sliding film strip that places different numbered film densities in the window of the device. Proper density is established when machine and processing are known to be correct. Deviations of two of the numbered step densities in subsequent radiographs signal a machine or processor problem.

THE OFFICE QA SYSTEM

Every dental office should have a description of its quality assurance system. The basic elements can be outlined as: (1) Daily evaluation (condition of x-ray room, machine dials, arm and tubehead movements, and performance of the film processing system). (2) Every three months (x-ray machine performance). (3) Every six months (inspection and darkroom light safety). (4) X-ray machine calibration at times required by local laws (some professional groups have recommended yearly inspections).

An office quality assurance system must be quick and simple for dental auxiliaries to utilize, if it is to be practical and acceptable by individual dental practitioners. While machine calibration has to be conducted by technicians trained in radiation physics, all other quality assurance procedures can be carried out by an auxiliary. Of all the auxiliary inspection procedures, the greatest need is the development of simple, inexpensive and quick tests for film processing and x-ray machine performance. Such tests, unified into a single test for both processor and machine performance will be described next.

A Processor-Machine Performance Test. The test object is an aluminum stepwedge that can be inexpensively obtained from a machine shop. The wedge has a base approximately 10 x 30 mm. There are 8 steps (approximately 4 × 10 mm) consisting of 2, 4, 6, 8, 10, 12, 14, and 16 mm of aluminum in thickness (Figure 20–15).

A standard reference radiograph is prepared at the time the machine is installed or whenever the machine has been inspected, calibrated and determined to be functioning properly, and when the processing solutions are newly prepared and the processor is functioning properly. The radiograph is made with the type film being used and the kVp, TFD and exposure time used for the maxillary central incisors using the aluminum stepwedge as the object (Figure 20–16). The radiograph will clearly show all eight steps when viewed on an x-ray viewbox.

Whenever the processing solutions are changed prepare a series of "exposed films." The films are exposed with the same machine and radiographic factors, using the aluminum stepwedge object, as with the standard radiograph. The number of films must be greater than the average number of days of the working life of the solutions; this can be identified when solutions have been changed a few times. The exposed films are stored in a light tight container in a cool dry place, away from x rays (Figure 20–17). Process one of the exposed films in the fresh solutions and compare the film with the standard radiograph. If the step densities are two

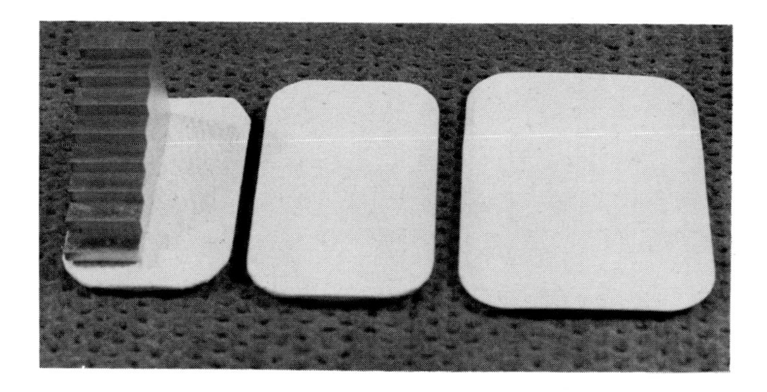

Figure 20–15. An eight step aluminum stepwedge placed on a size 0 intraoral film adjacent to a size 1 and 2 film

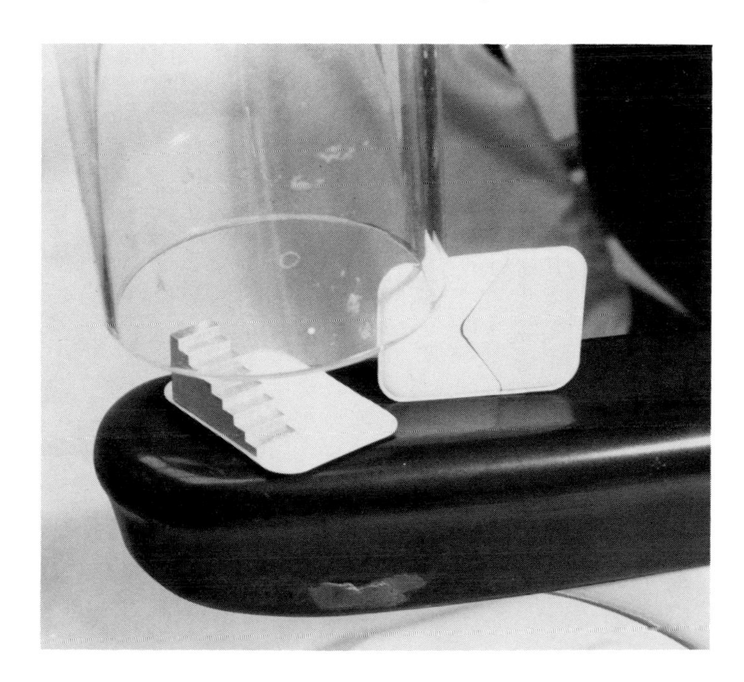

Figure 20–16. Film, stepwedge and x-ray beam (PID) positions during film exposure for the quality assurance test. The cone film distance can be standardized through the use of the long or short dimension of a periapical film.

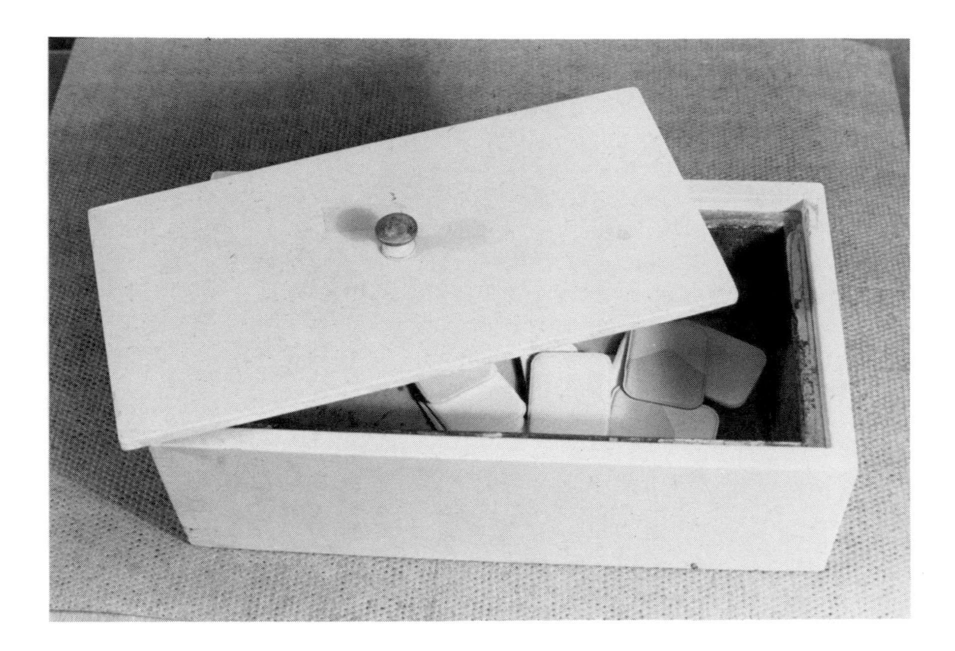

Figure 20–17. A lead lined box used for storing exposed test films.

steps more or less than the standard radiograph, the x-ray machine needs to be checked for proper dial settings and/or calibration (Figure 20–18). A processed radiograph that closely matches the standard radiograph it becomes the series reference radiograph for the series of exposed films. At the start of each day, process one of the exposed films. Compare the radiograph with the series reference radiograph. If the stepwedge image of the test film is two or more steps less in density than the series reference radiograph change the processing solutions. When the solutions are changed, prepare a new series of "exposed films" and use the first processed film with the standard reference radiograph to check the x-ray machine performance and establish a new series reference radiograph. A flow chart of the system is shown in Figure 20–19.

In the unified test, the auxiliary visually measures radiographic quality changes in the stepwedge image. Use of the test is based upon the concept that when the test indicates GO, loss of diagnostic information will not occur in radiographs made with the x-ray machine and processor in their present conditions since radiographic image changes can be detected much easier in a stepwedge image than in the images of teeth and bone. Cost, time, and effort in preparing the test

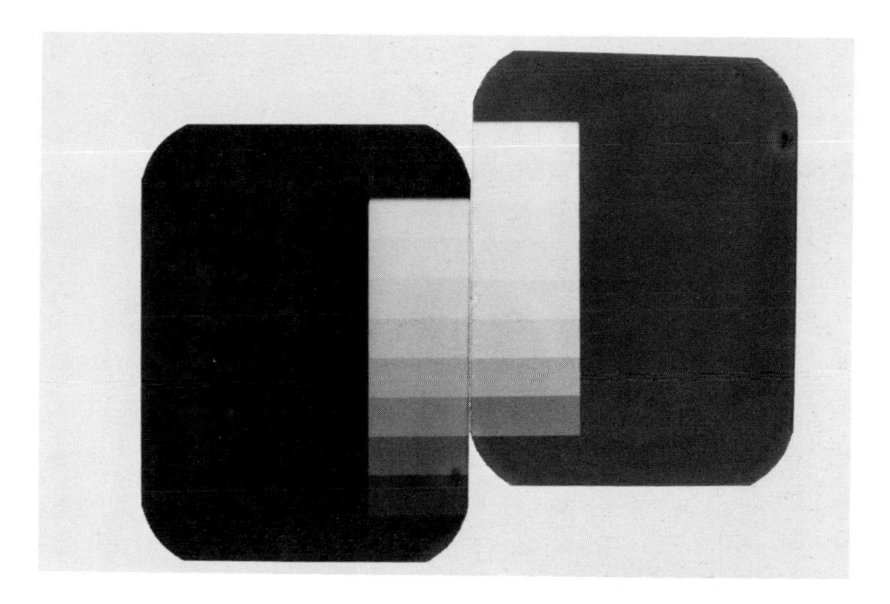

Figure 20–18. Standard reference radiograph (left) matched with a newly processed radiograph (right) for similar step densities. The new radiograph shows a two-step deviation from the standard.

materials is minimal. Processing one film daily does not interfere with normal auxiliary performance.

OPERATOR COMPETENCE

Objective evaluation of an x-ray operator's performance is at best difficult. This should be done by the dentist who has the responsibility for radiography quality assurance. Assessment of the quality of the radiographs produced in the dental office should be documented to identify repeated errors and the area of the operator's deficiency. Forms used by instructors who teach dental radiography students can be useful in developing an operator evaluation form for the dental office. A technic critique form presently being used in teaching dental radiography is shown in Figure 20–20.

The dentist may wish to test the radiography background knowledge of auxiliary personnel, initially or periodically. In addition, auxiliary personnel may wish to refresh and test their own knowledge while in the dental office. A series of multiple choice and true-or-false questions is presented for this purpose, and to assist in establishing operator competence in a quality assurance program. The correct answers are on the last page of this chapter.

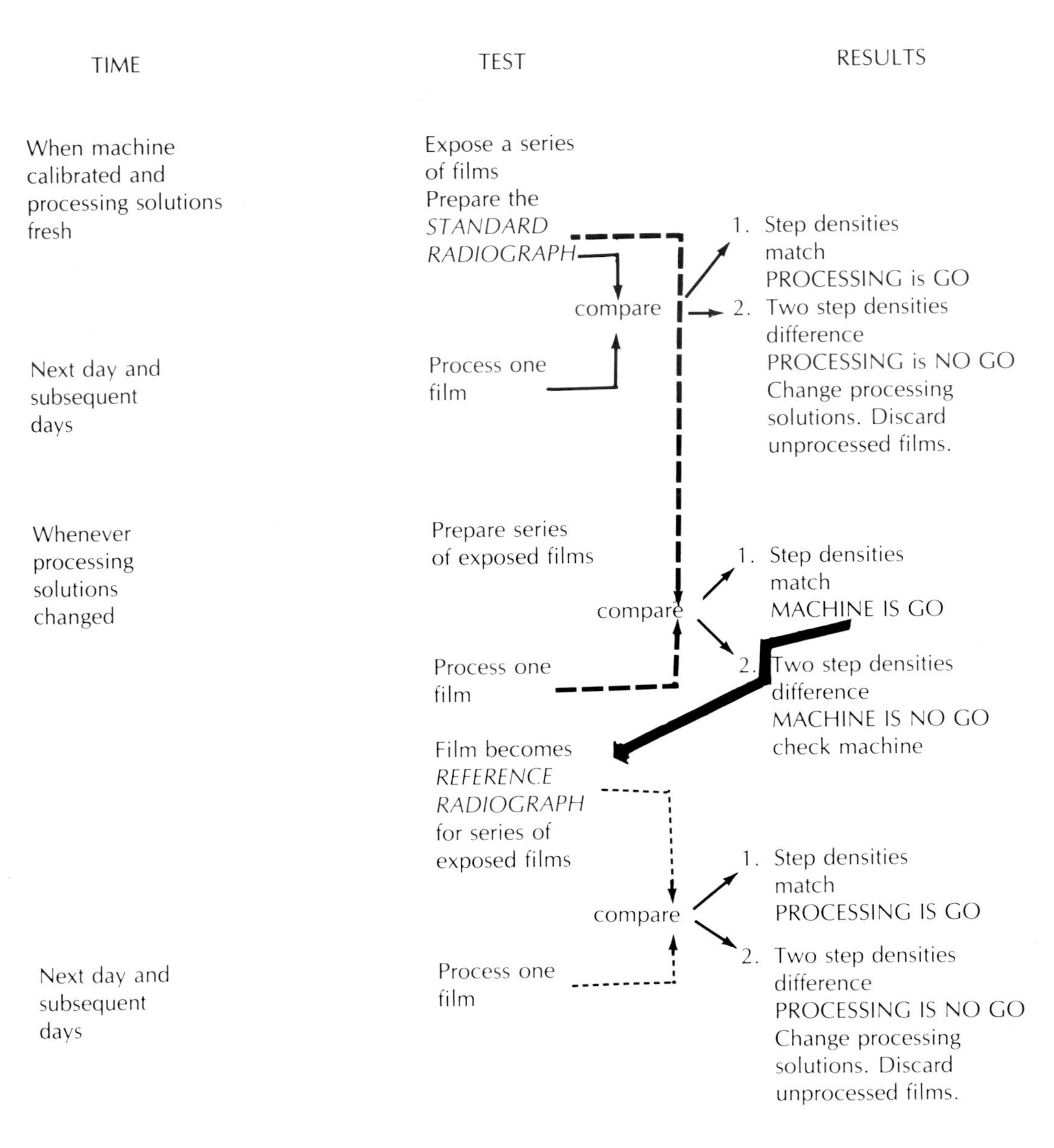

Figure 20–19. Flow chart of a simplified quality assurance test for both film processing and x-ray machine.

RADIOGRAPHIC TECHNIC CRITIQUE FORM

Student's Name ______________________ Date ______________

PATIENT Number

Sex: M F
Adult: Over 20 years
Adolescent: 12–20 years
Child: 6–12 years
<6 years

1	2	3	4	5	6	7	8	9	10

PATIENT CONDITION

	1	2	3	4	5	6	7	8	9	10
Gag reflex—excessive or moderate										
Tori—maxillary or mandibular										
Shallow palate or floor of mouth										
Edentulous										
Partially edentulous										
Complete dentition (third molars not included)										
Stretcher										
Hyperactive										
Poor tongue or musculature control										
Physically handicapped										
Mentally handicapped										
Poor cooperation of patient										

Number = Times Retaken

Letter = Error Type

ERRORS

A. Density
   a. High density
   b. Low density
B. Contrast
   a. High (short scale)
   b. Low (long scale)
C. Cone cutting
D. Vertical overangulation
E. Vertical underangulation
F. Horizontal angulation
   a. Too much from posterior
   b. Too much from anterior
G. Film placement
   a. Too far posterior
   b. Too far anterior
   c. Too far superior
   d. Too far inferior
   e. Slanting
H. Movement (patient, film, or tube)
I. Double or multiple exposures
J. Backward film placement
K. Missing film or film not taken
L. Processing failures
M. Wrong projection
N. Curved film
O. Improperly bent film
P. Film fogging
Q. Static electricity
R. Failure to remove dental appliances
S. Failure to remove eyeglasses
T. Other ______________

Figure 20–20. Radiographic technic critique form used in identifying problem areas of individual students.

Test Questions

1. An exposed radiographic film should remain in the fixer solution
   a. as long as it remained in the developer.
   b. until the film first clears.
   c. for 5 minutes at 70°F.
   d. at least 10 minutes.

2. The ideal developing time when a fresh developing solution is used is
   a. 3 minutes at 70°.
   b. 4 minutes at 65°.
   c. 5 minutes at 68°.
   d. 4 minutes at 68.5°.
   e. dependent upon when an image becomes visible on the film.

3. In most states, radiation protection laws require that the size of the dental x-ray beam at the patient's face be of a diameter of no more than
   a. 2¾ inches.
   b. 3¼ inches.
   c. 3½ inches.
   d. 4 inches.

4. The central ray of an x-ray beam
   1. has the shortest wavelength of any photon in the beam.
   2. has greater speed than other photons in the beam.
   3. is composed of photons traveling in the center of the cone of radiation.
   4. is used to fix or locate the position of the x-ray beam.
   a. 3 and 4
   b. 1 and 2
   c. 1 and 3
   d. 3 only
   e. 4 only

5. The density of a radiograph is decreased by
   a. increasing the milliamperes.
   b. increasing the exposure time.
   c. increasing the developing time.
   d. increasing the tube-patient distance.
   e. increasing the washing time.

6. The hamular process is seen in a radiograph made of
   a. the lower incisor area.
   b. the lower molar area.
   c. the upper molar area.
   d. the upper incisor area.

7. The unit which describes the amount of x-ray exposure in air is the
   a. rad.
   b. rem.
   c. roentgen.
   d. pid.
   e. MAS.

8. A very light radiograph may be caused by
   1. too short exposure time.
   2. wrong side of the film being toward the tube.
   3. developing solution being too warm.
   4. removing the film from the fixing bath too soon.
   5. white light leaking into the darkroom.
   a. 1 and 2
   b. 1 and 3
   c. 1 and 4
   d. 2 and 3
   e. 2 and 5
   f. 3 and 4
   g. 3 and 5
   h. 4 and 5

9. Which of the following structures appear radiolucent on a radiograph?
   1. median palatine suture
   2. anterior nasal spine
   3. mandibular canal
   4. genial tubercles
   5. hamular process
   a. 1 and 3 only
   b. 1, 3, and 5
   c. 1 and 5 only
   d. 2 and 3
   e. 2 and 4

10. Which of the following statements about radiation are correct?
   1. X rays can affect all living biologic forms.
   2. Developing, young, biologically active cells are more susceptible to x rays.
   3. In dental radiography, only the primary, direct beam of radiation is a potential hazard.
   4. Changes in normal adult cells that may be caused by radiation are of short duration and the effects are soon dissipated.
   a. 1 and 2
   b. 2 and 3 only
   c. 2, 3, and 4
   d. 1 and 3
   e. All of these

11. Which of the following structures appear radiopaque on a radiograph?
    1. nasal fossa
    2. mylohyoid ridge
    3. maxillary sinus
    4. external oblique line
    5. coronoid process of the mandible
        a. 1, 2, and 3
        b. 1, 3, and 5
        c. 1, 4, and 5
        d. 2, 3, and 4
        e. 2, 4, and 5
12. The x-ray tube-to-film distance is increased from 8 to 16 inches. What fraction of the original radiation intensity at 8 inches is the film now exposed to at 16 inches?
    a. one fifth (1:5)
    b. one quarter (1:4)
    c. one third (1:3)
    d. one half (1:2)
13. The x-ray beam is collimated to
    a. remove the less penetrating x rays.
    b. avoid delivering unnecessary radiation to the patient.
    c. reduce the size of the beam to facilitate easier visualization of the central ray.
    d. reduce the exposure time.
14. Restorative materials which appear radiolucent on an intraoral radiograph include
    1. silicate cements.
    2. zinc oxide and eugenol.
    3. plastics.
    4. zinc oxyphosphate cement.
    5. gutta percha.
        a. 1 and 5
        b. 2 and 4
        c. 1 only
        d. 2 and 3
        e. 1 and 3
15. When the mA on an x-ray machine is reduced from 15 mA to 10 mA
    a. the wavelength of the x rays produced will be decreased.
    b. the number of volts in the filament circuit will be decreased.
    c. the shape of the electron beam will be changed.
    d. the number of x rays produced will be increased.
    e. the number of x rays produced will be decreased.
16. The size of the x-ray tube focal spot influences radiographic image
    a. density.
    b. contrast.
    c. sharpness.
    d. magnification.
17. A good radiograph was made using a tube-film distance of 16 inches and an exposure time of 4 seconds. If the tube-film distance is decreased to 8 inches, what would be the correct exposure time?
    a. 1 second
    b. 2 seconds
    c. 6 seconds
    d. 8 seconds
18. An x-ray film subjected to great changes in temperature between different processing solutions may exhibit.
    a. a herringbone pattern.
    b. blurred images.
    c. chemical stains.
    d. reticulation.
    e. linear streaking.
19. Filters are used in the x-ray beam to
    a. reduce film density.
    b. correct the x-ray beam size.
    c. reduce the exposure time.
    d. remove low energy x rays.
    e. increase contrast.
20. After removing a film from the developer and before placing it in the fixer, the film should be washed in running water to
    a. remove the developer.
    b. harden the emulsion.
    c. dilute the fixer.
    d. neutralize the fixer.
21. Unsharpness of the radiographic image is increased by
    a. using a larger focal spot.
    b. increasing the tube-patient distance.
    c. decreasing the object-film distance.
    d. immobilizing the patient.
22. The radiation protection guide advocates that the x-ray dose to operators of dental machines should not exceed
    a. 100 milliroentgens per week.
    b. 10 roentgens per week.
    c. 100 roentgens per week.
    d. 300 roentgens per week.

23. The metal foil backing in an intraoral dental x-ray film packet
    a. increases the amount of secondary radiation that reaches the film.
    b. reduces the exposure of tissues behind the film.
    c. keeps the film from being bent or curved when placed inside the mouth.
    d. increases the flexibility of the film packet.

24. The rays which are most likely to be absorbed by the skin and cause an x-ray injury are the
    a. central rays.
    b. deep penetrating x rays.
    c. aluminum filtered x rays.
    d. x rays of long wavelength.
    e. x rays of short wavelength.

25. Elongation of the image on a maxillary radiograph may be caused by
    1. insufficient vertical angulation.
    2. excessive vertical angulation.
    3. poor patient position.
    4. improper placement of film.
    5. extended target-film distance.
       a. 1, 2, or 3
       b. 1 or 3 only
       c. 1, 3, or 4
       d. 2 or 4
       e. 2 or 5

26. The paralleling technic using the long cone, compared with the bisecting-the-angle technic uses
    1. greater vertical angulations.
    2. greater object-film distances.
    3. faster film.
    4. greater anode-film distances.
       a. 1 and 2
       b. 1 and 3
       c. 2 and 3
       d. 2 and 4
       e. 3 and 4

27. The speed of dental intraoral x-ray films
    1. is related to the rapidity with which the films can be processed.
    2. is determined mainly by the size of crystals or grain size in the emulsion.
    3. can vary by a factor of 12 from the slowest to the fastest.
    4. is determined by the thickness of the opaque packet covering material.
    5. is greater with large crystals than with small ones.
       a. 1, 3, and 5
       b. 2 and 5 only
       c. 4 and 5
       d. 1 and 5 only
       e. 2, 3, and 5

28. The bite-wing radiograph clearly identifies
    a. gingival changes.
    b. periodontal pocket formation.
    c. interproximal carious lesions.
    d. pulp exposures.
    e. periapical pathology.

29. X-ray operators must wear a film badge or radiation monitor if their average weekly x-ray exposure is more than
    a. 100 mR.
    b. 10 mR.
    c. 25 mR.
    d. 1 mR.
    e. 1 R.

30. The greatest total amount of radiation a worker is permitted to be exposed to at any age is expressed by the
    a. REM.
    b. MAD.
    c. RBE.
    d. RAD.
    e. MPD.

31. A film is properly exposed at 10 mA and 60 impulses. With 15 mA the film should be exposed with
    a. 90 impulses.
    b. 30 impulses.
    c. 40 impulses.
    d. 50 impulses.
    e. 45 impulses.

32. A raised dot is placed on the film to indicate
    a. where it should be held by the operator.
    b. where it is attached to the film clip.
    c. the corner where the film packet is opened.
    d. the exposure side of the film.
33. A radiolucent shadow is cast by
    a. enamel.
    b. canals and foramina.
    c. cortical bone.
    d. dentin.
    e. metal restorations.
34. In a radiograph of the maxillary molar region it is possible to see the
    a. coronoid process.
    b. anterior nasal spine.
    c. incisor foramen.
    d. mylohyoid ridge.
    e. genial tubercles.
35. An Angstrom unit is used to measure
    a. ionization.
    b. electron speed.
    c. amount of radiation.
    d. electricity.
    e. photon wavelength.
36. When no radiation shield is available the operator should stand out of the x-ray beam and a distance from the patient's head of at least
    a. 2 feet.
    b. 4 feet.
    c. 6 feet.
    d. 8 feet.
    e. 10 feet.
37. The purpose of the fixing solution is to
    a. shorten the film processing time.
    b. complete the development of the latent image.
    c. remove silver halide crystals not exposed by the x rays.
    d. remove silver halide crystals exposed by the x rays.
    e. fix the developed silver to the gelatin.
38. The material most effective in absorbing x rays is
    a. Tungsten.
    b. Copper.
    c. Aluminum.
    d. Lead.
    e. Enamel.
39. A low or long scale contrast radiograph is produced by
    a. increased kilovoltage.
    b. increased milliamperage.
    c. decreased filtration.
    d. decreased tube patient distance.
    e. decreased beam size.

40. When film density is related to film radiation exposure on a graph the resulting curve is called
    a. a characteristic curve.
    b. a sensitometric curve.
    c. a Hurter-Driffield curve.
    d. all of the above.

41. Automatic film processors require:
    a. a controlled water supply and cold solution temperatures.
    b. daily and periodic maintenance.
    c. solution to be changed every week.
    d. processing speed to be increased when a greater number of films are to be processed.

42. Reverse or ghost images are produced in panoramic radiographs by:
    a. radiopaque objects in the path of the x-ray beam on the other side of the patient being examined.
    b. defective rollers in the automatic film processor.
    c. gremlins in the cassette.
    d. static electricity discharges.
    e. tears in the film's emulsion.

43. The ALARA concept means:
    a. always lower amperage requirements with age.
    b. always lower all radiation absorption.
    c. always leave atomic radiation alone.
    d. as low as reasonably achieveable.
    e. as low as radiation allows.

44. Which of the following results in the greatest reduction in radiation to the patient?
    a. Quick film processing.
    b. Low kilovoltage.
    c. A wide circular beam of radiation.
    d. A long cone.
    e. Film with a fast emulsion.

45. With long or short cones, incorrect horizontal angulation results in:
    a. no change in teeth images.
    b. overlapping of teeth images.
    c. elongation of teeth images.
    d. foreshortening of teeth images.
    e. blurring of teeth images.
46. The paralleling technic must use a long cone to:
    a. avoid using the patient's finger to hold the film.
    b. reduce exposure time.
    c. reduce patient radiation dose.
    d. increase image magnification.
    e. decrease image magnification.
47. The focal trough in panoramic radiography is:
    a. the zone of sharpness.
    b. the collimated beam area.
    c. the slit in the scatter guard.
    d. the location of the electrons in the x-ray tube.
48. The teeth on the patient's right side in a panoramic radiograph are magnified and on the left side are excessively small. This is due to the patient's head being positioned in the machine:
    a. to the left of the midline.
    b. to the right of the midline.
    c. too far anteriorly.
    d. too far posteriorly.
    e. with the chin too far downward.
    f. with the chin too far upward.
49. Which of the following is NOT a classification of infectious microorganism?
    a. Bacteria
    b. Fungus
    c. Leukocyte
    d. Virus
50. What is the preferred method of infection control for the x-ray machine control panel?
    a. Steam autoclave
    b. Disinfecting wipe
    c. Spray with aerosol disinfectant
    d. Barrier protection
51. Which of the following is a chemical method used for disinfection/sterilization?
    a. Dry heat oven
    b. Diluted bleach solution
    c. Steam autoclave
    d. Ultrasonic bath
52. The anode is the negatively charged electrode during x-ray production. True or False
53. Electrons are positively charged particles. True or False
54. An electron cloud is produced by the cathode filament. True or False
55. Cells undergoing rapid mitosis are more sensitive to x rays. True or False
56. A kilovolt is one thousand volts. True or False
57. Placing the film in the fixer before the developer will fog the film. True or False
58. X-ray attenuation and x-ray absorption are the same process. True or False
59. The film emulsion is a mixture of sensitive crystals and gelatin. True or False
60. A cassette is a light proof container equipped with screens. True or False
61. A cone cut artifact is caused by the x-ray beam not covering the entire film. True or False
62. Higher kilovoltage produces a more black and white or high contrast image in the radiograph. True or False
63. Ionization occurs when an electron is removed from an atom. True or False
64. Erythema is an early sign of overexposure to x rays. True or False
65. Radiation damage to a chemical molecule occurs only through direct action of a photon on the chemical molecule. True or False
66. An AC electric current is an anode cathode current. True or False
67. When a photon produces many electrons by ionizing many atoms the process is called photoelectric absorption. True or False
68. Half value layer is a method of measuring the penetrating quality of an x-ray beam. True or False
69. A Hurter-Driffield curve shows the biologic response of living cells to varying doses of radiation. True or False
70. X rays travel with the same speed as light, i.e., 186,000 miles per second. True or False
71. All x-rays in the beam from a dental x-ray machine have the same penetrating power. True or False

72. The intensity of radiation is proportional to the square of the distance (from the x-ray source to the film). True or False
73. X rays can cause ionization of atoms. True or False
74. Collimating the x-ray beam reduces the amount of tissue being irradiated. True or False
75. X rays are emitted in 120 "bursts or impulses" of x rays per second when a 60-cycle electric current is used. True or False
76. The source of electrons in the x-ray tube is the target. True or False
77. kVp controls the penetrating power of the x-ray beam. True or False
78. Exposure time is the only control the dentist has over the amount or quantity of x rays generated. True or False
79. X rays are emitted by the patient for a few seconds after the x-ray machine has been turned off. True or False
80. Embryonic tissues and rapidly multiplying cells are more sensitive to x rays. True or False
81. X-radiation given to patients over the child-bearing age has no deleterious effects. True or False
82. Small interproximal carious lesions are more easily discovered through clinical examination than through the use of radiographs. True or False
83. Increased kVp (other factors constant) increases the density of a film. True or False
84. Fog on a film is responsible for poor image sharpness. True or False
85. In panoramic radiography one examines a layer or slice of tissue and thereby eliminates the superimposition (through blurring) of overlying structures. True or False
86. There is no safe dose of x-radiation. True or False
87. X rays are similar to light rays and radio rays, but they have shorter wavelengths. True or False
88. The dental assistant should hold the film in the patient's mouth when the patient is unable to hold it steady. True or False
89. The unprotected operator should not stand closer than 6 feet from the patient's head. True or False
90. The use of "fast" film is an effective means of reducing x-ray exposure to both patient and operator. True or False
91. The occlusal film is larger than the periapical film. True or False
92. With manual film processing, if the film is not washed for 20 minutes after fixation, a brown stain will form at a later date. True or False
93. The rays that pass from the x-ray tube through the filter and enter the cone are called secondary x rays. True or False
94. "Screen" x-ray film is used in a cassette and requires less exposure but yields a grainier image. True or False
95. Short wavelength x rays have less energy. True or False
96. The paralleling intraoral radiographic technic can be used on all types of patients. True or False
97. All panoramic radiographs examine the same layer of tissue in the patient's head. True or False
98. Commonly used panoramic radiographs are made with machines using the principle of tomography. True or False
99. The patient's radiation exposure stated in "roentgens" is a good indication of the total amount of x-ray energy that the patient receives. True or False
100. A bent film can show a white or a black line artifact when the film is processed. True or False
101. Handicapped patients must be treated with empathy. True or False
102. The latent period related to radiation effects is the period between exposure to radiation and the appearance of radiation damage. True or False

Answers

1. d
2. c
3. a
4. a
5. d
6. c
7. c
8. a
9. a
10. a
11. e
12. b
13. b
14. e
15. e
16. c
17. a
18. d
19. d
20. a
21. a
22. a
23. b
24. d
25. c
26. d
27. e
28. c
29. c
30. b
31. c
32. d
33. b
34. a
35. e
36. c
37. c
38. d
39. a
40. d
41. b
42. a
43. d
44. e
45. b
46. e
47. a
48. a
49. c
50. d
51. b
52. False
53. False
54. True
55. True
56. True
57. False
58. False
59. True
60. True
61. True
62. False
63. True
64. True
65. False
66. False
67. False
68. True
69. False
70. True
71. False
72. False
73. True
74. True
75. False
76. False
77. True
78. False
79. False
80. True
81. False
82. False
83. True
84. False
85. True
86. True
87. True
88. False
89. True
90. True
91. True
92. True
93. False
94. True
95. False
96. False
97. False
98. True
99. False
100. True
101. True
102. True

Index

Page numbers in italics refer to figures.